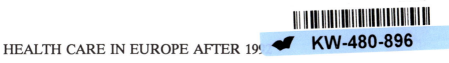

Published by
Dartmouth Publishing Company Limited
Gower House
Croft Road
Aldershot
Hants GU11 3HR
England

Dartmouth Publishing Company Limited
Distributed in the United States by
Ashgate Publishing Company
Old Post Road
Brookfield
Vermont 05036
USA

Typing and lay-out by
Contekst vof
Oudeland 55
3335 VH Zwijndrecht
The Netherlands

A CIP catalogue record for this book is available from the British Library and the US Library of Congress

Printed and bound in Great Britain by
Billing and Sons Ltd, Worcester

ISBN 1 85521 245 5

Contents

List of Contributors

- Dr. P.H. Admiraal, Faculty of Economics, Erasmus University Rotterdam, The Netherlands
- Prof. Dr. Christa Altenstetter, M.A., Professor of Political Science, City University of New York's Graduate Centre and Queens College, United States of America
- D. Bégué-Aboulker, Maitre de Conférences, Faculté de Pharmacie, Paris V, France
- Th. M. G. van Berkestijn, M.D., Secretary General of the Royal Dutch Medical Association, The Netherlands
- Dr. A. Berlin, Head of the Public Health Unit, Health and Safety Directorate, Commission of the European Communities
- P.F. Broere, M.A., Department of Marketing, Faculty of Economics, Erasmus University Rotterdam, The Netherlands
- Ronald V. Buise, LL.M. M.D. Deputy Head International Health Affairs Division, Ministry of Welfare, Health and Cultural Affairs, Rijswijk, The Netherlands
- M. Campari, Centre Diagnostico Italiana, Milan, Italy
- Prof. Dr. A.F. Casparie, Professor of Social Medicine, Department of Health Care Policy and Management, Erasmus University Rotterdam, The Netherlands
- F. Courcelle, Président de l'Association Recherche - Europe - Santé
- D.J. Doherty, M.I.P.M., Chief Executive Officer, Midland Health Board, Tullamore, Co Offaly, Republic of Ireland
- Prof. Spyros Doxiadis M.D., President, Foundation for Research in Childhood, Athens, Greece

Health Care in Europe after 1992

Edited by
H.E.G.M. HERMANS,
A.F. CASPARIE
and
J.H.P. PAELINCK

ERASMUS UNIVERSITY ROTTERDAM

Dartmouth

Aldershot · Brookfield USA · Hong Kong · Singapore · Sydney

- G. Duru, Directeur du Groupement de Recherche Santé, CNRS, University of Lyons, France
- Dr. E. Elsinga, Ministry of Welfare, Health and Cultural Affairs, The Netherlands
- W.J. van der Eijk, M.A., National Hospital Institute, Utrecht, The Netherlands
- Werner G. Fack, Dipl. -Kfm., German Hospital Institute, Duesseldorf, Germany
- M.J.M. Gerritsma B.Sc., National Hospital Institute, Utrecht, The Netherlands
- Prof. dr. W.J. de Gooijer, Professor of Hospital Management, Member of the Hospital Comittee of the European Community, Department of Health Care Policy and Management, Erasmus University Rotterdam, The Netherlands
- Prof. dr. J.-Matthias Graf von der Schulenburg, Professor of Insurance Economics, Institut für Versicherungsbetriebslehre, University of Hannover, Germany
- Chris B. Grimes, Head of Health Services, Chartered Institute of Public Finance and Accountancy (CIPFA), London, United Kingdom
- Clark C. Havighurst, William Neal Reynolds Professor of Law, Duke University School of Law, Durham, North Carolina, United States of America
- Dr. H.E.G.M. Hermans, Associate professor of Health Law, Department of Health Care Policy and Management, Erasmus University Rotterdam, The Netherlands
- R. van den Heuvel LL.M. Ph.D, M.Sc., President of the International Association of Mutualities, Belgium
- Shirley McIver, Kings Fund, London, United Kingdom
- H. Kaal, National Hospital Institute, Utrecht, The Netherlands
- P.J. van de Kasteele M.A., Ministry of Welfare, Health and Cultural Affairs, The Netherlands
- Bradford L. Kirkman-Liff, Dr. P.H., Professor of Health Administration and Policy, College of Business, Arizona State University, Tempe, Arizona, United States of America
- N.S. Klazinga, M.D., CBO, National Organization for Quality Assurance in Hospitals, Utrecht, The Netherlands
- H.J.E. Krol, M.A., National Hospital Institute, Utrecht, The Netherlands
- Prof. B.H. ter Kuile, LL.M., Professor of European Law, Faculty of Law, Erasmus University Rotterdam
- Sandra Lewis, J.D., M.H.S.A., Assistant Chief Examiner Arizona Department of Insurance, Phoenix, Arizona, United States of America
- Prof. dr. B. Leijnse, Emeritus Professor Faculty of Medicine, Erasmus University, The Netherlands
- J.C. Matthews, Director Commercial Affairs, Association of the British Pharmaceutical Industry, United Kingdom
- Alan Maynard, Professor of Economics and Director of the Department of Health - Economic and Social Research Council, Centre for Health Economics, University of York, United Kingdom
- J.H. Moerkerk M.A., Secretary National Commission on AIDS Control, The Netherlands
- C.K. Musch, C3 Hospital Consultancy b.v., Soesterberg, The Netherlands
- Anke Oosterman- Meulenbeld LL.M., Department of Health Law and Justice, State University of Limburg, Maastricht, The Netherlands
- Prof. dr. J.H.P. Paelinck, Faculty of Economics, Erasmus University Rotterdam, The Netherlands
- F.M. du Pré LL.M., Faculty of Law, Erasmus University Rotterdam, The Netherlands

- Prof. Povl Riis M.D., Chairman of the Danish National Research-Ethics Committee; Professor of Internal Medicine, University of Copenhagen; Chief, Med. Dept. C., Herlev University Hospital, Hellerup, Denmark
- (Mrs.) Prof. dr. H.D.C. Roscam Abbing, Department of Health Law and justice, State University of Limburg, Maastricht, The Netherlands
- Sybille Sahmer, Assessorin, Verbandssyndikus, Association of private health insurances Cologne, Germany
- Fernand Sauer, Head of Pharmaceutical Unit III/B/6, Commission of the European Communities, Brussels, Belgium
- Prof. K. Schutyser, Secretary-General, Hospital Committee of the European Community, Leuven, Belgium
- K. Sevinga LL.M. Faculty of Law, Erasmus University Rotterdam, The Netherlands
- W.H. Stikkelbroeck, National Hospital Institute, Utrecht, The Netherlands
- Mrs. Dr. Susanne Tiemann, Vice President of the European Association of Professionals (SEPLIS), Member of the Economic- and Social Committee, Brussels, Belgium
- Prof. Dr. Wynand P.M.M. van de Ven, Professor of Social Health Insurance, Department of Health Care Policy and Management, Erasmus University Rotterdam, The Netherlands
- Dr. M.A. Verkerk, Faculty of Philosophy, Erasmus University Rotterdam, The Netherlands
- Prof. Dr. Hans Rüdiger Vogel, General Director of the Bundesverband der Pharmaceutischen Industrie e.V.
- M.G.E. Welle Donker M.A., Foundation of the Dutch Council for the Disabled, Utrecht, The Netherlands
- Prof. dr. C.J. van der Weijden, Faculty of Economics, Erasmus University Rotterdam, The Netherlands
- Dr. P. de Wolf, Faculty of Industries, Erasmus University Rotterdam, The Netherlands
- Prof. dr. H.J. van Zuthem, Professor of Social Management, Twente University, The Netherlands

Preface

The congress 'Health Care in Europe after 1992', held in October 1989, drew more than 400 participants from 17 countries to discuss that theme in a scientific and logical environment. The contributions presented here have been organized into seven relevant topics:

1. The European and American perspective of the realisation of a common market;
2. Competition in health care;
3. Medical ethics;
4. Quality of care and the position of the patient;
5. Pharmaceuticals;
6. Health care management and health care professionals;
7. Public and private health insurance.

Dr. Alexander Berlin, head of the European Commission's public health unit, touched on several of the major themes in an introductory presentation. He mentioned the rising costs due to tensions between national autonomy and EC cooperation, health care being in fact the largest industry in Europe in terms of finance and size of workforce. He listed the ageing population, AIDS and drug abuse among the most important factors for the immediate future. Another problem he and other speakers mentioned was the surplus of general practitioners across the Community, even in overprovided countries, while nurses shortages are universal, it being vital in the future to expand the nurses' roles.

As *Professor Benno ter Kuile* pointed out, national health care systems may not only be affected by the Community's social security legislation, but also by the rules governing the free movement of goods and free provision of services. It is still very difficult to give a general statement on the influence of Community law on national public health care schemes, but it certainly sets a code of norms. It is clear enough however that development is tending towards integration, and this may cause more competition in all Member States.

The papers on competition provide an analysis separating it into behaviour and structure; behaviour cannot be forced, as will be pointed out in Chapter 2 of this book, but can be restricted, structure being measured in terms of market shares and evaluated by quality and quantity.

Lessons from the United States, with its federal and state structure, are another recurring theme; *Professor Clark Havighurst*, from Duke's University School of Law, notes great differences between the US and the EC, but federal government powers are very similar to EC law.

In Chapter 3 the ethical debate is concentrated on the necessity for European ethical guidelines. Informed consent issues and AIDS policy are shown as examples of the existing differences between the European countries, there being also a difference between ethics and morality.

It is striking that quality of health care and quality assessment (Chapter 4) are not found as items on the Brussels agenda for the internal market; it is even more striking that in the area of changing health care provision attention is still not being paid to the position of the individual patient and of patient organizations. This chapter, tackling one of the main and central issues during preparatory discussions, will raise the question of whether quality will play a key role in the realization of a more uniform European health care system, and to what extent patients will influence this system after 1992.

Discussion on pharmaceuticals is, as foreseen, the most controversial. In chapter 5 the major conflicts of interest between producers and consumers, as well as between mainstream and generic manufacturers, are revealed. *Mr Fernand Sauer*, head of the pharmaceutical unit at the European Commission, describes the new directives on quality, safety and efficacy, and gives an outline of the EC policy on approval, marketing authorization and pricing. What are the main opportunities and risks for the pharmaceutical industry after 1992? What role is to be played by the Transparency Directive of the European Commission?

In chapter 6 the case will be argued whether the single market will test managerial skills. A lack of consensus for political actions, the need for non-ambiguous European (health) care statistics and data registration, the growing shortage of health care personnel, the improvement of salary and labour conditions and the development of worker participation are the main themes.

Chapter 7 comes to the conclusion that, as far as doctors are concerned, Europe 1992 has already started; the social security systems however have been excluded from the establishment of the internal market. To some contributors Europe 1992 is limited to private activities and the influence of national governments may weaken in the long run. The importance of Europe 1992 lies also in the creation of a change in hospitals' strategic environments; will there be an expanding role of the nurse as manager in Europe?

The questions relating to public and private health insurance in Europe after 1992 (Chapter 8) are many and partly unrevealed. How should 'social health insurance' be defined? The public or private character of health insurance could have far-reaching consequences in Europe after 1992. Is 'medical tourism' possible in the future Europe? Will the EC market lead to a convergence of health insurance premiums and benefits? The last and probably most important question is this; is a European Health Insurance System possible? Lessons from the US experience could also clarify some questions and *Professor Kirkman-Liff* from Arizona State University does a remarkable job in making a comparison between the developments in the US and the options for public and private health insurance in Europe after 1992.

This congress-based book could not have been realized without the support of the Erasmus University Congress Office; in particular Marijke Vos, Jannis Kostoulas and Ans van de Pavert should be mentioned and thanked here. We should also like to thank most sincerely the Municipality of Rotterdam, the Goethe Institut Rotterdam and the group of sponsors without whose financial support our initiative could not have been realized:
- Department of Health Policy and Management, Erasmus University Rotterdam;
- Erasmus University Congress Office;
- Faculty of Economy, Erasmus University Rotterdam;
- Faculty of Medicine, Erasmus University Rotterdam;
- Faculty of Law, Erasmus University Rotterdam;
- Stichting Universiteitsfonds Rotterdam;
- Nieuwe Nationale Verzekeringssociëteit N.V., the Netherlands;
- European Health Care Management Association;
- Gesellschaft für Versicherungswissenschaft und -gestaltung e.V.;
- Ministry of Welfare, Health and Cultural Affairs, the Netherlands;
- Nefarma
- Thorn EMI Computer Software;
- National Council for Public Health, the Netherlands;
- Nashua

Herbert Hermans
Jean Paelinck

1 Realization of the Common Market

Contents

1 Realization of the Common Market

1.0 Introduction
B.H. ter Kuile

If one glances through this book, it reflects a great number of subjects dealt with at the Erasmus University Congress on 'Health Care in Europe after 1992'. The most striking reflections are health care's exceptionally numerous aspects. Some of which are inextricably mixed, others totally unrelated. But they all belong to health care and health care policy.

As the Congress theme already suggests, two aspects out of many spring forward: 'Europe' and 'economy'. These two elements are not always an acknowledged part of the health care organization, which as a third element in a dominant role, is very much a national affair and, as a result, varies to a large degree from country to country. Not only in Europe, but also worldwide.

The European Community, firstly, is an economic community striving for a common market, where supply and demand can meet freely, and where a system ensures that competition is not disturbed. The EEC Treaty does not contain specific provisions for health care. An approximation of national laws concerning this complex subject, is not high on the European Commission's list of harmonization activities for the Community, which are in its White Book for the establishment on the internal market after 1992. Not surprisingly, although the theory of economic markets is not altogether alien to health care, the normal interplay between supply and demand does not apply when the health care market is of a tripartite nature. Next to supply and demand, the financial agents (health care cost insurers and budget holders) play a dominant role as well. The market situation in most countries is complex in that supply and demand are to a large degree unaware of the price mechanism that applies to the services rendered or the goods supplied to patients and consumers. Price competition and incentives to improve efficiency in the health care market, are of a limited scope. In general, neither the provider agent (hospitals, pharmaceutical suppliers, medical and paramedical services) nor the patient cares very much about costs, as long as the public and private insurers pay for it. The latter can hardly affect the setting of the price of the transactions on the health care market. Moreover, the system ensuring that competition in this market is undistorted does not have the prime attention of the authorities, either within the Community itself or its Member States.

Since health care, historically, is purely a national affair and its organization is, Community-wise, so divergent, one may expect that 'Europe after 1992' will affect the national health care organizations in each Member State quite differently.

However, as we learn from the various papers read at the Congress, health care and health care policy are not immune to the Community and its rapid developments in the internal market. As an area without internal frontiers, the free movement of goods, persons, services and capital is ensured in accordance with the provisions of the EEC Treaty.

It seems only natural that the authorities of the Member States, will not take the initiative to arrive at an approximation of national health care laws. One may, however, expect measures to be taken by individuals, be it patients, consumers or providing agents, who are both competent and able to force upon the Community - step by step - a harmonization of health care legislation and rulings. It may start with a request from a natural or legal person to a national court of law, to order (after the receipt of a solicited decision of the European Court of Justice) certain services rendered or goods provided to an individual living in Member State A, by a provider agent established in Member State B, and paid for by a health care cost insurer, established at some place within the Community, whose insurance policy with the patient is deemed relevant in this respect.

We also learn from the Congress papers in this book that once this development is under way, no aspect of health care remains immune to the avalanche of events that will occur.

Before that can happen we are in need of an approximation of minds in the rich domain of health care, health care organizations and health care policy. The Erasmus University did well to organize the first steps towards this type of harmonization of the minds. It was one of the first steps taken. We will need many more if health care in Europe is to remain efficient after 1992. What is needed first of all is a general acknowledgement throughout the Community, that Europe does affect health care, and will eventually affect all of its numerous aspects.

The authorities should realize that the direction of this play is largely in the hands of individuals and independent courts of law. If not limited to the role of spectator, then the authorities are but the producer's assistant.

1.1 Current Trends likely to affect Health Care in Europe after 1992
A. Berlin

1.1.1 Introduction

The Health Care Enterprise in the European Community, as a single scope sectorial activity in the Community providing health care, is the single largest industry in Europe both in economic and manpower terms.

I will not attempt to assess the magnitude of health care costs in Europe, a preoccupation of all governments, who directly or indirectly manage most of the available funds. However in terms of manpower used by this enterprise I will hazard a figure - professionals alone represent probably over four million workers - around four per cent of the total labour force of the Community. Health care in Europe after 1992 will, of course, be affected by European integration, but it is obvious that other factors will play the major role:

a) the changing health status of the population related to natural circumstances
b) technological progress
c) economic factors

1.1.2 Changing Health Status of the Population

Ageing, AIDS (Acquired Deficiency Immune Syndrome) and possibly hallucinogenic drugs are the three factors which are most likely to change the potential health status of the population, leading to the need for more health care after 1992.

The demographic evolution is inexorable - the population of the European Community is ageing rapidly, particularly the age group over 75 which, with more than 20 million persons, already represents six per cent of the total population, against 12 per cent for the 0 - 10 age group. At present this group often requires special care due to lack of independence.

The AIDS epidemic is like a tropical hurricane - we have developed sophisticated tools to track down its course but have only been able, for the moment, to alter this path marginally. The current number of 25,000 cumulated cases of AIDS in the Community will certainly exceed 100,000 in 1992 - 1993 and, with the increased sophistication of treatment and availability of drugs, it is to be hoped that most of the new cases will be still alive, but they will require appropriate health care, along modalities probably still to be developed. In public health terms, if the effectiveness of AZT as a prophylactic tool for asymptomatic HIV carriers is fully substantiated the need for additional screening efforts will have to be reconsidered.

The negative health impact of the increasing use of hallucinogenic drugs is the third element of this tryptique. We seem to be now awaiting in Europe the tidal wave of cocaine and crack, possibly to be rapidly followed by designer drugs. The catastrophic health and social impacts which, in particular, crack has had in North America are well known to all of us, as are the very serious financial difficulties which certain cities encounter as a result of it.

There are however some hopeful factors. The increasing public awareness that both secondary, but especially primary, prevention can reduce cancer incidence is already leading to some changes in personal habits and acceptance of outside constraints -

3

notably a reduction in smoking. It is to be hoped that this trend will increase. Here I must add the European note 'The Programme of the Community - Europe against Cancer' has certainly helped unite and galvanize health authorities confronted with the pressures of the tobacco lobby.

Cardiovascular diseases are another area where prevention in the next few years may lead to a decrease in incidence. It is unfortunate that the programme 'Euroheart' proposed by the Spanish Presidency during the first semester of 1989 could not be adopted by the Council of Health Ministers, but 'Eurohope' is a slow process.

Systematic vaccination against certain benign diseases, such as measles, with an estimated quarter to half a million cases in the European Community annually, should contribute to reducing the burden on the health care system.

1.1.3 Technological progress

The technological impact on health care after 1992 and the public demand for the newest available technology have to be considered in terms of diagnostic, monitoring and treatment tools, which will influence the quality of care, costs and manpower needs. Increasing sophistication in diagnostic tools should help to establish early unequivocal diagnosis. However, the costs are high and have to be assessed in terms of long term benefits. Increased complexity of radiological diagnostic tools (tomography, scanner, NMR) requires high investment, a concentration of facilities and very specialized manpower. An example of the costs involved is reflected in the income of radiologists as compared with other medical practitioners in independent practice. A recently published study in France by the 'Caisse Nationale d'assurance maladie des salariés' shows that while the gross annual income of medical practitioners in general varies between 50,000 and 140,000 Ecus, for radiologists the average is over 300,000 Ecus.

The continuous discovery of new biological tests is obviously of considerable help for health prevention and care, but is also a significant cost. Two examples will illustrate the potential dilemma: HIV seropositivity tests and Hepatitis C for blood supply safety. Since 1985 the use of the HIV seropositivity test for all blood donations has become a necessity; probably more than ten million tests are performed each year. With the pre-exclusion of individuals from high risk groups as donors the number of positive findings has decreased considerably, increasing the apparent cost per positive finding to a level which may soon be out of proportion, in spite of the fact that absolute safety of blood supplies is a dogma, any tampering with which will not be easily accepted by public opinion. As a result, although blood donations in most Member States of the European Community are unpaid and voluntary the cost of blood transfusions will increase with the testing requirements for safety and also insurance liability.

Remote monitoring of patients and telemedicine represent another technological development of considerable future impact, it is to be hoped of a positive economic nature, in terms of increased autonomy of aged persons and provision of sophisticated medical services in geographically remote or less accessible areas of the Community - similar to the future medical advice on board ships.

Finally, technological developments and simplification in microsurgery should help spread its use from highly specialized centres. Similarly, the need for organs for transplantation, already in rare supply, is likely to increase.

1.1.4 Economic factors

In all Member States the rapid rise in health-care costs supported directly or indirectly by public funds has become a major preoccupation for the authorities. One of the early health councils of the Community, about ten years ago, was already devoted to this subject. The growing public awareness of health has increased the demand for health care services. In turn this, together with technological development and the increase in available medication has been able to provide a better service, resulting in a further increase in demand for the best service available in absolute terms, not necessarily possible locally. The dilemma of providing the best care possible while containing costs must be resolved.

1.1.5 Human Factors

The demographic problems of the health care profession are of growing concern in most Member States as expressed at a very recent seminar organized in Paris by the French Presidency. Overall in the European Community's medical profession there seems to be a surplus of general practitioners. This surplus is very unevenly distributed geographically. Even in countries with considerable surpluses there are remote areas with a deficit, and in some countries manpower limitations cannot be imposed for constitutional reasons. At the other extreme, there is the problem of nurses, or rather the lack of them. A considerable deficit exists in many countries and there are currently many experimental ideas in progress to try to resolve the problem. This deficit seems to be due not only to economic reasons (low pay) but also to working conditions and the role of nurses in the provision of health care. Nurses have gained a new assurance and voices are being raised for their role in the provision of health care to be developed and made more independent.

The changing health status of the population in the 1990's mentioned earlier, with the provision of ambulatory and home care, will see automatically the expansion of the role of nurses and consequently an increasing need for them in a system where there is already a deficit. Recent data provided by Member States on the number of doctors and nurses show some striking differences. The ratio of nurses to doctors varies from 0.8 in Portugal to 2.5 in Belgium with, in between, figures for Spain of 1.05 and for Germany 2.0. This range probably reflects differences in services provided which merit further research.

1.1.6 European Integration

The process of European Integration, with one of its major peaks in 1993, completion of the internal market, will have an effect on health care, the amplitude of which is difficult to evaluate. At present, health as an entity - like defence - is outside the scope of Treaties, and only the fringe elements related to the completion of the internal market are covered. The Treaties even specify that restrictions on the movement of goods and people by Member States can be justified on grounds of public health. Little by little, Community legal instruments and the European Court of Justice have narrowed down Member States' freedom of manoeuvre in the application of this provision. However, there is a growing willingness on the part of most Member States to adopt a flexible and open view in order to embrace some important health subjects which could benefit - as an added value - from a Community approach. The best example is the 'Europe against Cancer' programme already in operation for four years. Let us first consider direct and obvious consequences derived from the Treaties and Community legislation: freedom of movement of goods and people.

The freedom of movement of goods includes drugs, medical instrumentation and even preventive devices such as condoms (AIDS and sexually transmitted diseases). The aim is to ensure that only goods meeting commonly agreed safety requirements, of the highest possible standard, circulate freely in the Community. Due to the technical complexities involved, the European Standards Committee is charged by the Commission to elaborate the technical standards (qualified majority vote). The possibility for self-certification or the need for certification by third parties depends on the potential danger presented by the device. The present differences in the situations between Member States can be considerable, as a recent study on condoms, the main prevention device for HIV transmission, shows:

a)   three Member states have compulsory standards and testing;
b)   four Member states have professional standards, but which do not prevent the sale of condoms not meeting the standards;
c)   five Member states do not have any standards.

Thus of the nearly six hundred million condoms sold annually in the European Community, at present one can only be sure that less than twenty per cent meet the quality/safety standards. Hopefully this situation will change radically even before 1993.

Regarding the free movement of people, the Treaty currently covers only workers. Of course in an emergency treatment is provided, but permission to obtain treatment in another Member State is not automatic; the differences in Health Care costs between Member States largely explain these difficulties. However, the freedom of movement for doctors has recently been extended to all health professionals. The available data show that the number of persons who have taken advantage of this freedom has been small and without any major problems except in a few local circumstances in border areas. Can one extrapolate this to the future? The question is difficult to answer.

Health care services, and more specifically hospitals, will be affected by the directives currently being developed on health and safety at work, which apply to them and by the Community Charter of Fundamental Social Rights, the draft of which has been just submitted by the Commission to Council. More attention will have to be devoted to the safety of the workplace and working conditions. For example, a specific directive is presently being finalized on the handling of heavy loads, of special relevance to hospitals. Workers will have to be informed and consulted and must participate in particular in:

a)   all safety related matters;
b)   circumstances involving technological changes having major implications for the work force.

In addition it is likely that circumstances will lead to cooperation in fields such as:

a)   the more rational use of sophisticated expensive medical technology and services near internal border areas of the Community (A resolution on Poison Centres tabled by the Commission to Council moves in this direction);

b)   increased availability across the Community of organs for transplantation.

Finally a number of recent events in the European Community should help with the emergence of a European consciousness towards health among citizens. They include:

a)   European Emergency Health Card,
b)   Single Emergency Telephone Number,
c)   Emergency Health Care Card,
d)   Self-sufficiency of Blood Supply in the Community,
e)   Eurobarometer.

I shall expand briefly on the last item.

The next European Public Opinion Poll (*Eurobarometer*) will be almost exclusively devoted to Europe - the European Citizen and Health. Eurobarometer surveys through personal interviews of persons selected on the basis of a household survey approach take place simultaneously in all Member States. The present survey (number 32), each involving an interview of about one hour, will cover 22,000 persons. It will include questions on:

a)   health status of the person
b)   environment and health
c)   nutrition and health
d)   emergency health care (including poisoning)
e)   health education
f)   cancer
g)   AIDS
h)   Drugs
i)   Alcohol
j)   Ageing
k)   Health and the Single Market

1.1.7 Conclusion

In conclusion: slowly but surely health questions are becoming part of the Community scene. It is likely that with the completion of the internal market there will be necessarily a gradual equilibration in spending on various activities between Member States and this will automatically affect National Health policies, and, **de facto**, a debatable proposition requiring the development of common approaches. The main issue that will have to be tackled is the reduction, or at least slowing down of, the increase in health care costs, with particular attention being devoted to the health care of the aged.

1.2 Health Care in Europe after 1992: The European Dimension
B.H. ter Kuile, F.M. du Pré and K. Sevinga

1.2.1 Introduction: Health Care in the Perspective of a Changing Europe

1) Health care and health care organization have always been exclusively national affairs by nature and indeed still are in each of the twelve Member States of the European Community. In general, this is also true for any health care policy of national authorities in the Member States. However, this scene is likely to change rapidly in the near future. National policies, like health care, may no longer be immune from the radical developments taking place within the European Community approaching 1992. Experts of the Member States discussing problems of common interest concerning health care organization should, therefore, take this into account.

One of the central questions inspiring this Congress is, to what extent national authorities of the Member States will remain free to pursue their own policies and to organize health care in their separate countries the way they deem appropriate, or whether, due to direct or indirect effects of Community law, national health care policy will be set by current or future Community rules by 1992.

2) Although the practical importance of this question cannot be denied, the central theme of the Congress is of a more general character and concerns more aspects of health care organization. The agenda of the Congress includes subjects such as health care institutions, the supply of health care services, the pharmaceutical industry and trade as well as insurance in the Member States of the European Community. The Congress is meant to promote a stage for free discussion by experts of several disciplines on all of these topics, inextricably mixed in the perspective of a changing Europe. It is obvious that lawyers should not and cannot monopolize that discussion, but it is important to stress that in a democratic society any development of health care organization is both set and limited by the rule of law. What law? National law, Community law, or perhaps both?

3) The purpose of the following presentation is to explain the possible direct or indirect effects of Community law on health care and health care organization and to discuss its scope and limitation. This subject touches upon basic questions of national powers and sovereignty, therefore it is delicate and extremely complicated. There is no reason to circumvent this discussion that has only just started. Even if the outcome would be that by 1992 the national powers of the Member States in the domain of health care will be limited because the Community has taken over, it would be useful to know. Whatever the outcome may be, it can never be the result of a single presentation by a single lawyer.

1.2.2 Two Legal Systems and their Relationship

1) The birth of the European Community in 1958 created a kind of international organization that is different from any other. Indeed, the material and the constitutional scope of its legal rules affect the life of people in the Member States in a way that was never seen before. Will the Single European Market by 1993 really affect health care and health care organization, by offering the opportunity to all participants - patients, physicians, dentists, (veterinary surgeons), pharmacists, nurses, medical and pharmaceutical faculties at the universities, hospitals, laboratories, pharmaceutical research establishments, pharmaceutical trade and industry, insurance companies and public sickness benefit funds - to go and ask for, and, as the case may be, to offer or to finance health care assistance and education abroad, or to offer health care assistance and education to citizens of other Member States?

2) To put this question does not imply that, one day, we could have a uniform health care scheme throughout the Community, although theoretically that might perhaps be conceivable. What may happen, all the same, is that the national authorities who are organizing, managing and administering health care, will find themselves confronted with other and probably narrower margins of action. How may national authorities become aware of those margins? In general there are three ways to find out.

If national authorities already are conscious of the necessity to discuss at a national level the very question as to the existence of possible margins, a glance at the Treaty and the Official Journal of the European Communities should suffice. In other cases, a confrontation may occur through administrative and legal procedures that are instigated by the European Commission before the European Court of Justice, and directed to any Member State. The Member State might be sued by the Commission before the European Court in a procedure that makes it possible for the Court to establish that the Member State has acted in breach of its obligations under the Treaty.[1] And there is a third way.

Experience shows that more often the citizens (for example, physicians and patients) and the enterprises simply are getting to know the relevant provisions of Community law. Consequently, in an increasing number of cases, national courts in the Member States are being asked to guarantee the rights that Community law provides to the individuals. The national courts are doing just that, with a degree of help from the European Court.[2]

The points briefly stated above are not new. They are characteristics of the Community law system as it has developed since its birth and through its adolescence.

3) Community law can be found in the Treaty of Rome (1957) and in the legislation that has been issued by the legal acts (regulations, directives and decisions)[3] adopted by the Community's law-making Institutions, that is, the Council, the Commission and - to a lesser degree - the European Parliament. Community law is binding upon both citizens and Member States. So far the Common Market may be seen as a market that is common both to the Member States and their citizens. As subjects of Community law they are equal, in that the Community's legal rules are equally binding for both of them. Nevertheless, there is a difference in the range of the binding effect, according to the type of provision that is relevant. This may be illustrated as follows (4) and 5)):

4) When the **Treaty** states: thou shalt treat male and female workers equally and thus pay them equal wages for equal work (the Treaty says that, more or less, in its article 119), women may sue their employers to induce them to do exactly that. They may sue their employer, because the obligation is imposed by the Treaty itself. If the provision would have been stated in a **regulation**, the effect would have been the same. The regulation is the Community's legal act of a general character. It is binding in its entirety to both Member States and individual and it is directly applicable as a single rule of law;

it should be applied by all administrative authorities and courts in the Member States.[4] Its function is to create uniform law over all the Community.

5a) Something different however may happen when the Council issues a **directive** (a legally binding instruction) addressed to every Member State, to the effect, for example, that is should change within a certain time its legislation on access to the labour market and eliminate every discrimination between men and women in that respect. The purpose of a directive is to incite the Member States to conceive their laws in a parallel direction as to realize certain obligatory effects, without actually prescribing a uniform law system. Thus the function of a directive is harmonization of laws. When a Member State's competent legislative authority for some reason, by accident or consciously, does not follow that instruction in due time, women may sue the state; they cannot sue any private party, because the obligation under the directive only is binding upon the Member State.

5b) In this situation (5a)) something anomalous may occur. When the proper national legislation is lacking, any public authority in the state may be held responsible in law before a national court as to the consequences of that situation. The Member State is not only responsible as a neglecting legislator, but also as an employer [5] - and probably in any specific legal relationship to a private party. Consequently, any public authority could be involved, **including an authority that is managing national health care**. If the relevant provision in the directive is sufficiently clear and precise to be potentially applied by an national court, the court is bound to do so. The result may be that the citizen finds himself more or less in a situation as if the necessary national legislation (that was lacking) has been effectively passed.

6a) Nevertheless there still may be a problem, because the situations are not really comparable. The exact problem is about the remaining margins of action of the Member State. The binding effect of a Community directive being enforced through the courts instead of being implemented by legislation may have some awkward consequences for national administrative authorities, because it has been achieved within the **existing 'legal environment'**. The existing national legal environment has not been changed and that is what the politicians might have been intending (together with implementing the directive), but what they have been hesitating to decide.

6b) So within this situation (5b) and 6a)), the margins of action for the national administration have not been defined by the national legislative authorities in relation to the implementation of the directive; they are defined in relation to the existing national legislation. According to article 189 of the Treaty, a directive does not impinge on the power of the Member States to choose form and methods for implementing the binding provisions of the directive into their national legislation. The necessary legislation should have been passed within a certain time-limit, that in itself again is binding upon the Member States. In this legal analysis, the competent national legislative authorities had the freedom themselves to define the new legal environment within which the binding provisions of the directive should operate. However, they did not use in due time their power to choose, because they did not pass any legislation at all. It follows that after the judgement of the court, the final result may be that the margins of action for the national administration are even narrower or more inconvenient than the actual legal limitation imposed by Community law.

6c) Conclusions of paragraph 6):
First, the creation of proper legislation in due time should be stressed. It should be realised that it is not principally Community law that is restricting more than necessary the national margins of action: it is the failure of the Member State to fulfil its obligations under Community law. The real legal margins of action under a directive may be broader if the directive is properly implemented into national legislation.

Second, directives actually do impose some margins of action upon a Member State.

Third, it has to be remarked that, as a consequence of any national legislative authority's hesitancy to act, all kinds of administrative authorities that have nothing to do with legislation might find themselves involved in legal procedures, simply because all the Member State's public offices, in some of their specific legal relationships with individuals, are bound to execute the obligation that the directive imposed. Some lawyers even think that all specific legal relationships may be covered. Thus any administrative authority would be the ideal target for a lawyer to test before a national court the consequences of not correctly implementing a Community directive on any subject matter. In fact, one of those targets has been an office of the British National Health Service - so beware of directives! [5]

7) The legal technicalities demonstrated in the previous paragraphs can be summarized in terms of the relationship between Community law and national law in general.

8) The Court of Justice of the European Communities (established in Luxembourg) is, in the final analysis, the highest authority within the Community that decides on the interpretation of Community law and its relationship with the national law of the Member States.

9) The European Court has ruled that within each of the Member States two legal systems simultaneously apply:

a)   the traditional national system governed by the national Constitution and the laws of the country;
b)   a separate Community system, established by the rules of the Treaty of Rome and by its secondary Community laws (regulations, directives, decisions).[6]

10) The European Court also ruled that in case of a conflict between Community law and national law, Community law prevails in order to guarantee uniform law throughout the Community. Consequently, any legislation of a Member State - the Constitution included - in conflict with any rule of Community law has no legally binding effect whatsoever.[7]

11) A third basic ruling of the European Courts is the so-called direct effect of an important number of Treaty provisions[6] and of all Community regulations[4]. The provisions of a Community directive, even if these provisions are addressed and directed to Member States only, may have direct effect where the Member State has not adapted its legislation in due time or in the proper way to achieve the result that the directive bindingly imposes upon the Member States.[8]

11

12) Direct effect means that any natural or legal person may invoke the rights deriving from these Community provisions before any national court. The national court is bound to protect these individual rights of the person concerned.

Economic Rules of the Community

Community law may in several aspects be relevant for health care. The most relevant rules of Community economic law that are likely to affect health care are those on the free movement of goods, persons (including workers and establishment for the free professions), services and capital - all supplemented by the harmonization of national laws - and the rules on competition. The rules on free movement of persons again are supplemented by the Community's regulations coordinating the several national social security systems on behalf of migrating persons.

1.2.3 Professionals

1) Some of the fundamental rights that the Treaty gives to all 'EEC-citizens'[9] are the rights to pursue their professional activities anywhere in the twelve Member States of the Community. These rights aim at the mobility of the economic forces and they are dealt with in the three chapters of the Treaty on the free movement of workers (articles 48 e.s.), on the free establishment of the self-employed and the companies (articles 52 e.s.) and on the free provision of services within the Community (articles 59 e.s.). They may be considered as the embryo of a European Citizenship *in statu nascendi*.

2) First, any Member State should treat the migrating employed and the self-employed the same way as they treat their own citizens, without any (overt or disguised) discrimination on grounds of nationality, neither in law, nor in administrative practice, nor in fact. The non-discrimination rule does not only cover specific situations with regard to the professional activities themselves. It also affects any general powers that may be relevant to the pursuance of these activities, for instance, joining professional organizations or trade-unions, renting or buying offices from which to practise or residences to live in, the possibilities of obtaining credit, subsidies or possible tax reductions, or to enter into contracts. [10]

Second, as to the self-employed, **all restrictions to their activities, although applicable irrespective of nationality, should be abolished** if their effect is, exclusively or principally, to hinder the establishment of or the providing of services by non-national EEC-citizens. The scope of the rights of the self-employed therefore is wider than the mere rule of non-discrimination. Furthermore, it should be noted that these rights do not only cover the free access to, but also the free exercise of, these activities.[11]

It follows that there are two types of restrictions that should be abolished:

a) Restrictions that do not apply to persons established in the national territory. [12] However the Treaty allows two small exceptions to prevent restrictive measures **that specifically concern nationals of other Member States.** First there is the public policy, public security and public health proviso (articles 48, paragraph 3; 56 and 66 EEC). **This exception only applies to the person concerned and cannot be invoked by the Member State to restrict the access to or the exercise of the medical professions as an economic branch of activity.** [13] The second exception concerns

12

the exercise of public authority (articles 48, paragraph 4, 55 and 66 EEC). This exception can only be invoked as a restriction to the entry of certain activities, not generally for professions as a whole. When a non-national is effectively employed with a public authority, or has been allowed to take up such activities, the exception consequently does not authorize discriminating conditions of work. So EEC-citizens employed in a public hospital should have the same statute as the nationals, who are employed as civil servant.[14]

b) Restrictions that apply in principle to both nationals and EEC-citizens but that prevent or otherwise obstruct the activities of the EEC-citizens, without justification - that is: objectively necessary. [15] Thus the national rules for the medical and allied professions are subject to the tests of public interest, of non-discrimination and of proportionality if they have to be applied to EEC-citizens.[16] Their application to EEC-citizens should in certain cases be adapted, if unadapted application would amount to discrimination or to a forbidden restriction.[17]

Third, regarding the freedom to provide services, the customer may indirectly be entitled to these rights in his capacity as a recipient of services. Patients (and tourists) have been expressly qualified this way by the European Court.[18]

3) For whom do these rights of EEC-citizens involve an obligation to eliminate possible restrictions? According to the case-law of the European Court, the answer should be: not only for public authorities of every kind (social security institutions!), but also for all kind of private organizations, for instance, professional organizations (for example of the medical and legal professions), trade-unions and football-clubs.[19]

4) The above-mentioned rights that the Treaty gives to all EEC-citizens are, for the medical and allied professions, amplified in the directives on the elimination of restrictions and in the directives on the recognition of diplomas. [20] In addition, the directives give the EEC medical and allied professions the following rights, as summarized in the provisions of the directives and from the case-law of the European Courts.

a) Any EEC-citizen who presents a diploma mentioned in a directive should be admitted to the profession. This includes nationals who present a diploma from another Member State [21] and, in certain cases, nationals of a third country who are married to an EEC-citizen.[22] National authorities have no discretionary power to investigate or to decide whether the applicant fulfils the national professional qualifications, [23] neither can they otherwise impose additional conditions that are not mentioned in the directives.[24]

b) If registration with a professional organization is prescribed by law that lies within the power of a Member State to decide) or necessary in fact (in the Netherlands)[24] to practise the profession in the case of establishment and as an employed worker, registration should be open to any EEC-citizen who presents an EEC-diploma or an otherwise recognized diploma, without any discrimination on the grounds of nationality.[25]

c) EEC-citizens who are providing medical services in another Member State are exempted from registration with a professional organization and with a social security institution in the host country.[26] Patients and those providers of services may invoke that right before a national court if the Member State has not adapted its national legislation, because the exemption is given in the interest of the professionals **and** of the patients. So, a surgeon established in Paris could cooperate with an anaesthetist in Madrid and a radiologist in Amsterdam as a specialized team, to provide, for instance in a monthly scheme, operations and other medical services in London, Amsterdam, Brussels or Athens. A kind of 'European Flying Doctors Service' would legally be possible.

d) In border regions, cover schemes for the weekends or vacation periods could be organized by physicians cooperating on both sides of the border, as an application of the previous point.[27]

e) An EEC-citizen of the medical and allied professions who is practising in any Member State cannot be punished under penal law for illegal practice if the authority to practise has been refused (either by the Member State's public authorities or by the competent professional organization), as under Community law it should have been given.[28]

1.2.4 Institutions

1) There are no provisions of Community law which specifically apply to the institutions of health care such as the hospitals and clinics. But there are general directives that do affect activities of the institutions, for instance directives 71/304 and 71/305 (both on public works contracts) and directive 77/62 (public supply contracts).[29] Hospitals are specifically mentioned in those directives and they should apply these procedures. The award of public contracts will be the subject of new developments in the future, because the European Commission plans to introduce new Community rules in this field in their White Paper on the Internal Market.[30]

2) Cross-frontier establishment of institutions does not occur in daily practice, but this could change after 1992, particularly if there is a 'vacuum' of health care services just across the border in another Member State. National licence-regimes for the building of hospitals would not amount to discrimination, nor make the actual establishment of an institution from another Member State illusory. The same applies to cross-border services offered by an institution. At present, cross-border services probably only occur passively,[18] as far as patients from Member State A ask for the services of an institution in Member State B. Providing passive services should in principle be free on the internal market. In any circumstances, national restrictions should not discriminate as to the country of origin of the patient.

3) A national licence-regime for the purchase, by hospitals, of medical equipment may amount to a measure having equivalent effect as a quantitative restriction on imports and may thus contravene article 30 EEC. The exception of article 36 EEC will probably not apply, because it does not cover budgetary motives,[31] which are the reason for a licence-regime. But there may be another loophole (although only for publicly financed health care) and we will deal with this in the next chapter.

1.2.5 Pharmaceutical Products and Medical Equipment

1) Trans-national trade in pharmaceutical and medical equipment within the Community is trade in goods between Member States and is, therefore, governed by Community law. More specifically it falls within the ambit of the fundamental rules on the free movement of goods (articles 9-37 EEC).[32]

According to this Title of the Treaty, pharmaceuticals and medical equipment can freely be traded from one Member State to another as soon as these goods have been released on the market of any Member State.[33] Therefore national measures restricting *specifically* imports to or exports from a Member State infringe article 30 EEC. Such a measure can only be justified (article 36 EEC) on the grounds of - *inter alia* - the protection of health and life of humans, animals and plants. Restrictive measures that, on the contrary, are applicable without distinction both to national and to imported goods may also be justified on the grounds of consumer protection, of fairness in the trade, for ecological reasons and for combating inflation in health care (see next paragraph).[34] In addition, these measures have to meet the general principles of non-discrimination and of proportionality.[35] The burden of proof lies with the Member State. Where Community directives approximating national law on these public interests have been issued, the protection of these interests has been transferred from national to Community level. In this case, national authorities generally no longer have the power to issue any rules contrary to Community law on these subjects (the so-called Tedeschi-rule).[36]

2) On the basis of the provisions on the free trade of goods, the European Court ruled that a national measure, intended to control the increase in price of pharmaceutical products and the differentiation between domestic and imported products, contravened article 30 EEC.[37] The Court acknowledged that Member States have the means to combat inflation, but national price-restricting measures cannot place imported medicines at a disadvantage. Furthermore the reimbursement systems for medicinal products may combat inflation, but they should be compatible with article 30 EEC. As the European Commission stated in the communication on the compatibility with article 30 of the EEC-Treaty of measures taken by Member States relating to price controls and reimbursement of medicinal products, published on 4 December 1986, and paraphrasing the Duphar judgement:

> measures adopted within the framework of a compulsory national health care scheme with the object of refusing insured persons the right to be supplied, at the expense of the insurance institution, with specifically named medical preparations **are compatible with article 30 of the EEC-Treaty, if** the determination of the excluded medicinal preparations involves no discrimination regarding the origin of the products and is carried out on the basis of objective and verifiable criteria (..),[38] and provided that it is possible to amend the lists whenever compliance with the specified criteria so requires. (...) These principles apply *mutatis mutandis* to positive lists (listing medicinal products which are approved for reimbursement).[39]

In the first months of 1989, the Council of the European Community issued a directive relating to the transparency of measures regulating the pricing of medicinal products for human use and their inclusion in the scope of national health insurance systems.[39a] The directive elaborates these principles and will affect national policies. The Commission plans to introduce several proposals for the elimination of restrictions to trade in pharmaceutical products in the White Paper-project.[40]

3) So far, in the health care sector, only a very limited number of trade restricting measures of each of the twelve Member States have been tested under Community law. That this number may increase as soon as nationals in the Member States are more aware of their rights under Community law, is illustrated by two recent judgements of the European Court, that concern the trade in pharmaceuticals. In the Schumacher case, [41] the Court ruled that a German law prohibiting any private individual to import any pharmaceutical product, even if it is for his personal use and if it has been bought at a pharmacist's in another Member State, infringed the Treaty. The patient had bought the product in another Member State at a quarter of the price than in his local pharmacy. Another recent judgement (Royal Pharmaceutical Society of Great Britain)[42] on parallel imports of pharmaceutical products, shows that fundamental questions, such as the relationship between doctors and their patients, may be relevant for the interpretation of the rules on the free movement of goods.

1.2.6 Private and Public Health Insurance

1) The way that the Member States of the European Community organize the financial substructure of their health care schemes shows a great variety.[43] Although in most Member States a majority of the goods and services in the health care sector is provided from public funds, in most Member States private commercial insurance companies play a certain - and sometimes considerable - role also.[44] Community law may affect those types of insurance, public and private, in a different way. As far as public health care schemes in the Member States are part of the social security regime of that country, Community law as to social security applies.[45] On the other hand, private insurance companies may fall within the ambit of the chapters of the Treaty concerning services and establishment.[46]

2) The objective of the Community's social security rules being mere coordination of the existing national schemes, these rules do not as such affect the content of the national social security legislation. However, they may have a certain influence on the national systems. The best known example is perhaps article 22 of Regulation 1408/71. This provision enables insured persons (that is, persons affiliated to a national public sickness benefit fund) to receive treatment in another Member State than their normal state of residence. Provided that such a treatment has been authorized by the competent national health care authority, the costs of the treatment are at the expense of this authority. In its Pierik cases,[47] the European Court ruled that the power to refuse authorization was limited by the requirement that the insured person should be guaranteed the opportunity to receive a treatment appropriate to his state of health in any Member State, whichever the Member State of his residence or of the competent social security authority might be.[48] National health care authorities have not often used the possibilities offered by article 22. Could effective use of this provision not be helpful to avoid unnecessary investment at a national level, in particular investments in highly specialized and very expensive medical equipment or services in, for instance, a border region?[49]

3) The national health care systems may not only be affected by the Community's social security legislation, but also by the rules on the free movement of goods[50] and on the free provision of services, as has been illustrated above.[51] As far as the services are concerned, in the view of the European Court the patient can invoke certain rights as a customer.[18]

4) It remains very difficult to give a general statement on the influence of Community law on national public health care schemes. The main point is that Community law is relevant and sets a code of norms; the national authorities of the Member States may not be fully aware of this. National public health care schemes could be tested under Community law on both discrimination and proportionality.

5) For the private insurance sector the situation is different. Community law affects this sector under the service chapter of the Treaty. If an insurance company established in a Member State meets the conditions that apply to insurance under the national law of another Member State, the company cannot be barred from doing business in the latter state. These companies may fall under the scope of the first and second directive on direct insurance.[46] According to the preamble of directive 88/357, an internal market for insurance services had to be achieved by July 1990. This means that for the insurer the opportunity to render services (to offer a health insurance policy) is to be facilitated. On the other hand, the insured (the 'patients') may have the opportunity to ask for the services of insurance companies abroad.

6) Although all the implications of Community legislation in the insurance sector may not yet be known, it is clear that development is tending towards integration. This may cause more competition among the insurance companies in all the Member States. It is unrealistic to assume that those developments will not have any effect upon the public health care sector.

1.2.7 Notes

Remarks:
Case-law of the European Court is quoted from the English version, the European Court Reports, as follows: Case-number, party or parties, [year] E.C.R. page number. Year and page number are the same in all other linguistic editions of the Courts Case-law.

OJ stands for Official Journal of the European Communities, quoted as follows: OJ (year), L (L-series, as opposed to C-series), number/page. The numbers are the same in all other linguistic versions.

1   Article 169 EEC.
2   Article 177 EEC reads (essentially): The Court of Justice shall have jurisdiction to give preliminary rulings concerning a) the interpretation of this Treaty; b) the validity and interpretation of acts of the institutions of the Community; c) 'Where such a question is raised before any court or tribunal of a Member State, that court or tribunal may, if it considers that a decision on the question is necessary to enable it to give judgement, request the Court of Justice to give a ruling thereon.'
3   Article 189 EEC.

4   Article 189 EEC; Case 43/71, Politi, [1971] E.C.R. 1039; Case 84/71, Marimex, [1972] E.C.R. 89; Case 93/71, Leonesio, [1972] E.C.R. 287; Case 39/72, Commission v. Italy, [1973] E.C.R. 101.

5   Case 152/84, Marshall v. Southampton and South West Hampshire Area Health Authority, [1986] E.C.R. 732.

6   Case 26/62, Van Gend & Loos, [1963] E.C.R. 3.

7   Case 6/64, Costa/ENEL, [1964] E.C.R. 1143; Case 106/77, Simmenthal, [1978] E.C.R. 629; see also footnote 4.

8   Case 148/78, Ratti, [1979] E.C.R. 1629; Case 8/81, Ursula Becker, [1982] E.C.R. 53; Case 102/79, Commission v. Belgium, [1980] E.C.R. 1473.

9   We will use this expression as a shorthand term for the citizens of the Member States when they are pursuing their economic activities in a way that is relevant under the EEC-Treaty.

10 General Program (Establishment), OJ.1974, Special Edition, Second series, p.7; General Program (Services), OJ.1974, Special Edition, Second series, p.3. See also Case 63/86, Commission v. Italy, [1988] E.C.R. 29 and Case 221/85, Commission v. Belgium, [1987] E.C.R. 719.

11 Article 52, second alinea EEC; Case 197/84, Steinhauser, [1985] E.C.R. 1819.

12 Case 33/74, Van Binsbergen, [1974] E.C.R. 1299; Case 2/74, Reyners, [1974] E.C.R. 631. See also: conclusions of Advocate-General Darmon in Case 292/86, Gullung, [1988] E.C.R. 111.

13 Case 131/85, Gül, [1986] E.C.R. 1573.

14 Case 307/84, Commission v. France (nurses), [1986] E.C.R. 1725; See also: Wyatt and Dashwood, *The Substantive Law of the EEC*, London 1978, 209.

15 Case 33/74, Van Binsbergen, [1974] E.C.R. 1299; See also: conclusions (of 18-11-1987) of Advocate-General Darmon in Case 292/86, Gullung [1988] E.C.R. 111.

16 Case 279/80, Webb, [1981] E.C.R. 3305; Case 110/78, Van Wesemael, [1979] E.C.R. 35; Case 205/84, Commission v. Germany (insurance), [1986] E.C.R. 3755.

17 Examples: a condition on residence is not allowed, Case 33/74, Van Binsbergen, [1974] E.C.R. 1299; neither a condition on reciprocity, Case 11/77, Patrick, [1977] E.C.R. 1199; to subject the provision of services by a physician - established in another Member State - to the condition that each professional activity only may concern one patient within a period that is not exceeding two days is an infringement of the Treaty; the same applies to the condition that an EEC-citizen cannot be registered in the register of the *Ordre des Médecins* without withdrawing all previously existing registrations (in particular in the Member State of origin): Case 96/85, Commission v. France (physicians and dentists), [1986] E.C.R. 1475.

18 Case 286/82, Luisi and Carbone, [1984] E.C.R. 377; Case 186/87, Cowan, [1989], E.C.R. 195; See also: Case 205/84, Commission v. Germany (insurance), [1986] E.C.R. 3755. These cases illustrate that in the last few years it became clear that the rights to the free provision of services do not only apply in the situation of the **active** type, implying a temporary movement to another Member State of the person providing the service. The Court, in the first case just quoted, made a distinction to the effect that these rights also apply in the situation of the **passive** type (the recipient of the service moving temporarily to another Member State) and of the **neutral** type (providers and recipients of the service stay in their respective Member States and communicate by post, telephone, telefax, computer etc.). These different

types of services may be governed by different types of legislation in the several Member States, that may be affected in their turn by Community law.

19 Case 90/76, Van Ameyde, [1977] E.C.R. 1091. The Court ruled that 'for discrimination to fall under the prohibitions (..) it suffices that such discrimination results from rules of whatever kind which seek to govern collectively the carrying on of the business in question. In that case it is not relevant whether the discrimination originates in measures of a public authority (..)'. See also: Case 71/76, Thieffry v. Conseil de l'Ordre des Avocats, [1977] E.C.R. 765; Case 271/82, Auer v. Ordre national des Vétérinaires, [1983] E.C.R. 2727; Case 107/83, Ordre des Avocats et Barreau de Paris v. Klopp, [1984] E.C.R. 2971; Case 5/83, Rienks, [1983] E.C.R. 4233; Case 292/86, Gullung, [1988] E.C.R. 111.

20 These directives, that may in certain cases have been subsequently amended, can be listed as follows:
a) physicians: directive 75/362, OJ 1975, L 167/1; directive 75/363, OJ 1975, L 167/14;
b) nurses: directive 77/452, OJ 1977, L 176/1; directive 77/453, OJ 1977, L 176/8;
c) dentists: directive 78/686, OJ 1978, L 233/1; directive 78/687, OJ 1978, L 233/10;
d) veterinary surgeons: directive 78/1026, OJ 1978, L 362/1; directive 78/1027, OJ 1978, L 362/7;
e) midwives: directive 80/154, OJ 1980, L 33/1,; directive 80/155, OJ 1980, L 33/8;
f) pharmaceutical professions: directive 85/432, OJ 1985, L 253/34; directive 85/433, OJ 1985, L 253/37;
g) general practitioners (specific education); directive 86/457, OJ 1986, L 267/26;
h) certain other allied professions may be affected by the recent Council Directive 89/48 of 21 December 1988, on a general system for the recognition of higher education diplomas awarded on completion of professional education and training of at least three years duration, OJ 1989, L 19/16.
Note the changes in these directives following the accession of Portugal and Spain: Act of Accession of Portugal and Spain, OJ 1985, L 302.

21 Case 246/80, Broekmeulen, [1981] E.C.R. 2311; Case 115/78, Knoors, [1979] E.C.R. 399; Case 292/86, Gullung, [1988] E.C.R. 111.

22 In virtue of Regulation 1612/68, these rights also may be invoked by a national of a third country who is married to an EEC-citizen to whom article 48 EEC applies. He has a right to be authorized to exercise a regulated profession in a Member State, provided that he holds a medical degree under Directive 75/363. The Court ruled this in the case of a Cypriot doctor with a Turkish and a German medical degree, who wanted to practise as an anaesthetist in Germany, where his British wife was a worker, as in article 48 EEC. Case 131/85, Gül, [1986] E.C.R. 1573.

23 Case 29/84, Commission v. Germany (nurses), [1985] E.C.R. 1661.

24 Case 246/80, Broekmeulen [1981] E.C.R. 2311.

25 Case 246/80, Broekmeulen, [1981] E.C.R. 2311; Case 11/77, Patrick, [1977] E.C.R. 1199; Case 96/85, Commission v. France, (physicians and dentists), [1986] E.C.R. 1475; Case 292/86, Gullung, [1988] E.C.R. 111.

26 Articles 16 and 17 of Directive 75/362. Article 17 reads: 'Where registration with a public social security body is required in a host Member State **for the settlement with insurance bodies of accounts related to services rendered to persons insured**

under social security schemes, that Member State shall exempt nationals of Member States established in another Member State from this requirement, in cases of provision of services entailing travel on the part of the person concerned'.

Just as food for thought: that provision may be invoked (Advocate-General Reischl in Case 246/80, Broekmeulen, [1981] E.C.R. 2311) before German social security authorities and courts, for instance, both by a Belgian or a French doctor established in Belgium and providing a medical service in Germany and, in our view, also by the patient treated in Germany. See also footnote 17.

27 Case 96/85, Commission v. France. (physicians and dentists), [1986] E.C.R. 1475; the Court mentioned expressly replacement services.

28 Case 5/83, Rienks, [1983] E.C.R. 4233. See also the Gullung case.

29 Directive 71/305, concerning the coordination of procedures for the award of public works contracts, OJ 1971, L 185/5; directive 71/304, concerning the abolition of restrictions on freedom to provide services in respect of public works contracts and on the award of public works contracts to contractors acting through agencies or branches, OJ 1971, L 185/1; directive 77/62, coordinating procedures for the award of public supply contracts, OJ 1977, L 13/1 (recently amended by directive 88/295, OJ 1988, L 127); directive 72/277, concerning the details of publication of notices of public works contracts and concessions in the Official Journal of the EC, OJ 1972, L 176/12.

30 Proposals of the Commission in the branches of water, energy, transport and telecommunication.

31 Case 238/82, Duphar, [1984] E.C.R. 523, paragraph 23.

32 The influence of Community law on the trade in each of these goods is not identical, as there exist specific Community rules on the distribution of pharmaceutical products; such rules do no exist for medical equipment. See footnote 33.

33 The licence is to be granted by the national authorities on the basis of Community directives, guaranteeing that the conditions for admittance are similar for national and imported products: directive 65/65, on the approximation of provisions laid down by law, regulation or administrative action relating to proprietary medicinal products, OJ 1965, L 369/65, as lastly amended by directive 87/221, OJ 1987, L 15/36. See also directives 75/318, OJ 1975, L 147/1 and 75/319, OJ 1975, L 147/13, as amended subsequently.

34 Case 238/82, Duphar, [1984] E.C.R. 523; See also the fundamental Case 120/78, Rewe 'Cassis de Dijon', [1979] E.C.R. 664.

35 Proportionality implies that these measures must be mandatory for the achievement of the legitimate purpose that they have been issued for; they may not go any farther than is necessary and other - less restricting - measures that may have the same result should not be available.

36 Case 5/77, Tedeschi, [1977] E.C.R. 1555.

37 Case 181/82, Roussel, [1983] E.C.R. 3849.

38 Case 238/82, Duphar, [1984] E.C.R. 523; the Court mentioned three examples of objective criteria which could justify a decision to exclude a medicinal product from reimbursement:

   a) the existence on the market of other, less expensive, products having the same therapeutic effect,

b) the fact that the preparation in question is freely marketed without the need for any medical prescription, and

c) reasons of pharmaco-therapeutic nature justified by the protection of public health.

39 OJ 1986, C 310/7, 9 - 10.

39a OJ 1989, L 40/8.

40 Fourth Report from the Commission to the Council and the European Parliament of 20 June 1989, doc. COM(89)311 def., Appendix 3, 4.

41 Case 215/87, Schumacher, [1989] E.C.R. 617.

42 Joined Cases 266 and 267/87, Royal Pharmaceutical Society of Great Britain, [1989] E.C.R. 1295.

43 Comparative Tables of the social security schemes in the Member States of the European Community, Commission of the EC, Luxembourg 1988; Papers prepared for the preliminary sessions of this congress, 20-22 June 1988; C. de Klein en J. Collaris, Sociale ziektekostenverzekeringen in Europees perspectief, Wetenschappelijke Raad voor het Regeringsbeleid, 's-Gravenhage, 1986.

44 In those Member States where a kind of co-payment system (ticket modérateur) exists, private insurance companies often reinsure the financial risks of those systems, which may be considerable.

45 Article 51 EEC, amplified by Council Regulation 1408/71, OJ 1971, L 149/1, spec. ed. 1971 (II) 416, as amended and updated by Regulation 2001/83, OJ 1983, L 230/6; see also Regulation 574/72, OJ 1972, L 74, concerning administrative procedures.

46 The Treaty rights that have been mentioned above in the chapter on the Professionals, apply also to (insurance) companies. See Case 205/84, quoted in footnotes 16 and 18. See also the so-called First and Second Directives on the coordination of laws, regulations and administrative provisions relating to direct insurance other than life assurance: directive 73/239, OJ 1973, L 228/3 and directive 88/357, OJ 1988, L 172/1.

47 Case 117/77, Pierik, [1978] E.C.R. 825 and Case 182/78, Pierik, [1979] E.C.R. 1977.

48 The ruling was based upon the version of article 22, paragraph 2, that was applicable at that time. After these judgements, the text was amended by Regulation 2793/81, OJ 1981, L 275.

49 Patients in Zealand-Flanders in the Netherlands often visit hospitals in Antwerp, Bruges or Gand in Belgium, or are brought there by ambulance. In a serious emergency it seems to be faster than to try and reach a Dutch hospital. It may be wiser to take account of the existing standard of health care just across the border, than to invest at all costs in such a region.

50 See Duphar case, footnotes 34 and 38.

51 See for an example footnote 26; Would it be sensible in the future for a health care institution to refuse to authorize one of its affiliated patients to go abroad, if, on the other hand, the same institution is bound to accept the services of a foreign physician who comes to the country of this institution to treat the same patient there, at the expense of the same institution?

Appendix: Some Questions

1.   Could a patient choose within the Community:

a)   for medical and allied services in another Member State, since in his view these foreign services are of better quality and/or are supplied at a lower price?

b)   for any health care service and/or product which he deems appropriate (both within his country and in any other Member State) or is he limited to the choice of services and products that are supplied, paid for or reimbursed by the sickness benefit funds
- in the Member State of his nationality?
- in the Member State of his nationality **and/or** in the Member State where he lives as a migrating worker?
May the patient in this situation choose to travel back or to be brought back to his own Member State to be treated there when his illness may lead to a kind of 'medical homesickness'?

c)   to be insured by any insurance or any public sickness benefit fund in the Community?

2.   Could a public sickness benefit fund or any insurance company choose to make a contract with:

a)   any physician, pharmacist or hospital established in any Member State?

b)   a physician, pharmacist or hospital established just across the border in another Member State?

c)   any patient in the Community?

3.   Could a physician choose to (also) take part in any foreign public sickness benefit fund within the Community

a)   if he deems the conditions of this sickness benefit fund better then those in his own country and region?

b)   if he also wants to treat patients from any other Member State, and he is not established in a border area?

c)   if he also wants to treat patients from the Member State just across the border, and he is established in a border area?

4.   Could a physician choose to have his practice just across the border

a)   and treat only patients who are insured in his Member State at the other side of the border?

b)   and treat both patients insured in his Member State and patients insured in the Member State where he established the practice? (see also questions 1. and 2.)

5.   Could any administrative authority governing a hospital choose freely its architects, builders, constructors and suppliers of (expensive) medical and other equipment all over the Community? Are they free to limit their choice to enterprises established in their own Member State?

6. Is a Member State in all circumstances free to issue measures restricting the sale of pharmaceutical products that is allowed to be sold in any other Member State?

7. Is a Member State in all circumstances free to issue measures restricting the sale of pharmaceutical products at the condition of a physicians prescription, if that/those product(s) may be freely sold in any other of the Member States?

8. Can a Member State issue any measure of its own choice restricting the price of (all) pharmaceutical products sold in its territory?

9. Could a pharmacist establish his pharmacy in a border region, with a view to selling his goods in the whole geographical area and not only to clients in his Member State?

10. Could a patient take a prescription from his physician to a pharmacist established in another Member State, if this pharmacist would supply identical pharmaceuticals at a lower price (including the costs and time spent for the patient's voyage abroad, for instance in border regions)?

11. Could insurance companies, including national public sickness benefit funds, be obliged under Community law to guarantee the payment of these pharmaceuticals?

12. If so, could they make payment or reimbursement conditional to buying at the cheapest pharmacy within a certain distance of the patient's residence?

1.3 European Community and the Right to Health Care: an agenda for the future
H.D.C. Roscam Abbing

1.3.1 Introduction

Recently, Dutch newspapers focused attention on trade in human organs between member countries of the European Community. The transport, for industrial purposes, within the EC of cerebral membranes and placenta, without knowledge let alone consent by the person concerned (or his relatives), was another event, highlighted by the media.
So far, the EC has not undertaken particular action in this field. Yet these and other developments involving bodily material touch upon the legal position of the person from whom the material is taken, and has likely implications for the health of the donor as well as the recipient. So far, only one relevant field in this respect has been covered by EC action, namely the field of blood products. The 1989 directive on blood products introduces - though hesitantly - the principle of self sufficiency and of non-commercialization. Because of the growing international exchange of organs and other bodily material either for implantation purposes or for industrial processing, there is every reason from a quality and safety viewpoint in health care (and therefore health protection) to put these items on the Brussels agenda. The Dutch Government has already taken some initiatives to this end, as well as one of the Dutch Euro parliamentarians. Indeed, within a Europe without borders, national policies alone can no longer cope with these and similar problems. Thus, for instance, the recent English ban on organ commercialization cannot prevent an English national from travelling to

another EC Member State to sell one of his organs. This is just one example of areas which touch upon health protection and health care for which national action alone is inadequate in the perspective of an integrated European Community. There is even more reason for EC action because there is also an availability aspect involved.

As we all know, the EC-Treaty does not form a legal basis for a common policy in the field of health, unlike in the social field, regarding occupational health, which I will not discuss, and, since the European act, the environment, which equally falls outside the scope of my presentation. As, for instance, expressed in 1977 by the then Commission member, Vredeling, before the European Parliament, there is no basis for the development within the EC of a comprehensive health service at Community level, let alone of one free of charge. Although, therefore, harmonization of health services will not be pursued, the Commission will, according to the same speaker, attempt to improve the health care of citizens of the Community by coordinating and harmonizing certain existing arrangements. Since that date, it has become more and more apparent that EC undertakings not only have to take into account consumers' rights to protection of health and safety, but also directly or indirectly promote the realization of the right to health care throughout its Member States. In respect of the latter the realization of the European Market offers ample possibilities. Recent undertakings regarding a 'Social Charter' are a clear proof that the EC is aiming at further implementing socioeconomic rights of European citizens. In my opinion this means, in fact, implementation of the Council of Europe Social Charter at Community level, adherence to which Charter could well be envisaged by the EC.

Despite the fact that the realization of the right to health care, which is one of the rights included in the Council of Europe Social Charter, is not directly covered by the Treaty of Rome, the attainment of the objectives of the EC has direct impact on national health care systems. Thus, for instance, the free movement of persons and services (doctors, nurses, paramedicals, pharmacists and the like) as well as goods (pharmaceuticals, medical devices, but also bodily material) presupposes that minimum quality standards and requirements are laid down at the EC level. This clearly influences the level of quality in health care in the Member States.

Furthermore, the social policy of the Community calls amongst other activities for containment of growth of social expenditures, in particular those in the health care sector. Measures for cost-containment have been suggested frequently in the frame of the EC. Suggestions include price- and tariff-control, measures at the supply side (as for instance health care planning on the basis of need estimates) and the demand side (ranging from health education to review of coverage through health care insurance schemes).

The fact that since 1977 the ministers for public health of the Member States and the EC-Commission have met regularly, to discuss various major health issues, also indicates that health care is one of the fields of concern of the EC. Among the more or less permanent items on the agenda are the economics of health care, health education policies, measures to combat illnesses (such as AIDS, cancer, cardiovascular diseases) and alcohol and drug addiction.

In 1978, the items which were declared priority fields included pharmaceuticals, specialized manpower, harmonization of definitions and statistical data relating to health care. Present research projects include the fields of genetics, pre- and postnatal care, the handicapped and health services. Also the European Parliament has focused attention on the health care sector, with particular emphasis on the immaterial aspects. The latter has for instance resulted in the drafting of a charter for the rights of the child in health institutions, in texts related to the position of the elderly in health care, on the rights of the patient and regarding the AIDS problem. The European Parliament also has initiated the introduction of a European health card and has asked for rules governing organ transplantation, the latter, so far, without tangible results.

1.3.2 Summary of Achievements

A pressing question is the one on the state of the art of the consequences of the EC for the health care sector. A next question is, with the 'magic' date of 1 January 1993 on the horizon, what we can expect from the EC to further implement the right to health care. I will try to give some answers from the viewpoint of a health lawyer to both questions. There are, and always have been, qualitative and quantitative disparities regarding health services in the EC Member States. However, trends regarding quality of care, structure, organization and financing of health care equally show similarities. The same applies to ethical questions which have become more and more pertinent in health care, to the legal position of the individual in health care as well as to health legislation in the various countries.

The undertakings of the EC in the field of the free circulation of persons, services and goods have clearly had its harmonizing effects on the health care sector. I will present some of the major points:

1) Health Care Professionals In the field of the free movement of persons, progressive abolition of restrictions on the establishment (and employment) of members of the medical, pharmaceutical and other health professions has been achieved. The latest directive to impact on the field of health care is the one on mutual recognition of diplomas of higher education, which is of importance for paramedical professions. The endeavours of the EC now more or less cover all aspects of free establishment and of rendering services in the health care sector. In the foreseeable future, possibilities of access of medical professionals to governmental services will also be amplified. This activity area follows jurisprudence of the Court of Justice, which gave a restrictive interpretation on the possibilities to refuse free access to governmental services (article 48, 4 of the Rome Treaty). Only those occupations which involve public authority or protection of general state interests will be excluded from the free access. The latter restriction might for instance apply to health inspectors. By now at least (minimum) standards apply throughout the EC regarding the competence to enter the health care market as a health professional.

The EC rules on qualitative requirements, which have resulted in harmonizing to some extent medical and allied curricula, also have an indirect quantitative influence on national health policies. National measures restricting admittance to medical faculties and other related educational facilities as part of a manpower planning policy in health care have now to take into account the European dimension. These measures, therefore, can only be efficient if supplemented by measures focused upon the admittance to the health care market, such as a licence system or measures in the frame of the health insurance system, appropriate to contain the number of health care professionals entering the health care market. It is standing jurisprudence that such national measures which are clearly directed towards cost containment in health care, are compatible with EC law as long as they do not have a discriminative effect on qualified health care professionals from other EC member countries.

2) *The Product Sector* The protection of health naturally also calls for strict quality requirements for goods destined to circulate freely within the community. The removal of trade barriers in respect of goods presently calls for close attention because of the majority vote which was introduced in this respect with the European Act, in which framework the Commission strives at a high level of protection. Once a directive has been accepted on this basis, exceptions on the basis of article 36 (national departing measures on ground of protection of health) will only be possible on a very limited scale. They are moreover subject to scrutiny by the European Commission and the Court of Justice.

Because of the present harmonization policy of norms and standards regarding the product sector, an obligatory information procedure applies **inter alia** to national draft rules regarding pharmaceuticals, medical devices and blood products. This procedure enables the Commission not only to check conformity with Community law, but also to consider whether the subject requires Community action (as was done in the frame of the blood products directive).

Other aspects of a common market for products include the development of GMP's, GLP's, certification of test laboratories, mutual recognition of inspection systems and the like. Indeed, there is hardly any room left for deviant national policies regarding goods, products and apparatus to be introduced to the health care market.

Thus, it is crucial for national governments to formulate their own level of safety requirements and health protection prior to discussions on EC directives. On the other hand, like in the case of health care professionals, a national licence system regarding specific medical technologies for financial and/or quality reasons as applied in the Netherlands is compatible with EC law provided it does not present (hidden) discrimination regarding manufacturers from other Member States.

Various directives in the pharmaceutical sector have been issued for the purpose of approximation of laws based on Article 110 of the EC-Treaty. These measures are also concerned with health and safety control of imports coming from third countries. Proprietary medicinal products, sera, vaccines, radiopharmaceuticals and blood products are covered by the directives. Uniform rules for tests and trials have been formulated. Conditions for suspension of licence and revocation of medicines are also established. However, the efforts in the pharmaceutical sector have not yet resulted in a real common market. Registration requirements are still based on various national systems. In the future, there will most likely be a combination of systems for admittance to the EC market: mutual recognition of registration of products, the so-called multi-state procedure, (hence a decentralized system) and central registration, the latter for at least bio-technological products and so-called 'high tech' products. Other items still under consideration include information leaflets, OTC's and only on prescription medicines (POM), for which latter purpose 'minimum lists' will be elaborated.

A recent achievement in the field of pharmaceuticals is the so-called Transparency directive. This directive enables the Commission to examine national measures on price-setting and refunding of pharmaceuticals in the light of the purposes of the common market. A databank including not only technical essentials, but also economic aspects is a next step. At the national level, the possibility to exclude medicines from insurance coverage for public health reasons remains, provided the measures are not discriminatory and are taken on basis of objective, controllable criteria. Regarding blood products, the manufacturer is required to give proof of safety (in particular regarding infectious diseases, such as AIDS and Hepatitis-B) and has to obtain a licence for marketing purposes.

Discussions on good clinical practice in clinical research (= clinical trial data) are presently ongoing. Standardization of European requirements for clinical research (documentation and GCP trials) is to be expected at least for pharmaceutical products. The consultation of ethics committees will certainly be part of the requirements. This will also have a bearing on the position of the individual who takes part in experimental research. Norms for acceptability of experiments involving human beings, in particular regarding the incompetent, information, consent- and privacy issues (to be laid down in national law and regulations) will thus (in)directly be influenced by EC requirements in this respect. Individual human rights in health care to be applied in particular when a third party interest is involved will then enter the domain of EC law. It might well give an impetus to further coordinating or harmonizing national rules governing medical research involving human beings.

In the field of medical devices, activities have been speeded up after the decision had been taken (in 1985) on a new approach, which limits legislative harmonization to the adoption of essential safety requirements, with which products put on the market must comply, technical norms being formulated by European Normalization Institutes (CAN and CENELEC).

Regarding the safety requirements for medical devices, the industry is in favour of a classification according to the risks involved: for low-risk medical devices a mere declaration and administrative registration of marketing is considered sufficient; for a middle-risk category a declaration of conformity with GMP's should be added; for high risk products an approval of the fabrication file would in addition be necessary. The fields to be covered by EC directives are active implantable electromedical devices, active medical devices, non-active medical devices and 'in vitro' diagnostics. As in the case of medicines, it should be considered by the EC to introduce regulation along the lines of OTC and POM's also in the field of 'in vitro' diagnostics. This in particular because some so-called 'do-it-yourself kits' if directly available might harm the consumer (genetic tests, HIV test).

Whereas most of the activities in the field of medical devices are presently concentrated on marketing requirements - with its bearings on experimentation and the legal position of the individual involved - the postmarketing surveillance equally calls for attention. As in the field of medicine, an early warning system, conditions for licence suspension and product recall are necessary to protect the health and safety of the consumer throughout the Community. A databank on particulars of the device, its costs and also possible negative implications, as well as an appropriate EC data system on faults and near accidents which have occurred are a prerequisite, not only at the national but also at Community level. This presupposes the standardization of national incidence reporting and notification systems.

Liability rules on products have already been laid down by the EC. A proposal for a directive on product safety is presently being discussed. This directive aims at guaranteeing safety of products in addition to the requirements laid down in specific directives; it may constitute a useful additional instrument for the protection of the consumer and is therefore worthwhile to follow up.

3) Health Insurance Schemes The health insurance sector has also been subject of some regulation, in the sense that coverage of expenditure incurred in another member country is provided by their own national insurance scheme, in particular in case the expenses if incurred in their own country, would also have been refunded. As long as the health insurance falls under the national social security system, there are not other EC rules applicable. However, the EC reciprocal health insurance refunding rules, together with increasing mobility within the EC might well result in alignment of national health insurance schemes. Private health insurance schemes clearly fall within the scope of EC rules. The latter might complicate ongoing changes in national health care insurance systems, as is the case in the Netherlands. Moreover, within the framework of a social health insurance scheme, price and tariff agreements have to comply with EC competition rules.

1.3.3 A Health Agenda for the Future

1) Health Protection Most of the activities of the European Community which were briefly summarized, strive at balancing the economic objectives of the EC with the right to the protection of health and safety of the consumer. The very possibilities for the free movement of persons and goods within the EC also call for a common approach to prevent the spread of communicable diseases: thus, conditions for entrance at the outer borders (vaccination requirements and so on) cannot any more be subject to national rules, but have to be formulated at community level. This has indeed been realised in the case of AIDS (in a negative sense). The same applies to measures such as obligatory (nominative) notification of diseases, isolation and quarantine as well as to vaccination schemes in member countries. Policies regarding communicable diseases cannot be left any more to national authority. Because of this consequence of the Common Market, the EC will not only bring about a common level of health protection, but will also have impact on the legal position of the individual (in particular regarding the right to physical integrity and the right to privacy).

Equally from the perspective of health protection, a Community policy is needed regarding the exchange of organs and other bodily material: indeed, with the abolition of national borders, there should be uniform requirements to prevent transmission of diseases through bodily material destined to be used in man, both at the outside frontiers and within the EC. Indeed, the 'high protection level' in the frame of majority decision taking directly touches upon the health and safety of the European citizen, but also has impact on individual human rights in health care. Isolated actions within (parts of) Member States are henceforth incompatible with EC law.

2) Quality of Care Unlike the product sector, where safety requirements and early warning systems for marketed products have been or are being laid down or considered, health professionals are not subjected to uniform standards of care and treatment. However, the more mobility of health professionals within the EC increases (for which, as I will indicate later on, there is every reason from a perspective of availability of health care facilities and services), the more coordination and harmonization of standards of treatment and care will follow. In fact, with the internationalization of medicine, the technical professional standard is already increasingly set at an international level. In addition, the free movement within the EC will have a unifying influence on the professional standard, which also contains duties towards the patient and social obligations. The same holds also for norms and standards applied in the framework of national disciplinary law. In the long run, certification schemes for health professionals and health care facilities might well be developed at the EC level. There might even be a necessity to do so as soon as health care delivery increasingly will cross national borders and patients will more readily seek treatment in other Member States. National disparities in quality of care will then clearly hamper the free market.

3) Availability of Health Care Services and Other Possibilities One of the main targets of the realization of the right to health care is the equitable distribution of available possibilities for medical care. Despite the fact that a common health policy does not fall within the objectives of the EC, there is still every reason to aim at an appropriate infrastructure of health services throughout the EC, thus increasing efficiency, quality of care and cost-effectiveness. Activities might encompass various undertakings, such as the exchange of specific health services according to a fixed scheme ('the flying health care team'), the creation of 'Centres of Excellence' by a common effort, and the repartition among member countries of training facilities for high tech specializations: international pooling of scarce resources will thus broaden the possibilities for treatment. There is in fact no reason to have at the disposal of citizens every highly specialized and sophisticated medical possibility in Maastricht, in Aken, in Brussels and in Ghent. The EC disposes in fact, as I indicated already in 1979, of all the prerequisites to pool scarce possibilities. Organ banking at European level is another example of solidarity in health care to be pursued by the EC.

I do recognize that within such a system of pooling of resources and equipment, the problem of selection of patients still remains. A careful set of objective and rational criteria as well as a built-in system for supervising the application of these criteria should be part of such a supranational scheme.

4) Human Rights It is also to be expected that in the field of immaterial aspects related to health technology a common approach will develop from the common market. Medical technology assessment with its social, ethical and legal aspects will undoubtedly become part of community endeavours. Common research projects within areas which touch upon the individual's position, like those in the field of genetics and AIDS, will also at least indirectly result in a common approach to the legal position of the individual. The guarantees for and implementation of individual human rights in health care as included in the Council of Europe European Convention on human rights will indeed eventually become more and more a matter of concern at the level of the EC. The right to life, to bodily integrity and to privacy, but also the non-discrimination principle have to be respected at the same level throughout the Community. Common problems in fact need a common approach. The EC might well function as a clearing house regarding developments in medicine, technology, health services and the like. It should ensure a constant intercountry transfer of knowledge and information through databanks. For this purpose uniformity of definitions and statistical data relating to health care is necessary.

In respect to the right to health care the EC should seek to promote equity and social justice. To this end it might give impetus not only by further expanding its activities in the field of quality of care, but also in creating further guarantees for financial accessibility of health facilities and in promoting international availability through pooling of existing resources.

A study on the possibilities which offers the EC in this respect should be carried out as soon as possible in order to develop a plan of action for a coherent approach to health care within the EC, covering all relevant aspects involved (including the immaterial ones). Such a study should be performed in close cooperation with the WHO (Regional Office for Europe) and the Council of Europe.

It is my conviction that the EC offers ample possibilities for guaranteeing throughout its Member States individual human rights in health care as well as for further realizing the right to health care. The perspectives in this respect are in principle positive. It is the task of the health lawyer and of politicians to pursue the aim of individual human rights as well as of socio-economic human rights, not only at a national, but also at an EC level.

1.3.4   References

Gertis, L. (May 1989), Good clinical practice in clinical research, *The Lancet*, 1008 - 1009.
Leenen, H.J.J. (1986), Pinet, Prims, *Trends in health legislation in Europe*, Masson: Paris.
Roscam Abbing, H.D.C. (1979), *International Organizations in Europe and the right to health care*, Kluwer: Deventer.

1.4   The Effects of European Policies on Health and Health Care
Chr. Altenstetter

1.4.1   Introduction

Health issues touch on every aspect of human existence of the 322 million people living in the European Community. In consequence, national and Community policy-makers face numerous challenges in responding to old and new health threats in the future. However, the development and implementation of supranational and national problem-solving strategies are influenced by scientific knowledge but, above all, by the comparative politics of health governance of the Member States in EC institutions as well as by domestic politics. A considerable diversity of cultural, social, political, administrative as well as legal and economic traditions prevailing in the Member States come into play in EC policymaking.

1.4.2   Four 'Freedoms'

Behind the idea of a Single European Market to be established by 1 January, 1993, and sanctioned by the Single European Act (SEA 1986) is the provision of four 'freedoms': the freedom to move goods, services and capital, and the freedom to move within the European Community. The realization of these four freedoms is surrounded by many uncertainties, but one thing is clear. The Single European Market is likely to generate dynamics with medium term and long term impacts on health and health outcomes. However, for health, 1992 is not going to be the 'magic date', nor will it be a milestone in health policy development of the European Community. Rather, if we need a date which marks a watershed in health policy development and health innovations in European societies, it is 1980 and 1984 respectively, when the European version of a

Health-For-All (HFA) strategy and the 38 regional targets were adopted by the 32 Member States of the European Region of the World Health Organization (EURO), which includes the Twelve among its members.

This common European health policy is binding on the European region only. It is not binding on individual nation-states nor the European Community. The policy rests on four pillars: lifestyles, the elimination of risk factors affecting health and the environment, a reorientation of the health care system itself, and finally, in every society an improved macro- and micropolitical management capability, including the use of new biomedical and information technology and research.

It is true that this pan-European policy was adopted outside the political, institutional and legal framework of the European Community and that it, therefore, lacks a clear legal and constitutional basis. But it hardly lacks legitimacy, credibility, acceptability nor political support of the Member States and the Community at large. A narrow and all-inclusive professional definition, that is a biological definition of health, valid for most population segments throughout the history of the western world, was challenged to give way to a broader social-ecological paradigm with which it co-exists today. National and Community policymaking as well as efforts carried out by the WHO Regional Office for Europe (EURO) bears traces of both orientations. Health issues are internationalized, and international and national agenda-setting and problem definition are no longer the sole prerogative of the politico-administrative and professional establishments.

Unquestionably, a Community health policy and/or policy responses (legislative, administrative and judicial) to specific and diverse health risks or to new diseases such as Acquired Immune Deficiency Syndrome (AIDS) by EC institutions will eventually have to be measured against the core philosophy, the criteria of health inherent in the European Strategy for Health for All by the Year 2000 and, above all, against the first of the 38 outcome targets set for the European Region, namely equity in health. Equity in health means the reduction of differences in health status between countries and between groups within countries.

This year, a leading health expert in Europe assessed 'Health for All in Europe at the Midpoint' this way. The successes and the strength of the approach adopted in the 1980s are now clear:

a limited technocratic understanding of planning has evolved into a politically, socially and economically sensitive concept of health policy development which can be adapted by all Member States

the sense of vision, the adherence to the central UN ethic of social justice (equity), the long term perspective, and the comprehensive character of health policy have been retained through the adoption of the HFA Strategy and Targets. This is particularly emphasized by the stress on outcomes, pursued through an interlocking set of focused substrategies (disease prevention and control, promotion, environment, appropriate care, supportive measures), countering short term effects whether related to political or economic instability or to a dominant preoccupation whether social (AIDS) or economic (health services cost containment) (Barnard, 1989:38)

If the intention exists in the European Region in 'turning HFA policies into action by society' ('from paper to people') (World Health Organization, 1989:9), actions taken by

31

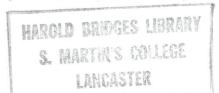

the European Community will have to be inspired by the same credo. But will EC measures be counterproductive to these activities and insights? Will a Community health policy, whatever it may be and whenever it may emerge, clash with the content and the substantive components underpinning the common European HFA-policy? Are the values underlying a fledgling Community health policy compatible with those underlying the common European health policy? Are the values underlying other EC policies compatible with creating equity or reducing it? Only in-depth examinations and careful observation will tell.

1.4.3   Market Forces versus Traditions

Two key questions arise for health comparativists and practitioners of health care organizations. Will free market-forces and competition set the direction of future developments? Or, conversely, will the European tradition of granting universal access to health care, regardless of economic means and social status, and the philosophy of solidarity between the sick and the healthy, be retained and set the direction in which future health policy will be developed and health care organizations and subsectors may move? If it is the latter, state interventions and regulations remain crucial. They also remain essential, if the new poverty and its social distribution as well as gender issues are to be addressed seriously. Neither the traditional thinking which inspired the development of social policy in the welfare states in European countries in the past nor the political forces which have fostered welfare state developments in the past are sensitive enough to these new and salient issues. However, what matters most in the emerging developments after 1992 is the fact that Member States find themselves at different stages of development in relation to a broad range of issues ranging from health care and health care organizations to health promotion and health protection policy issues outside and beyond the traditional health care delivery system.

Uniquely European traditions in health and social policy remain alive in most societies organized within the Community. They continue to stress workers' political and economic rights and universal access to health care, financed by different national health schemes. These rights and their portability when migrating to another country are secured in the provisions concerning the 'social dimension' (Commission, Title V, **Bulletin**, 1986: 13-14; Commission 1988b). How real the dangers of social dumping and regional and local dislocations are going to be, is as uncertain as the possibility that collective bargaining and workers' participation will be sacrificed in the future. In addition to social provisions on the free mobility of workers and the liberal professions which existed previously, the Single European Act explicitly stressed the need for maintaining and improving occupational health and safety requirements in worksites, as well as environmental health.

1.4.4   From Economics to Coalition and Organizational Politics

Changes will occur, but which theoretical insights help predict future developments? Drawing on macro-or micro-economic theories of the market and competition is most attractive in input - output modes of thinking. But they also have a price because they exclude from their analytical focus a) political processes which convert inputs into outputs inside the black box of governance and the political system and b) the effects (intended, unintended, direct or indirect, short-term or long-term) on health outcomes.

Even though economic theories explain the economic dynamics, most likely the initial driving forces in the European Community, they have these limitations. The development of creative problem-solving strategies inside the black box are contained by time-honoured traditions, established policies and policy networks or organizational actors as well as coalition politics of the Member States in the relevant EC decision-making bodies. The following considerations are based on three premises which have a high degree of plausibility and are rooted in experience and confirmed knowledge in the policy sciences. In policy processes 'institutions matter' (March and Olsen, 1984), 'different kinds of policies matter' (Lowi, 1972) and, last but not least, supranational coalition and national (coalition) politics matter.

1.4.5 The European Community: Authority and Responsibility in Health

Prima facie, the European Community lacks authority to decide on health (services) policies and it lacks operational responsibilities to implement policy decisions. Policy-making in health care and health care organizations continues to be a national responsibility. Therefore, health hardly figures prominently in the Single European Act nor in the Treaty of Rome (1957). Yet, health and health-related areas have not entirely remained outside the purview of policy-making by the institutions of the European Community. European health law is set in some distinct areas. For example, the Community has authority to legislate on the free mobility of labour and self-employed professions, a healthy living and working environment, and occupational health and safety. The European Coal and Steel Community (ECSC) became involved in industrial hygiene and safety as early as 1951. The European Atomic Energy Community (EAEC) created in 1957 took on responsibilities for nuclear fission energy, controlled thermonuclear fusion, biology and health protection in 1957 (Baert and van Etten, 1985). Today, these areas, occupational health and safety and the working environment (Article 118A, Commission of the European Communities 2/86:13) and environmental protection (Title VII, Commission of the European Communities 2/86: 13) are not only basic pillars of the 1992 project but are also European law amended by the Single European Act. However, as a leading scholar in Community health law argues, the Single European Act has not broadened the scope of fairly restricted responsibilities in health which the European Community has had in the past (Bélanger, 1989). National sovereignty is defended and national law applies to most health issues.

1.4.6 The Need for Policy Coordination and International Cooperation

The Commission (of the European Communities) intends 'to avoid as far as possible any overlap or duplication of the activities of other international organizations in matters of health, and to consult with these organizations with the aim of achieving mutual compatibility and thus making maximum use of limited resources' (Commission, 1989:13-14). This may - but need not - mean that the Community is open and willing to endorse a social - ecological orientation rather than a restrictive public health approach dominant in many European countries in the past. Will mixes of both approaches be applied in the future, as they have been in the past? Quite likely. However, one prerequisite is essential. International coordination and cooperation presupposes internal, that is, intra-European Community policy coordination and the elimination of internal contradictions of concerted efforts pursued by separate

Directorates-General. These contradictions have a bearing on health and health outcomes explicitly or implicitly.

International cooperation between the European Community and the World Health Organization bore fruit in the past. Several EC concerted action programmes in health are directly traceable to HFA concerns. The European Community, in collaboration with the WHO Regional Office for Europe, is active in environmental protection and health, a 'smoke-free Europe', 'Europe against Cancer', pleas for the development of a common European public health policy to fight Acquired Immune Deficiency Syndrome (AIDS) and many other programmes. This involvement is feasible, even though the Community mostly lacks explicit and comprehensive powers to formulate a Community health policy. But more cooperation is needed, if the European Community wants to utilize the possibility that 'in the area of health as in others, the European Community can demonstrate the unique value of its "multiplier effects" ' (Commission, 1988c: 15). This may require major efforts and political will both of supranational and national actors.

1.4.7 The Single European Market and Health

As previously mentioned, the Community's legislative powers for developing a Community health policy are severely limited and the Single European Act has not created a possibility to broaden the authority of EC institutions over health matters. In citing the WHO preamble, Bélanger (1989:14; 1985) points out: 'The governments have the responsibility for their peoples' health'. While these constitutional, legal and procedural issues will occupy the Member States, the EC institutions and the European Court of Justice and legal scholars for some time to come, the creation of the Single European Market by 1 January, 1993 will set in motion dynamic processes which simply will not wait until agreements on the fine constitutional or political points are reached, or until judicial policy-making sets final European law.

At the same time, these processes which, among others, may result in the adoption of problem-solving strategies and policy choices, need to be recognized as setting the preconditions and the conditions for leading a healthy life in safe home and working environments and for repairing illness in each Member State. The only reasonable and equitable benchmark for supranational and national concerted efforts, at least in theory, is the 38 regional targets and the European HFA strategy with equity as a main focus. On the other hand, the transnational origin of health hazards will further put pressures on the European Community and national decision-makers to support 'an interlocking set of focused substrategies (disease prevention and control, promotion, environment, appropriate care, supportive measures)' (Barnard, 1989:38) globally, regionally and nationally.

The Commission of the European Communities, after decisions on priorities were taken by the European Council, recognized three priority areas as having a direct bearing on health (Commission, 1989:3-4).

a) the abolition of physical frontiers within the Community;
b) the harmonization of technical standards, including uniform standards for testing and certification;
c) the abolition of physical checks on animal and crop products which require disease prevention strategies.

A fair number of exhaustive and not so exhaustive directives are already in existence for implementation by the Member States. When all directives are implemented, they will affect key industries in general and the biomedical and pharmaceutical industries (including marketing, production, labelling, processing and sales) in particular. They will also touch on elements essential to the provision of quality health care which include health specialities, pharmaceuticals, veterinary medical products, hightech medicine, implantable electromedical devices, single use devices (disposable), 'in vitro' diagnostics and many other items (Calingear, 1988:108-113).

The removal of fiscal barriers is another top priority for 1992 (Commission, 1985:41-56). The intended harmonization of value added tax, excise taxes on alcohol and tobacco, may be counterproductive to all ongoing anti-smoking and anti-drinking campaigns in countries which have used taxation as a tool to discourage smoking and drinking by imposing high taxes on these products (World Health Organization, 1988c).

1.4.8   The Single European Market and Health Care Systems

How will the established health care systems be affected by the unified market? The precise answers will be provided in the papers presented to the conference devoted to this topic. Here I will only draw on past experience. Historically, the state in European countries has been an extensive regulator of the health care system whether paid through taxes, public or private insurance premiums, out-of-pocket payments, or a combination of all these approaches. In addition, the state in most countries of the European Community extensively has controlled the registration of pharmaceutical and biomedical products and their price controls.

Short-term few things will change, but medium- and long-term the single market can reasonably be expected to bring about other changes of consequence to each national health budget, independent of its specific form. For example, price differentials of products and health care (which have a direct bearing on individual out-of-pocket funds) can cause some patient migration to those areas and countries which offer quality but less expensive care. The Single European Act secures the migration of labour and health professionals (Hurwitz, 1989) and the 'mutual recognition of diplomas' rather than the antecedent concept of the 'harmonization of diplomas' (Orzack, 1989:31-32). However, the precise impact of intra-European migration of health workers and care givers will be known only in years to come. By way of summary, the clusters of policy packages, most of which are in the non-health areas adopted by 1992, are likely to induce slow structural changes in the nature of the health care organizations, the public - private interactions in health, and the relations of state and society in health matters in each Member State.

1.4.9   Summary and Concluding Comments

The momentum for the creation of a Single European Market and the further pursuit of the long-term and comprehensive goals and objectives of the regional HFA strategy is irreversible. The regional targets provide the yardstick for measuring the impact of policies on health and, by analogy, any progress or deterioration in health outcomes. Whatever changes occur, from within or from outside the health sector, health experts and laypersons increasingly will have to reckon with a predictably increasing interpenetration of supranational health policies and programmes and national health policies and programmes. The reverse is also true. However, national political and organizational traditions unique to each Member State and society will determine the speed of this evolutionary process of interdependence, its magnitude and nature.

The challenges for European societies and the European Community as a whole in the future are considerable. As transnationalism takes hold in Europe, or as health threatening developments occur, Community and national policy-makers will have to face up to new political struggles and cope with new diseases and demographic changes or with their consequences. Eventually a non-health issue arises which has to be dealt with. How can a need for policy responses to health threats and disease and the effects of transnational dynamics be balanced out against national political and electoral politics as well as social and economic circumstances in individual countries?

The Single European Act introduced changes in the *modus procedendi* of EC policymaking, notably inside the Council of the European Community. The change is from unanimity to majority policy-making in several though not in all areas. Coalition building of the governments of the Twelve may lead to the adoption of joint policies and action programmes in some areas faster than in the past. In politically and socially sensitive areas unanimity in decision-making will be retained and, in consequence, progress may be slow.

In conclusion, four patterns of intra-European developments with regard to health and health policy come to mind. Mentally, their development - not necessarily their implementation - can be envisaged as trains travelling on railway tracks which allow for unequal speed and which are connected with different railway junctions. The TGVs in France (*Trains à Grande Vitesse*) will travel at fast speeds and possibly entail swift changes. The rapid ECs (European-wide inter-City trains) will travel at fairly high but steady speeds and will have multiple connections to national ICs (Inter-City trains). The national ICs, while they link up with the ECs, are somewhat slower. And, finally, the locals (the *omnibus* in French) will stop at every station on the way. The dilemma - others would say a chance - is that only a few of the 12 Member States dispose of railway tracks which allow for all four speeds. But all kinds of trains are fairly reliable in arriving on time and making the necessary connections in Europe. Which track will the train generating change in relation to health and a Community health policy travel on?

One thing is clear. Evolving transnational processes and the ways in which EC policies may affect health issues are less tangible than the consequences of the transfer of goods, services or capital. Health policy and health services research can make important contributions to our understanding of unfolding developments and how these bear on health outcomes. Researchers are called upon to signal developments which are less than desirable in time. Systematic, applied and problem-oriented policy studies can identify and trace crucial links between public (health and non-health) policies and health outcomes.

1.4.10 References

Baert, A.E. and G.M. Van Etten (1985), *The Future of Health and Health Systems Research in the EEC*, paper prepared for the International and Interdisciplinary Meeting on the Future of Health and Health Systems in the Industrialized Societies, Belagio, Italy, 27-31 May.

Barnard, K. (1989), *Working for Health for All. Health Policy Planning and Management in Europe: An Evolution*, Copenhagen: Regional Office for Europe, March (P6/24/1 PWDG-4554N).

Bélanger, M. (1989), *The Legal Foundations of a European Health Community*, prepared for delivery at the Inaugural Conference of the European Community Studies Association, George Mason University, Fairfax, VA, May 24-25.

1985, *Les Communautés et la santé*, Bordeaux: Presses Universitaires de Bordeaux.

Calingaert, M. (1988), *The 1992 Challenge from Europe: Development of the European Community's Internal Market*, National Planning Association, Washington, D.C.

Commission of the European Communities.

1985, *Completing The Internal Market*, white paper from the Commission of the European Council, Office for Official Publications of the European Communities, Luxembourg.

1986, Single European Act, *Bulletin of the European Communities*, Supplement 2.

1988a, *Completing the Internal Market: An Area Without Frontiers. The Progress Report Required by Article 88 of the Treaty*, presented by the Commission, Brussels, 17 November (COM988 650 final).

1988b, *Social Europe. The social dimension of the internal market*, Special Edition, Directorate General for Employmment, Social Affairs and Education, Office for Official Publications of the European Communities, Luxembourg.

1988c, *Europe against Cancer. Target: 15% Fewer Victims by the Year 2000*, Office for Official Publications of the European Communities, Luxembourg, 5-6 March.

1989, *Employment, Social Affairs and Education*, Directorate General, Directorate General Health and Safety, 10 April.

The Commission's Programme of Work for 1989 in the Health Related Fields, Luxembourg (internal document).

Dijck, van J. (1989), Towards Transnationalization of Economic and Social Life in Europe, *European Affairs* **1**, 73 - 80.

Hurwitz, L. (1989), *The Free Circulation of Physicians Within the European Community*, Grower, Avebury.

Lowi, Th. J. (1972), Four Systems of Policies, Politics and Advice, *Public Administration Review*, 288 - 310.

March, J.G. and J.P. Olsen (1984), The New Institutionalism: Organizational Factors in Political Life, *Am. Pol. Sci. Rev.*, **78**, (4), 734 - 49.

Orzack, L.H. (1989), EC Progresses on Mutual Acceptance of Diplomas, *Europe*, **284**, 31 - 2.

World Health Organization

1988, *A 5 Year Action Plan. Smoke free Europe*, Regional Office for Europe, Copenhagen.

1989, Document on Programme Budget Main Orientations: EURO's Priorities for 1992-1993 (1995).

1.5 American Federalism and American Health Care:
Lessons for the European Community
Cl. C. Havighurst

The assumption behind the invitation to prepare this paper was that experience in the United States, where responsibility for health care policy is divided between the federal government and the states, might offer some guidance to the European Community in allocating health policy responsibilities between the Community as a central authority and the individual national governments. On the basis of some limited research into Community law, I have tried to identify some American experiences that might yield useful lessons in federalism for Europe. Despite the very great political and institutional differences, I believe that several aspects of the US experience shed at least indirect light on problems that the European Community will encounter as it proceeds toward increased political as well as economic integration.

1.5.1 American Federalism in a Comparative Perspective

The American Constitution is a grant of power to the federal government directly by the people themselves and not by the states as intermediate governments. It is therefore distinguishable from the several treaties among sovereign states that provide the foundations of the European Community. The difference between the two systems is fundamental, with the American federal government being free from any direct control by the states as such and having, in turn, only limited authority to direct the states to take particular actions.

The American Constitution of 1787 granted only limited, enumerated powers to the federal government. Within its proper sphere, however, federal law is supreme and state laws that are inconsistent with it may be held invalid. In the European Community, the procedure for modifying or overriding specific laws of the Member States is different, but Community law appears to enjoy roughly the same supremacy as federal law in the US. There may be subtle differences, however, in the degree of compunction felt by legislators, officials and courts in the two systems about overriding the acts of a constituent state's elected legislature.

One of the powers expressly granted by the Constitution to the federal government is the power to regulate interstate commerce. A corollary of that grant of authority to Congress is that the states themselves are barred from regulating in ways that adversely affect interstate trade. The Constitution was thus construed, in accord with the clear intent of its framers, to create a true 'common market', with the federal government in charge of its regulation. The parallel to the Treaty of Rome, as amended by the Single European Act, is clear.

One of Congress's specific powers under the Constitution - the power to impose taxes for the general welfare of the United States - was expediently interpreted during the Depression to allow it to create redistributive income-maintenance and other welfare programmes. Since that time, although the states are not prevented from taking welfare initiatives of their own, Americans have looked primarily to Washington to finance redistributive measures. This has been true in part because the federal government is a more effective revenue raiser than the states, some of which are relatively poor. In addition, the states have more reason than the federal government to fear that disproportionate tax burdens will drive industry and productive persons elsewhere. The European Community should perhaps bear in mind that one of the disadvantages of a common market is that its governmental subunits may be constrained by competition for private investment in exercising their powers of taxation - and thus in maintaining liberal welfare programmes. The American experience suggests how this competition may lead to centralization of revenue raising and welfare spending.

Although the US federal government has possessed the power to initiate welfare programmes since the 1930s health care remained almost exclusively a state responsibility until 1965, when the Medicare and Medicaid programmes were created to finance care for the elderly and the poor respectively. As is well known, these programmes leave many Americans still without adequate private or public protection, and the federal government is showing little inclination to widen their scope. In these circumstances, the states are currently making significant, although uneven, efforts to fill some of the gaps in a mixed, poorly coordinated federal/state, public/private system of health care financing. In striking contrast to the US, the European Community is proceeding from a situation in which the Member States, rather than the Community as such, are virtually the only sources of funds and direction for health and social security programmes.

Notwithstanding the federal government's lack of constitutional authority to direct the states as such, its broad power to tax and spend allows it to place virtually any substantive condition it wants on grants it makes. Although some federal assistance to the states takes the form of categorical 'block grants' that the states may use without appreciable accountability, the principal US welfare programmes for the poor take the form of offers by the federal government to assist the states in meeting specific welfare needs on the condition that they abide by very extensive (and constantly changing) federal requirements. The Medicaid programme is the paramount example of a federal welfare programme that is administered by the states under detailed direction from Washington. Under it, the states are offered 'matching' funds - based on a formula significantly more favourable to the less prosperous states - to assist them in offering coverage that meets minimum federal standards but that may, if a state so chooses, be more generous. Some states, primarily the richer and more liberal ones, do indeed provide more extensive benefits for broader categories of low-income persons, while one state, Arizona, has never participated in Medicaid at all.

The variations among state Medicaid programmes in the US are frequently decried by adherents to the 'solidarity' principle that inspires in varying degrees the national health care systems of Europe. It is notable, however, that the state-by-state differences in per capita spending on Medicaid beneficiaries in the US are substantially less than the variation in per capita health care spending between Member States of the European Community. It will be interesting to see whether, in time, the principle of solidarity will be invoked in Europe on a Community-wide basis, leading to some wealth sharing such as one already finds in the American federal system.

With only modest constitutional limits on their powers, the states retain most of their sovereignty and have governmental responsibilities throughout a wide field. In the health care sector their many functions include - in addition to administering the Medicaid programme - educating and regulating health professionals; licensing hospitals and other institutional providers; authorizing the health care functions of local governments; regulating private health insurance; paying for or directly providing additional health services for the poor; financing long-term nursing home care; controlling costs through economic regulation and maintaining legal remedies for medical malpractice. A number of states have taken creative steps to expand the availability of private health insurance or otherwise to make services available to persons lacking private or public coverage.

Americans debate endlessly the relative merits of the federal government and the states for performing various functions. Although the states are constantly chided for their inevitably uneven performance, there are some areas in which they have been quite innovative - in Medicaid cost containment, for example. Numerous other examples could also be cited to demonstrate the strengths that flow from diversity in a federal system in which the various Governments learn positive lessons from each other and in which the mistakes from which they also learn are less consequential than if they had been made by the central government. In general, the states may be the better vehicles to use when conditions differ materially from place to place and when there is no consensus on the correct policy objective or on the best strategy for achieving it.

The peculiarities of the American federal system have strongly influenced the configuration of health care financing and delivery in the US. Sometimes the division of responsibilities between the two levels of government has been beneficial in allowing alternative policy ideas to be developed and tried. Also, however, federalism has sometimes made it difficult to implement a sound or coherent policy.

1.5.2   Regulating Health Care Professionals

One area of significant federal/state interaction in the US is professional licensure and discipline. Under their inherent 'police powers', the states rather than the federal government have long regulated health care personnel and institutions. This arrangement, under which each state independently licenses health professionals practising within its borders, has been less than ideal in a number of respects. An obvious problem is fragmentation of the regulatory effort. However, informal collaboration by and among state officials and national occupational groups has overcome some of the inefficiency, redundancy and restrictiveness of maintaining as many as 50 separate licensing authorities for each occupation.

Despite such cooperation, however, decentralized regulation of health care professionals in the US has not been regarded as a success. Although there have been recent improvements in state disciplinary mechanisms, the federal government has been moved to take some independent responsibility for policing physicians under the Medicare programme. The vehicles employed for this purpose are called Peer Review Organizations. PROs are private organizations operating under contract with the federal government. Each of them has the medical capability and the exclusive responsibility for reviewing the services received by Medicare beneficiaries in a single state. A PRO is empowered to suspend a physician from the Medicare programme for providing substandard care.

The federal PRO initiative is an important break with the tradition of state oversight, one that occurred only because the federal government felt responsible for the quality of care given through its own programmes. Among the unanswered questions surrounding PROs is whether they will implement a uniform national standard of care or will recognize that conditions and standards may vary from place to place even within a single state. A constant dilemma in any federal system is how to raise local standards where they are clearly deficient without enforcing artificial or misguided uniformity. The federal PRO programme, employing local physician reviewers and local standards to some degree but also capable of introducing exogenous improvements, may be a way of achieving an appropriate degree of diversity.

In the European Community, the regulation of physicians and other health care personnel is most likely to remain the exclusive responsibility of the Member States. Unlike the American states, however, these governments will also probably remain primarily responsible for financing or otherwise providing personal health care for their residents. Thus, the European Community seems unlikely to encounter the problem of divided responsibilities that has caused the US federal government to assume a greater role in policing individual physicians.

Among the basic principles of the European Community is the commitment to allow free movement of persons. American constitutional law similarly prohibits states from interfering with citizens' decisions to relocate themselves. Some important differences exist, however, in the attitudes taken towards free movement. The Europeans, by taking a more instrumental approach in pursuit of a relatively clear economic objective, may have achieved a superior result than the Americans, with their predominantly rights-based, legalistic approach to such problems. I gather, however, that a tendency exists in Community law to move away from a purely functional view of the free movement guarantee of the Treaty of Rome.

Consider first the free movement of professionals. Most American states, in carrying out their licensing functions, readily recognize professional credentials granted by other states. Free movement by professionals is not unrestricted, however. Several states, especially those with attractive climates, have maintained entry barriers that few established professionals can easily surmount. Because federal courts, being sensitive to state sovereignty, are disinclined to recognize state protectionism for local professionals, there is no guarantee in the US that professional credentials are transportable from one state to another. The European Community may be addressing this problem more successfully.

Viewing free movement of professionals primarily as an economic policy - as in Europe - or solely as an aspect of personal freedom - as in the US - may obscure what may be its greatest significance, namely, the practical limitation it imposes on the ability of a single political subdivision to take unfair advantage of professionals practising within its borders. If professionals are free to move their practices to another jurisdiction, a state would face a loss of trained personnel - a 'brain drain' - if it should seek to impose substantially more burdensome regulations or to set substantially lower compensation levels than apply in other places. Although some might view any inhibition on a Member State's ability to control its own professionals as a reason for going slow in promoting their free movement, free movement can also be seen as an essential feature of a true common market. Each Member State, acting in effect as a kind of purchaser of professional services, establishes the conditions of work and competes against other States to obtain just the services that its citizens require.

A particular defect in the American pattern of professional licensure has been the ability of individuals disciplined for improper practices in one state to enter practice in another without having the record of their earlier difficulties follow them. Federal legislation in 1986 addressed this problem by creating a federally financed databank, with mandatory reporting. The databank is currently being implemented amidst concerns in the medical community about the potential for errors in reporting and interpretation and about the programme's overall flavour of Big Brotherhood. Such a databank would seem as desirable in the European setting as it is in the US.

Although the European Community has provided for free movement of persons seeking to accept employment in another Member State, it recognizes no general freedom to relocate. The Community's dominant purpose is the instrumental one of widening the labour pool and relieving pockets of unemployment. In contrast to this approach, US courts have converted an implied constitutional right to travel into a prohibition against a state's requiring a period of residency before an individual is eligible for the state's welfare and Medicaid benefits. Such vigilance on behalf of individual rights could, however, have the perverse effect of causing states to provide less liberal welfare benefits - either in the hope that the poor will emigrate to obtain better benefits elsewhere or out of fear that more liberal benefits will attract more poor people. Because freedom of movement creates a kind of market in which governments compete for citizens, it can be highly advantageous for those who seek freedom and opportunity - such as skilled East German workers fleeing their homeland and physicians migrating in search of better conditions under which to practise. But an unlimited right of free movement may also interfere in some measure with a state's or nation's efforts to care for its less fortunate residents. Although poorer Europeans are even more closely tied to their communities by culture and language than are Americans, the European Community might be wise to adhere to an instrumental view of free movement guarantees and not to create a right to travel and relocate as extensive as the right created by the US Supreme Court.

1.5.4 Competition Policy

Next, I come to the important subject of competition policy. Unlike the EEC-Treaty, the American Constitution declares no substantive economic policy regarding the maintenance of competition and free markets. Indeed, the preservation of competition became an affirmative federal policy only with the passage of the Sherman Antitrust Act in 1890. That statute applies, however, only where interstate commerce is affected and governs only private persons, not the states as such. As a result, it has not been easy to maintain competition throughout the American economy. For various reasons, the states have often subverted competition within their borders, and federal law has had only limited success in altering such policies. The European Community will undoubtedly encounter similar restrictions in national legislation, and will have to decide whether and when to challenge them.

In the US, many of the states' strongest anti-competitive impulses have affected the health care industry and private insurance, including health insurance. Both of these fields were regarded historically as more appropriate for regulation than for competition and also as involving only interstate commerce, making them a state responsibility and putting them beyond the reach of federal law, including the Sherman Act. A major feature of US health care since the 1970s, however, has been a struggle to introduce competition in the health care and health insurance fields, which were finally held to involve interstate commerce after all. Some of the complex federalism issues that have been encountered in this struggle are described in the paper as illustrations of pitfalls that the European Community should seek to avoid.

The predominant effect of much state regulation of professionals has been to foreclose potentially beneficial competition - by maintaining high entry barriers, by limiting the role of alternative providers, and by preventing such 'commercial' practices as advertising, the use of trade names and salaried or corporate practice. Because state regulation has often reflected the disproportionate political influence of the occupational groups being regulated, there is reason to wish that paramount federal power could be brought to bear to promote consumer welfare by allowing competition a larger role. In the late 1930s, however, the Supreme Court essentially ceased defending individuals commercial and property rights against state economic regulation. As a result, the federal courts today nearly always respect the actions of state legislatures in the commercial realm, upholding regulatory legislation as long as some plausible police-power rationale for the challenged regulatory measure can be imagined. An illuminating exception to this generalization is the Supreme Court's willingness to invalidate anti-competitive state restrictions on truthful professional advertising - but only because such restrictions violate free-speech rights, not because they infringe individuals economic freedoms.

The Federal Trade Commission, an independent federal agency with anti-trust and consumer-protection missions, has recently issued regulations asserting federal power to override state laws discouraging the commercial practice of optometry. This initiative by federal bureaucrats to invalidate anti-competitive local legislation is perhaps as close as the US has yet come to using the approach that the European Community might use in similar circumstances. Apparently directives from European bureaucrats in Brussels can be used directly to effectuate Community policies over the heads of national legislatures. On the other hand, the Treaty of Rome opposes restrictions on competition only insofar as they 'may affect trade between Member States', and thus may leave policy on competition in health care and health insurance to be determined by national legislatures, at least until these fields become more international and more commercial than they now are.

An especially interesting problem has been the application of federal anti-trust law to various kinds of state action. Although federal anti-trust law is the 'supreme Law of the Land', the Sherman Act has not been construed to override any state law that happens to restrict competition in interstate commerce. Instead, its prohibition against trade restraints is understood to govern only private parties, not the states. Nevertheless, it has been necessary to reconcile the conflicting commands of state and federal law when a private party claims that its anti-competitive actions were expressly authorized by a state. This problem has been addressed by a sophisticated federal rule of comity which acknowledges that Congress, while asserting a strong policy in favour of competition, did not mean entirely to pre-empt the states' role in making policy on business organization and conduct in particular industry settings. Thus, when a state legislature has clearly concluded that competition is not the best policy in some specific area and has substituted another policy in its place, federal courts are likely to respect that judgment.

A particularly striking federalism problem is raised when a state regulatory agency adopts anti-competitive regulations not expressly authorized by state legislation. Several state boards adopting such regulations for professionals have been directly charged with violating the Sherman Act. This approach works legally because such boards, although created by a state, are not themselves sovereign entities and often have the earmarks of a state-sponsored but unsupervised cartel. The anti-competitive restrictions that have been challenged in cases of this kind include rules against advertising and against participation in competitive bidding.

These American experiences in implementing competition policy in a federal system may be instructive for the European Community only if it elects to treat health care - or some element of it, such as the dispensing of eyeglasses or pharmaceutical products - as involving a commercial 'undertaking'. Moreover, as the Treaty of Rome now stands, Community law cannot pre-empt national law unless the latter adversely affects 'trade between Member States'. American courts have found migration of patients across state lines to receive treatment, or a flow of medical supplies, capital funds, or insurance payments between state, to be enough to allow federal law to govern restraints of trade in local health care markets. It is hard, at least for an outsider, to predict whether the European Community will in due course first assert the inappropriateness of barriers to the free flow of patients, medical supplies and medical payments across national borders and then, as a consequence of the inter-Member trade thus established, assert the supremacy of the Community's competition policy over national legislation. If the Community should employ such rationales for widening its authority, its task might be somewhat less complicated than comparable efforts to assert central authority in the US, where the states' sovereignty is fixed and not readily subject to evolution toward fuller political integration. It is ironic that the federal structure in the US, in which the states are independent sovereigns and do not directly participate in the central government, may engender a greater need for inter-governmental comity than may ultimately exist in Europe, where the central authority's legitimacy flows from increasing cooperation among independent nations.

1.5.5 Health Care Insurance and Employee Benefits

Special attention has been given to the allocation between the US federal government and the states of responsibility for regulating private health insurance and health care financing. Federal legislation expressly delegates regulatory power in this area to the states and expressly exempts 'the business of insurance' from the federal anti-trust laws to the extent that a state regulates it. Historically, state regulation of insurance has been a serious barrier to innovation in private health care financing. A great deal of litigation has left the division of responsibility still unclear and the health insurance industry free from close scrutiny of it's sometimes questionable behaviour.

My impression of European Community law is that insurance is regarded as very much an object of 'trade between Member States', thus making it a potential object of the Community's competition policy. Insurance is also classed as a service to which the free-movement/free-establishment policy applies. It thus appears that the European Community has established clearer lines of responsibility and a more clearly pro-competitive central policy for the insurance industry than prevails in the US. It remains to be seen, however, whether health insurance specifically - including sickness funds and other public and private vehicles for financing health care - will actually be treated under the rubric of 'insurance' and thus as an intended target of the Community's pro-competitive initiatives.

There is also a question whether competition among European health insurers will be allowed, or required under Community law, to ripen into purchasing practices that foster real competition among health care providers. US experience has shown that local regulation of the business of insurance can easily shelter providers of insured services from the necessity to compete actively on the basis of price. An analogy can be drawn to the common European practice of letting health care providers bargain collectively with sickness funds. Because such collective bargaining by providers destroys competition, it might be placed in jeopardy if the Community's competition policy is ultimately applied to health care and health insurance.

Another area of federal/state conflict in the US has been the regulation of employee health benefits. Federal legislation in 1974 sought to provide some uniformity in the law governing employee benefits generally, so that multi-state employers would be relieved of the necessity for satisfying every state's special requirements. That law substituted federal for state regulation, pre-empting the states from regulating health (and other) benefits while leaving them still free to regulate and tax 'the business of insurance'. Because state insurance regulation and taxation can raise employer costs, many larger employers have elected to self-insure their employees' health care needs, so as to be subject only to federal law.

I am not aware of any movements as yet in the European Community to shift responsibility for prescribing and otherwise regulating employee benefits to central authority. As employers become more multi-national, however, one might anticipate pressures to substitute uniform requirements for those of the individual Member States. In the US at least, the assertion of federal authority has left employee benefits subject to less overall regulation than many state would choose to impose. On the other hand, some of the regulation that is pre-empted - for example, the mandate to cover particular health services or the services of particular classes of provider - are not obviously in the public interest, appearing to increase the cost of benefits without commensurate gain in value.

1.5.6 Health Planning and Regulation of Capital Investment

The history of US legislation dealing with health planning reveals some of the difficulty of making coherent health policy in a federal system. Federal legislation in 1974 created a complex network of local health planning bodies and state agencies with regulatory power to slow the growth of the health care system by requiring so-called 'certificates of need'. That legislation sought to enforce state cooperation by conditioning the grant of certain federal funds earmarked for health-related purposes on a state's adoption of certificate-of-need regulation meeting detailed federal standards. Nearly all states dutifully complied with the federal mandate by the end of the 1970s.

By 1986, however, Congress had become thoroughly disenchanted with central planning, and it repealed the federal health planning legislation altogether. Although this move brought to an end the era in which federally inspired state regulation was expected to bring health care and its costs under appropriate control, most of the regulatory laws that the states enacted under federal compulsion in the 1970s remain on the books today. The battle for deregulation must therefore be fought all over again in 50 state capitals, against the resistance of hospitals and other entrenched providers who benefit from regulatory barriers to new competition. Presumably the European Community will be able to avoid fiascos of this kind because, unlike the US government, it has an acknowledged right to prescribe the outline of some national legislation. Even if it should radically change some policy - as Congress did when it walked away from central planning for the health care industry -, the Community can give effect to its new policy by a new directive, not simply by retracting an earlier one.

1.5.7 Conclusion

The episodes I have related about federal/state conflicts over health care policy in the US do not reflect very well on the American Constitution and the political system it created. On the other hand, American federalism is not primarily responsible for the many well-known shortcomings of American health care policy. If anything, federalism has probably been a positive force in health policy development, allowing values that one level of Government might sacrifice to be reasserted at another level. Although American federalism lacks the neatness of an organization chart, it has not precluded constructive cooperation. Moreover, it facilitates creative experimentation, and the checks and balances it provides have probably frustrated more destructive policies than constructive ones. Although it is doubtful that the European Community will ever closely resemble the US federal system, it may learn from our experiences something about how to utilize the new pathways that federalism offers for effectuating desirable change in the face of inertia and political obstacles.

2 Competition in Health Care

Contents

2 Competition in Health Care

2.0 Introduction
P.H. Admiraal

Setting differences aside, what do economists agree on with respect to competition in health care? Maybe they agree on the following statement: A competitive equilibrium in a well-managed market will produce efficiency. In simple terms: in favourable conditions competition will lead to the right level of health care expenditure.

The most important questions raised regarding this, are dealing with:

a)   the economic efficiency of health care;
b)   the necessary market conditions for competition;
c)   the trade-off between goals;
d)   the European perspective.

2.0.1 Economic Efficiency

What is the right level of health care expenditure? There are different answers possible. It must be stressed that market competition does not guarantee cost containment. If consumers are willing to pay extra money for higher levels of quality, more services or new therapies, then the expansion of health care is contributing to welfare, because marginal productivity is relatively high. We are moving along the steepest incline of the total productivity curve. In contrast an inefficient health care system can be characterized by 'flat-of-the curve' medicine.

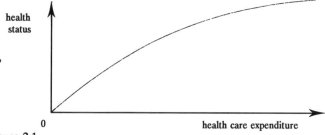

Figure 2.1

Given this approach it is reasonable to distinguish between EC-countries with a high and a low Gross Domestic Product (GDP). Probably countries with a low GDP are just starting to climb the slope of the productivity mountain. In these countries health care seems to be underdeveloped. Sissouras mentioned shortages of nurses and lack of efficient ambulatory care organization. This means that there is no adequate environment for well-managed competition in health care.

The position of EC-countries with a high GDP is not without dispute. Following Nonneman they find themselves on the flat part of the curve, because the share of GDP going to health care is relatively large. However Naaborg has arrived at the opposite conclusion by stressing equity. Probably it is wise to be reluctant to interpret very global statistical figures, indeed relatively high costs of health care may indicate inefficiencies. To be sure of our conclusions we need detailed information about marginal productivity, consumer preferences (see above) and policy goals (see later).

2.0.2 The Market Place

Competition can only be achieved if there is a bargaining arena and if there are parties willing to compete on price. This implies incentives for providers; they do not compete automatically. They only do so when the insurance companies select cost-efficient providers to keep their costs down, and the insurers in their turn only do their selection under market conditions, in which they have to compete for the consumer Ecu.

Now we reach a critical assumption with respect to a market-orientated alternative to heavily regulated or publicly-run systems. We have to assume that the consumer is able to make well-informed choices in medical markets, or we have to know which way the consumer will be carried through the insurance market. This last option is called 'pre-screened plan competition'. Here Enthoven's concept of sponsors applies,[1] and it is possible also to apply Pauly's idea of a two-part market.[2]

2.0.3 Policy Goals

Graf von der Schulenburg has drawn our attention to a dilemma of health care system modelling. In his view three major goals are proclaimed: solidarity, price competition and freedom of choice. In reality these three goals cannot be achieved at the same time; at least one of them has to be sacrificed.

The assumption implicit in this reasoning is that the choice of goals takes place in a yes-or-no fashion. Why is this? Because solidarity is not well defined, it will be limited somehow; competition is not pure and perfect; and so on. From our point of view every health care system is based on a trade-off between policy goals. However, within existing systems you cannot achieve a trade-off so easily. A health care system is characterized by a delicate balance of an organic whole and it is not possible to substitute parts on request. For instance, the introduction of price competition in the German statutory health care scheme would undermine the mechanism of flexible budgets.[3] The same situation will probably hold good for other regulated and publicly-run systems as well. The introduction of competition will change them fundamentally.

2.0.4 European Perspective

Havighurst has given us an outline of how the European integration process may create room for emerging competition. Most likely this will not be implemented by the European Commission or the Council of Ministers, it will depend on decisions made by the High Court in Luxembourg. Several speakers have advised the national authorities to play a waiting game, for reasons spelled out in the preceding paragraphs. The functioning of the market implies the decentralization of decisions, with the Government stepping back to give room for emerging competition in health care.

The outcome of these revolutionary changes is uncertain; the economists have no clear-cut ideas about an efficient market organization, neither are they sure how economic efficiency is related to other policy goals. Maybe a trade-off between goals cannot be avoided. In this respect some of the speakers are gravely concerned about the social dimensions of a competitive health care system in Europe after 1992.

2.0.5 Notes

1 A.C. Enthoven (1988), *Theory and practice of managed competition in health care finance, North-Holland, 113-119*.
2 M. Pauly (1988), Efficiency, equity and costs in the US: the health care system, in IEA, Health unit Paper no. 5, *American health care*, London, 35.
3 See in this volume: J.M. Graf von der Schulenburg, *Competition, Solidarity and Cost-Containment in Medical Care*.

2.1 Workable Competition versus Workable Monopoly
C.J. van der Weijden

The concept of workable competition is the explicit expression of the idea that competition is not an end in itself, but that in reality in a certain period there may be too much or too little competition from the point of view of certain results one wishes to be realized. The intensity of competition that more or less realizes certain goals may be called workable competition, effective competition or optimal intensity of competition. An implication of this approach to competition is that (what an economist calls) market imperfections are not always condemned but can be accepted. So, when there is no freedom of exit from the market as a result of high fixed costs (that is, a market imperfection) and demand for the product diminishes, an additional and compensating imperfection in the form of an agreement between suppliers that excludes price competition with the purpose of capacity reduction may be acceptable. Naturally this could not continue forever but only for a reasonable period of time.

Therefore the familiar question 'what do we want competition to do for us' is still relevant. Nowadays a great number of economists will say that we want static and dynamic efficiency. Static efficiency encompasses an efficient production of goods and services in a certain period, a reasonable ratio between price and cost, consumer-led production; dynamic efficiency encompasses the introduction of new products, new production and distribution techniques and organization structures.

In reality there can be a dilemma between static and dynamic efficiency. Low prices, that imply a small difference between price and costs per unit, may impede dynamic efficiency if profitability becomes too low. The introduction of new products and so on asks for a reward and so temporary monopoly profits are acceptable. It is not the purpose of the competitive process to eliminate all profits but to enforce an erosion of profits over a period of time. The competitive process is a process of moves and responses, a process of creation, erosion and recreation of profits. The result of innovative behaviour - the monopoly profit or rent - ought to be passed on in the form of lower prices to buyers and higher rewards for the means of production - not as a result of the benevolence, good will or an arbitrary decision of the individual producer or supplier, or as a result of a Government order, but as a result of a situation in which 'normal business motives' impel entrepreneurs to do so.

The choice for a market economy implies a choice for competition and thus for independent action in what we call the market sector of the economy. This is, however in the presence of workable competition not a choice at all costs, therefore in certain circumstances agreements regulating competition between suppliers are temporarily acceptable, in other circumstances they are undesirable. Market power - a dominant position in a market - of a supplier is acceptable under the condition that there is no abuse with respect to prices, terms of delivery, in the form of conditional sale or boycott.

The Dutch competition law of 1956 was founded on the idea of workable or healthy competition. Legally enforceable agreements between firms or members of certain professions (for instance the medical profession) regulating the competition between them can be dissolved if, and only if, they are contrary to the common good. This conflict ought to be evaluated - according to the law - by the Minister. According to the law there is also a possibility of a *per se* rule against certain types of agreements regulating competition. For instance, in the Netherlands the Government is considering a *per se* injunction against horizontal price agreements. Of course there is always a possibility of exemption. In accordance with the idea that too much competition is also a possibility, it is under Dutch law possible to make an agreement between certain parties concerning the regulation of competition mandatory for all the members of an industry. In recent years this possibility led to a minimum price rule - excluding price competition - for white sugar and bread. There are two conditions: the regulation must not only promote the interest of the industry but also promote the common good. A second aspect of Dutch law is a regulatory approach concerning misuse of a dominant position. In this case also the misuse has to be judged from the viewpoint of the common good.

Recently the Ministers of Health and Economic Affairs asked the Dutch monopolies commission whether the competition law could be enforced in the medical sector. The answer avoided the tricky question of whether the choice for competition in the medical sector would result in a better performance than the existing planning and regulation approach. There is a report of an *ad hoc* committee asking for more competition and it is the task of the Government to make a choice. The answer of the monopolies commission was rather laconic. Of course it is possible in principle to evaluate an agreement regulating competition between general practitioners in a city or a district; the same is true for a similar agreement between hospitals. It is possible in principle but not easy.

The competition law is applicable to general practitioners, medical specialists, dentists, pharmacists, physiotherapists and midwives. In principle any agreement regulating competition between members of these professions has to be reported to the Minister of Economic Affairs. However by decree of 14 May 1987 regulations of competition in the health sector were exempted from reporting to the minister if the regulation or the behaviour has been approved of or is under supervision according to provisions in special laws concerning health care. As a result, a number of agreements will not be reported and this means in practice that the possibility for evaluation under the competition act could be rather restricted.

In addition to this we need to realise that the foundation or closing of a hospital is only possible after a licence from the Government. The same is true for a general practitioner and a pharmacist who want to establish themselves, or for a medical specialist who wants a private practice at home. The freedom of entry in several branches of health care is severely restricted. Competition - actual and potential - with the exception of some quality competition, is non-existent. Instead of asking for the workability of competition the real question seems to be whether the different legally created or accepted monopoly positions are workable.

Let us look for a moment at this problem. In the broader sense, concerning health care we want: continuity, quality, accessibility, improvement and efficiency. Is there a need to change our regulated system because the results are bad? The only serious problem is the development of costs, especially those for medicines, for analysis in laboratories in hospitals and for the multitude of activities (requiring) medical examinations and expensive surgical operations (for instance heart-transplants). It is very difficult to reduce the volume component of these expenses because of the impact on incomes of specialists, on the responsibility for the quality of treatment and the pressure of the wishes of the patients. There is some doubt whether competition can reduce these costs, without negative effects on the other aspects of health care, that is, the other aspects of efficiency.

In economic theory the instrumental approach of workable competition - that is, the choice for competition not as an end in itself but as an instrument to achieve static and dynamic efficiency - has its limits. It is not acceptable to eliminate competition completely by individual agreements; this is only acceptable as a consequence of a political decision. This happened with respect to the medical sector in the Netherlands and led to regulated and workable monopoly (from the point of view of the results). The necessity of competition to realize better results has not been proved; it is rather a political choice at a time when regulation by the Government has to be reduced. The result will be regulated and perhaps workable competition instead of regulated and workable monopoly, and not necessarily a better performance in terms of efficiency.

2.2 Competition, Solidarity and Cost-Containment in Medical Care
J.-Matthias Graf von der Schulenburg

2.2.1 Introduction

Discussing 1992 and the future of the German health care system is like discussing the love affairs of our politicians: there is a lot of gossip but no one knows the details; what has happened and what will happen. We all know that the service sector in particular (and medical care belongs to the service sector) will be affected more by the EC harmonization process than any other sector of our economy, but we do not know what the changes will be. We do not even know whether European health insurance schemes will converge or not.

In this paper I will provide an overview of the German health care system and recent developments in medical care.

The health care system of the Federal Republic of Germany is characterized by comprehensive statutory insurance coverage, regulated fees for physicians' and hospitals' services, and strict separation between hospital care and ambulatory care provided by office-based physicians. The German health care system has managed to achieve a number of partly-conflicting goals at the same time: comprehensive coverage and equal access for everyone, freedom of choice, high quality medicine and cost containment. The reason for this success is the combination of a decentralization of power and decision-making, and the establishment of a negotiation scheme including negotiations at different levels; the national level (*Konzertierte Aktion im Gesundheitswesen*), the state level and the local level. The separation of hospital care and office-based physicians, however, results in excessively long hospital length-of-stay. A major task of German health politics during the next few years will be to remove the barriers between the ambulatory care sector, the hospital sector and the institutions providing nursing care for the elderly.

Currently, negotiations take place between the sickness fund associations and the providers associations, the outcome of which is binding for all providers and sickness fund members. To guarantee this, physicians and dentists have to join their own medical associations and employees are compulsorily insured in one of the sickness funds if they earn below a certain ceiling. The federal government is only supervising the statutory health insurance system, not setting budgets, fees, quality standards and so on. I think that this system appeals to newly-industrialized countries because it was introduced at a time when Germany was on its way to becoming an industrialized nation over a century ago and has shown great stability and ability in adjusting to new challenges in medical care.

2.2.2 Goals of the German Health Care System

Three major goals are proclaimed by politicians, providers, and consumers with regard to future health care systems.

a) The system should allow equal access to health care facilities for all citizens. This can be called the solidarity goal, because it implies a comprehensive social health insurance scheme covering the health care costs of all.

b) Competitive pricing should ensure efficiency and the best allocation of scarce resources in medical care. To develop price competition, providers must have the freedom to lower prices or increase them in the event of a demand surplus.

c) Consumers and especially providers call for freedom of choice. Everybody should be able to choose that physician or hospital he or she prefers.

In reality, as Uwe Reinhardt has pointed out and as Table 2.1 indicates, all of these three goals cannot be achieved at the same time. In this article we will show by a detailed description and analysis of the German health care scheme that at least one of the goals mentioned above has to be sacrificed. If we attempt to create a health care system which is characterized by equal access, freedom of pricing and freedom of choice, health care costs will explode.

Table 2.1
Dilemma of Health Care System Modelling

Type of System	Solidarity: Equal Access	Competition: Freedom of Pricing and Determining the Quantity	Freedom of Choice	Cost Control
What everybody wants and does not work	Yes	Yes	Yes	Impossible
Statutory health care scheme, e.g., Germany	Yes	No	Yes	By negotiations, price and quantity regulations
HMO-type insurance scheme	Yes	Yes	No	By negotiations, barriers to entry
Chicago-school pure market system	No	Yes	Yes	By market forces, but unsuccessfully thus far

The second option outlined in Table 2.1 is characterized by comprehensive insurance coverage, freedom of choice but no price competition. Prices for medical services are set by negotiated fee schedules, *per diem* rates, or other statutory pricing rules. The advocates of a pro-competitive strategy, however, prefer the third choice of having a number of competing insurance plans, PPOs or HMOs. In principle, providers are then free to charge any price. However, Preferred Provider Organization (PPO) and Health Maintenance Organization (HMO) members may only consult a doctor who is under contract with his or her insurer. If a provider is too expensive, the insurer will exclude him from providing care for its members. Gaining solidarity and price competition often limits the freedom to choose the health care supplier.

In contrast to this 'American view', health services were always considered as special goods in Germany. Everybody should have access to medical services regardless of the persons' income or willingness to pay. The governments's obligation is to guarantee a comprehensive health insurance coverage for everyone and to set the rules for an effective cost control. In the German interpretation, equal access also implies the freedom of choosing the physician and hospital. Obviously Germany had opted for the second choice of health cares system modelling, as described in Table 2.1. Equal access is guaranteed mainly by a very comprehensive statutory health insurance scheme, covering more than ninety per cent of the population. Under the pressure of rapidly increasing health care costs and the modern deregulation movement, reform proposals advocate modifying the German system in the direction of the third and fourth choices described in Table 2.1. Some small co-payments were imposed by recent cost-containment laws and some drugs for the treatment of minor illnesses have to be paid out of pocket. Before discussing recent developments in German health care policy, we will first begin with a general overview of the health care scheme. Second, we will explain in more detail the remuneration of providers. This section contains remarks about ambulatory care, hospital care, and pharmaceutical products. The last section summarizes the German method of controlling costs.

2.2.3 Historical Development

Most characteristic of the German system is the statutory sickness fund (*Gesetzliche Krankenkassen*), whose genesis was an address by Emperor Wilhelm I to the Reichstag in 1881. When the Health Insurance Act came into effect in 1883, blue-collar employees - and later other members of the population - had to be insured by one of the numerous sickness funds. Accordingly, the statutory health care scheme became the oldest part of the social security system, followed by acts concerning accident insurance (1884), retirement funds (1889), public assistance (1924), and unemployment insurance (1927). Contributions, benefits and other components of the statutory sickness funds are regulated in detail by the second code of the Social Insurance Act, the first draft of which dates from 1911.

After World War II, the West German legislature enacted numerous statutes concerning public health care, the most important of which resulted in the founding of the Federal Department of Health and Human Services in 1961. The Government established statutory fee schedules for physician services and dentist services in 1965, revised in 1982; specified employer's liability for continued payment of wages in case of illness; and created the Medical Profession Education Law in 1970. Also important were the 1972 laws concerning the financing of hospitals and the disputed Health Insurance Cost Containment Law of 1977, which was followed by the Second and Third Health Insurance Cost Containment Laws of 1982 and the Health Insurance Reform Law of 1989. With these regulations the German health care system became the most regulated sector in the entire economy.[1]

Table 2.2 provides some information about the general trend of health care expenditures (including cash-transfers).

If we plot the national health care costs (cash-transfers deducted) as a percentage of gross national product (GNP) for two very different health care systems, the heterogenous United States system and the solidarity-type system adopted in West Germany, we receive a striking picture of the German expenditure growth. There was a rapid increase from six point four per cent of GNP in 1970 to nine point four per cent in 1975, and a levelling off since then. The price explosion in the early 1970s was due to the social reform policies of Social-Democratic Chancellor Willy Brandt (who came into power in 1969), the need for constructing new hospitals and the relative increase in the number of elderly people.

2.2.4 Cost Trends

Discussions concerning German health policy are dominated by controversy over causes for the explosive increase in health care expenditures and proposals to stem spiralling costs.

Table 2.2
Health Care Expenditures in Germany

	1970	1975	1980	1985	1986	1987
total (in bill.DM)	70.6	134.5	196.3	241.3	251.3	263.4*
per person	1,164	2,175	3,188	3,954	4,116	4,313
Statutory health insurance (in bill.DM)	25.2	61.0	89.8	114.1	119.9	125.0*
in % of GNP	3.7	5.9	6.0	6.2	6.2	6.2
per insured	471	-	1,616	2,096	2,213	2,324
per member (including his or her dependants)	824	1,821	2,537	3,152	3,289	3,383
exchange rate DM/US $	3.65	2.46	1.82	2.94	2.17	1.80

* estimate

Source: K.-D. Henke, *Die finanzielle Situation im Gesundheitswesen*, September 1989 (Universität Hannover, FB Wirtschaftswissenschaften) and Statistisches Bundesamt (various publications).

If we plot the national health care systems, the heterogenous United States system and the solidarity-type system adopted in West Germany, we receive a striking picture of the German expenditure growth. There was a rapid increase from six point four per cent of GNP in 1970 to nine point four per cent in 1975, and a levelling off since then. The price explosion in the early 1970s was due to the social reform policies of Social-Democratic Chancellor Willy Brandt (who came into power in 1969), the need for constructing new hospitals and the relative increase in the number of elderly people.

In 1973 an intensive public discussion on the cost of medical care was initiated by Heiner Geissler, who was at that time Minister of Health and Social Affairs and became later on General Secretary of the Christian Democratic Party till 1989. The formerly moribund sickness funds discovered the power given them by the Social Security Act and insisted on conditions that would allow stable contribution rates (by percentage of income).[2] A public campaign and studies at the sickness fund-financed research institute provided support. As a result, regulatory measures taken by the state and federal Governments produced the Health Insurance Cost Containment Law in 1977, which introduced the National Health Conference (Konzertierte Aktion im Gesundheitswesen) and expenditure caps on ambulatory medical care as well as on prescribed drugs. It is interesting to note that once the increasing cost in medical care became a public concern the German health care scheme was quite successful in containing cost. The first cost containment law was followed by two cost containment laws in 1981 and the Strukturreform in 1989 which was also a measure to manage the cost of medical care.

The last section provides some more information on the miracle of German cost containment efforts. Still, Germany belongs to that group of countries with the highest *per capita* health care expenditure. As Table 2.3 indicates, Germany is placed second in the European Community if one considers 1989 *per capita* health care expenditures, and is placed fourth worldwide by the OECD report.[3]

Table 2.3
Health Care Expenditure in the EC in US $
(ranked by expenditure in 1989)*

	per capita		average annual growth rate
	1970	1989	
1. France	223	2 054	12.4
2. FR Germany	220	1 901	12.0
3. Netherlands	232	1 711	11.1
4. Belgium	147	1 406	12.6
5. Denmark	252	1 294	9.0
6. Italy	171	1 216	10.9
7. Ireland	122	1 111	12.3
8. Great Britain	161	1 089	10.6
9. Spain	102	824	11.6
10. Greece	70	475	10.6

* Portugal and Luxembourg are not included

Source: Institut der deutschen Wirtschaft e.V., Köln. The figures for 1989 are estimates.

Table 2.4 provides a general view of the components of national health care expenditures as they are reported in German health care statistics. Note that certain cash benefits are included in Table 2.4 but are not included in international comparative statistics. One criterion of decomposition is the type of expenditure. The German statutory health insurance normally provides benefits in kind, that means that the patient is consulting a doctor or an hospital with his or her sickness-certificate or referral-order (health insurance identification card). The providers are then reimbursed by the statutory health insurance and not by the patient. Only twenty-six point three per cent of total health expenditure are cash benefits: continued payment of wages in the case of sickness, reimbursement to the patient for certain services, grants for young mothers, new eyeglasses and medical appliances. A second criterion of decomposition is the type of benefits: very little is spent on preventive care. On the other hand the percentage of follow-up costs of diseases is extremely high because statutory sickness funds and pension funds also cover the costs of convalescence after a disease or to maintain health. The third criterion employed in Table 2.4 is the question of where the money comes from. Of course, every mark spent for medical care has to be financed by the people, that is either by contributions to sickness funds, insurance premiums to private health insurers or taxes or direct payment. In Germany the statutory sickness funds finance the largest part of all health care expenditures. The share of the private health insurance seems to be relatively low, because more than ninety per cent of the population are covert by one of the statutory sickness funds. But private health insurance is currently rapidly growing because it appeals to high income people especially if they have only a few or no children. This is because the contribution to the sickness fund is a fixed percentage of gross income and the sickness funds cover all services to the dependent children and spouse of the insured if they have no independent income. Private health insurers, instead, calculate premiums on an actuarial basis, so the whole family has to pay a single premium.

Table 2.4
Resource Allocation in Medical Care in bill.DM (%), 1986

Total Expenditure 251.3 (= 100%)		
by type of expenditure		
- benefits in kind	174	(69.3)
- cash in kind	66	26.3)
- administrative expenditure	11	(4.4)
by type of benefits		
- preventive and nursing care	15.4	(6.1)
- medical treatment	148.9	(59.3)
- follow up cost of diseases	71.5	(28.4)
- education	4.3	(1.7)
- other benefits	11.2	(4.5)
by type of financing institution		
- private health insurance	12.6	(5.0)
- social pension funds	20.3	(8.1)
- social accident insurance	8.2	(3.3)
- statutory sickness funds	117.2	(46.6)
- employees	39.8	(15.8)
- public budgets	33.3	(23.3)
- private households	19.8	(7.9)

Source: Statistisches Bundesamt, Ausgaben für Gesundheit 1986, in *Wirtschaft und Statistik* (1988) **8**, 546 - 53.

Table 2.5 presents a general survey of the German health insurance scheme. More than ninety-two per cent of the population are covered by one of the 1 214 statutory sickness funds. Those people are either compulsorily insured or are voluntary members of these funds. If someone earns above a certain ceiling (about $ 3 500 per month) he or she can stay voluntarily in a statutory sickness fund or opt out.

The sickness fund covers the health care costs of the whole families of its members. The costs of the sickness funds are financed by contributions (see Table 2.6). Half of the contributions are paid by the employers, half by the employees. The contributions are calculated by each sickness-fund individually, and are defined as a percentage of the gross-income of the members. If, for instance, a sickness fund needs thirteen per cent of the gross-income of its members to finance its current costs, a member with an income of DM 4 000 has to pay DM 260 to the sickness fund and his or her employer has to pay DM 260 in addition. The contributions are calculated on a pay-as-you-go basis, because the sick do not receive governmental subsidies or transfers and do not accumulate financial reserves.

Table 2.5
The German Health Insurance Scheme

	number of funds/insurers/ institutions	number of insurants (in millions)
Total population		61.0
Statutory health insurance	1 214	56.0
- local sickness funds	270	24.2
- professional sickness funds	927	11.9
- sailor's insurance	2	1.6
- substitute funds	15	18.3
Private health insurance	42	10.4
- fully private health insured		5.8
- additional private health insured to statutory health insurance		4.5
Other health service coverage (public assistance, police, army, federal mail etc.)		1.3
Uninsured or without any health service coverage		0.5

Source: *Statistik der Kassenärztlichen Vereinigung*; Mikrozensus 1982; *PKV, Die private Krankenversicherung*, Rechenschafsbericht 1988, Köln 1989.

Table 2.6
Financing of the Statutory Sickness Funds in 1988

Total revenues	132 533 million DM = 100%	
- contributions of the members and their employers		97.0 %
- other revenues		3.0%
- contributions of non-retired members		81.0%
- contributions of retired members		16.0%
Average contribution per member (average contribution rage)	DM 4 092	(12.9%)
- local sickness funds	DM 4 111	(13.5%)
- professional funds industry	DM 4 372	(11.5%)
- professional funds craft	DM 3 365	(12.8%)
- professional funds agriculture	DM 3 098	-
- professional funds sailor	DM 5 659	(12.8%)
- professional funds mining	DM 5 439	(13.3%)
- substitute funds blue-collar worker	DM 4 230	(11.9%)
- substitute funds white-collar worker	DM 4 067	(12.7%)
Lowest and highest contribution rate		
- local sickness funds		11.0% - 16.0%
- professional funds industry		9.0% - 15.0%
- professional funds craft		10.0% - 15.0%

Source: BPI, Basisdaten des Gesundheitswesens 1988/89, Frankfurt: Bundesverband der Pharmazeutischen Industrie 1989.

As a consequence, the contribution rates differ between sickness funds and between regions. In regions with a low income level and a high physician-population ratio the contributions are higher than in other regions. Those who opt out of the statutory health insurance scheme may buy private insurance coverage. However, even some of those who are covered by one of the statutory sickness funds buy supplementary private health insurance for special services not covered by the statutory sickness funds (for example a private bedroom in a hospital; full coverage for dentistry).

Unemployed people are covered by local sickness funds which are then reimbursed by the statutory unemployment insurance and the civil service's own health insurance arrangements. Less than one per cent are not covered by any type of health insurance; those are the very rich and the very poor who are homeless.

2.2.5 Price Control

As mentioned above, a comprehensive third party coverage and freedom of choice requires price control mechanisms. To understand the German system of price control, one has to remember two factors. First, more than ninety per cent of the German population are covered by one of the 1 200 statutory sickness funds providing full coverage for ambulatory, hospital and dental care. Second, there is a sharp distinction between ambulatory care of office-based physicians and hospital care. Office-based physicians do not normally have hospital privileges. Hospital-based physicians operate on a salary basis, and their salaries are covered by the *per diem* rates negotiated between the sickness funds and the hospitals. Only private patients (that is, patients who are not covered by a sickness fund or public assistance) have to make additional payments for physician services in a hospital.

Table 2.7
Supply and Demand of Services per 1 000 Population, 1988

physicians	
- total	2.81
- office based	1.15
- hospital	1.35
dentists	0.82
employees in drug stores	0.96
hospital beds	
- total	11.05
- public	5.62
- non-profit organizations	3.89
- private	1.54
hospital nurses	6.23
sick persons	
- total	163.0
- acute	52.0
- chronic	100.0
- accident	11.0

Sources: Various sources and own calculations

To summarise, most medical services costs are regulated in Germany, but costs are not set by the government. They are negotiated between the sickness funds associations and the suppliers associations. Table 2.7 shows that the density of physicians and hospital beds are relatively high in Germany, and that those regulated costs have not led to a shortage of medical supplies. The sickness funds and their members of course, fear an oversupply due to the ability of physicians and hospitals to attract demand for their own services. But the sickness funds have also a strong interest in an appropriate supply of services. Even so, the utilization rates in Germany, reported in Table 2.8, are quite high.

Table 2.8
Utilization of Medical Services

hospital bed days per 1 000 population	3 496
hospital discharges per 1 000 population	206
average length of stay in days	17.5
average number of ambulatory physician treatments per insured per year	7.36
average number of other ambulatory treatments including dental treatment	1.32
average number of physician contacts per person per year	11.4
average number of prescribed drugs per person per year	11.0

Source: Sachverständigenrat zur Konzertierten Aktion im Gesundheitswesen, Jahresgutachten 1989 and various other sources.

The sickness fund system has also led to relatively even regional distribution of health care facilities (see Table 2.9). However hospital bed and physician density is still higher in cities than in rural areas and in the south of Germany.

As in most other industrialized countries it is quite difficult to control expenditure for hospitals and for medical appliances. However, the expenditure for office-based physicians and dental care could be contained by negotiations between the sickness fund associations and the medical and dental associations.

Table 2.9
Regional Distribution of Health Care Suppliers

state	hospital beds per 10 000 population	inhabitants per pharmacy	physicians per 10 000 population
Schleswig-Holstein	104	3 608	26.4
Hamburg	104	3 337	41.4
Niedersachsen	94	3 672	23.8
Bremen	121	3 474	36.0
Nordrhein-Westfalen	108	3 467	26.4
Hessen	121	3 410	29.4
Rheinland-Pfalz	115	3 294	25.6
Baden-Württemberg	106	3 400	28.1
Bayern	111	3 376	28.2
Saarland	117	2 933	--
Berlin (West)	177	3 374	46.4
FR Germany (West)	110	3 435	28.0
FR Germany (East)	100	8 000	25.0

2.2.6 Physician Profile

In West Germany, office-based physicians play the dominant role in the health care sector as a whole. Every patient who is covered by a statutory sickness fund must first consult a physician in order to receive any type of medical care. Only office-based doctors may provide ambulatory care, prescribe drugs and medical appliances, and decide who is to be hospitalized. If the case is not an emergency, the hospital requires a referral order written by an office-based physician before the patient may be treated. However, the numbers of hospital physicians increased greatly during the last decades and has already exceeded the number of office-based physicians.

During the period 1960 to 1988, the number of physicians, and especially the number of office-based physicians, has increased rapidly (see Table 2.10). This amounts to two point eight physicians per 1 000 inhabitants, which is a higher physicians-population ratio than in most other countries (see Table 2.7). The number of physicians is expected to increase even more rapidly during the next few years due to the increased number of medical students. In 1970 about 4 400 students were registered at medical schools as first year students, increasing to 11 350 in 1983. Since then about eleven to twelve thousand students are accepted every year by German medical schools. Until now the medical associations have had little control over the medical schools, because these are part of the German state universities, financed by general taxes. To stem the rapid increase in physicians, the so-called physician glut ('Ärzteschwemme'), the medical associations as well as the sickness fund association, have proposed a reduction of students entering medical schools, a longer training period for young physicians, and a more difficult licensing procedure for foreign physicians. The federal government has recently enacted a decree that physicians have to spend a significant longer period of training at a hospital and a physicians's office before they may open their own office.

Table 2.10
Physicians and Dentists in the Federal Republic of Germany

	1960	1970	1980	1984	1988
Physicians					
Total number	79 350	85 801	118 726	156 593	171 784
Per 100 000 population	142	163	211	255	272
Per cent office-based	62%	51%	45%	44%	41%
Per cent hospital employed	29%	39%	46%	47%	48%
Per cent in administration or without occupation	9%	10%	9%	9%	11%
Dentists					
Total number	32 509	31 175	32 958	33 713	38 055*
Per 100 000 population	58	51	54	56	60
Per cent office-based	97%	95%	94%	94%	81%

* 1986
Source: Statistisches Bundesamt, Statistisches Jahrbuch, Wiesbaden.

The number of foreign physicians has increased significantly in the past few years. Most of these have studied medicine in Germany and have then succeeded in staying. Citizens from countries belonging to the European Community (EC) do not need a work permit and are free to practise in Germany. However, the number of physicians from EC countries is still relatively low due to the restrictive licensing procedure (see Table 2.11).

Table 2.11
Personal Characteristics of German Physicians
31 December 1988

	Foreign Physicians	Native Physicians
Total number of physicians	9 376	167 625
General practitioners		67%
Specialists		33%
Female physicians		27%
Age under 35		25%
35 - 39		16%
40 - 49		23%
50 - 59		12%
60 - 65		14%
Over 65		14%
Foreign physicians	100.0%	
EC countries	14.4%	
Other European countries	36.3%	
Africa	6.4%	
Asia	32.7%	
America	4.8%	
Others	5.4%	
Total number		177 001
Without speciality		80 036
Internists		20 834
General Practitioners		15 030
Gynaecologists		8 759
Surgeons		8 471
Anaesthetists		6 393
Paediatrists		6 032
Neurologists		4 711
Orthopaedists		3 986
Opthalmologists		3 954
Radiologists		3 190
Otolaryngologists		3 045
Dermatologists		2 466
Urologists		2 389

Source: Arnold, M., *et al.*, Der Beruf des Arztes in der Bundesrepublik Deutschland, Köln: Deutscher Ärtze Verlag: Bundesärztekammer 1984; Ärztestatistik, Die ärtzliche Versorgung in der Bundesrepublik Deutschland zum 31. Dezember 1988, Köln: Deutscher Ärzteverlag 1989.

In 1952 only thirty-four per cent of the office-based physicians were specialists; this segment had increased to fifty-eight per cent by 1988. A major reason for this increase is finance. Specialists have a much higher income (after deducting professional expenses) than physicians in primary care, that is paediatricians, general practitioners and gynaecologists. Since technical services have relatively high fees in comparison to personal physician services, specialists who provide more technical services gain higher incomes. Even recent reforms of the fee schedules which brought an increase in fees of personal services did not change the over-valuation of technical services: laboratory tests, electrocardiograms, electroencephalograms and X-rays. In spite of the increase, the percentage of specialists in the United States remains much higher than in West Germany. Unlike the United States, group practices are rare in Germany. In 1980 only 5 819 office-based physicians, that is about ten point three per cent of all physicians, were working in 2 844 group practices. However, the number of group practices is increasing. On 1 January 1988, as many as 5 363 group practices existed in Germany with 11 164 physicians. This is already sixteen point seven per cent of all office-based physicians.

2.2.7 Remuneration of Physicians

In the 1920s, the statutory health insurance scheme was in great disorder. Chancellor Brüning enacted an emergency decree in 1932, shortly before Hitler came into power, whereby medical associations, KV (*Kassenärztliche Vereinigungen*), were to be founded in each state, and every office-based physician treating sickness fund patients had to join the KV in his state. Since then, the remuneration of physician services has been subject to negotiation between the sickness funds and the KV. It is important to note that no direct negotiations or contacts take place between individual physicians and sickness funds. Physicians receive payment from their KV, which in turn is compensated by the sickness funds.

The medical associations and the dental associations were very successful in their negotiations with the sickness funds, so that physicians belong to the highest income classes of society. However, dentists even outstrip physicians and are now at the apex of the income pyramid. This in mainly due to the relatively constant number of dentists (see Table 2.7) and increased costs for dental care, which have been nearly fully covered by the sickness funds since 1975. Although physicians' incomes have increased over the past few years, the differential between the average income of all employees and physicians' incomes has diminished. The income of office-based physicians in comparison to the average income of all employees increased until 1971 but has decreased since that time. In 1971, German physicians earned 6.5 times the average income of German employees. Today this factor is only about 3.5. The physicians in the US fared much better in maintaining their relative income position.

This raises two questions. First, how are physicians and especially office-based physicians represented in Germany, and second, how are they reimbursed. Physicians are normally members of three or four associations. Every office-based physician who wants to treat sickness fund patients, and those are ninety-eight per cent of all physicians, have to be a member of the Medical Association of Insurance Doctors in his or her state (*Kassenärztliche Vereinigung*). In addition, every physician has to be a member of his or her Medical Chamber (*Ärztekammer*), which is responsible for licensing, quality control, education and professional honourship. Both the Medical Association of Insurance Doctors and the Medical Chamber are bodies of public law. Most physicians belong also to one of the professional organizations (*Internistenverband, Verband der*

Allgemeinmediziner and so on) and to one of the professional pressure group organizations (*Hartmannbund*, for office-based physicians and *Marburger Bund*, for hospital-based physicians). As a result, physicians are the most highly-organized profession in German society.

The medical associations as well as the chambers are represented in the National Health Conference (Konzertierte Aktion im Gesundheitswesen) with eight out of 64 being members of this conference.

All terms of remuneration of office-based physicians are negotiated between the sickness funds associations and the medical associations. On a federal level the fee schedules are negotiated. They consist of about 2 500 items and name for each item a certain number of 'points'. For instance, a telephone conversation with a patient has 80 points, a home visit has 360 points and a X-ray has 360 to 900 points.

On a state level the sickness funds negotiate with the state medical associations a flexible budget (*Gesamtvergütung*) which has to be paid from the 1 200 sickness funds to the 18 medical associations. Note that in Germany the office-based physicians are neither paid by the patient nor by the sickness funds. They receive their remuneration from their medical association on the basis of the negotiated fee schedule, that is the relative value scale, and the value of one point in German marks.

The German method of remunerating physicians uses positive incentives of a fee-for-service scheme but guarantees cost control, so that expenditure does not increase faster than salaries. It is also a system where full coverage of services is combined with a high degree of competition among physicians and professional freedom of physicians. However, the competition among physicians has also induced a rapid increase in services, so that the point value has decreased over the past few years. From the beginning of 1987 until the end of 1988 the point value decreased from 0.103-0.12 DM to 0.0915-0.935 DM.[4]

This devaluation of the point-value due to a more rapidly growing number of services compared to salaries is one reason for the decline of physician income in real terms; the growing overheads of physicians are another. Since 1975 when the cost containment policy started, the income of physicians remained relatively constant and declined in real terms, because the cost of running an office increased much more rapidly than the revenues of office-based physicians.

One may ask why the number of services of physicians has increased so rapidly. The reason is that the growing number of physicians has increased consumer demand for physicians services due to reduced waiting and travelling time. In addition, it has increased the efforts of physicians to encourage demand for services. In an empirical study we have estimated these effects.[5] The estimated elasticities of an increase of physicians are:

cost per visit	0.1596
visits per treatment	0.2899
treatments per person	0.6590.

To sum up, one per cent increase in physicians will lead to a one point one-one per cent increase in costs.

Some additional comments may help the reader to understand the negotiation process. The relative value scale for remunerating physicians is negotiated on a federal level between the sickness funds associations and the physicians associations. A constant working group with representatives of the sickness funds and the physicians has the task of making necessary revisions to the fee-schedule. The point-value, however, and the ceilings for certain services are calculated and negotiated at state level. The Government is only indirectly involved in those negotiations because it is represented by the National Health Conference.

2.2.8 Hospital Care

There are three characteristics of German hospital care which dominate the current discussion: the relatively long length-of-stay; the financing of hospital care and the explosive increase in hospital care expenditures; and the governmental planning of hospital facilities (*Krankenhausbedarfsplanung*).

1) Relatively Long Length-of-Stay In 1987 the average length-of-stay was 13.1 days. Although the mean length-of-stay came down from 18.3 in 1970, to 14.9 in 1980 and 13.1 in 1987 it is still quite long in comparison to other countries. A major reason for the relatively long length-of-stay in German hospitals is the sharp separation between the ambulatory care provided by office-based physicians and hospital care. This is because most hospitals are prohibited from offering outpatient care, even when the patient has previously been hospitalized. A committal order written by a private physician is required in order for a patient to receive hospital care. Both because of the poor flow of information between private and hospital physicians, and because office-based physicians do not have access to the (usually superior) hospital equipment, hospitals repeat many diagnostic examinations already performed by private physicians prior to hospitalization. In fact, such duplication is more the rule than the exception in Germany. Medical examinations which could be carried out before hospitalization are a standard part of hospital treatment itself, adding to length-of-stay and, ultimately, to cost-of-stay. This sharp separation between ambulatory and hospital care has another effect: patients stay longer in hospitals because hospital doctors, unsure about the nature of medical care after discharge, prefer to keep a patient in the hospital until a complete recovery has been made.

The solution to the above problem seems very simple. Hospitals should have the capability of providing outpatient care, and private physicians should be granted access to hospital facilities and allowed to provide hospital care. The powerful German medical associations, however, have succeeded up until now in hindering the passage of legislation that would have enabled a better cooperation between the ambulatory and hospital care sectors.

A second reason for the relatively long length of hospital stays in Germany seems to be the lack of incentives under the present hospital financing scheme for hospitals to shorten the length-of-stay, as is explained in the following paragraphs. However, many patients do also prefer a longer stay in a hospital after an operation or a baby's delivery because of increasing difficulties in providing home care due to the higher employment rate of women. A group of health economists, including myself, is currently undertaking a research project on the incentives of a diagnosis-related-group (DRG) remuneration. Since 1987 a hospital in Kiel is remunerated by DRGs. The mean length-of-stay has decreased to one third and the hospital has started to cooperate intensively with office-based physicians to reduce the duration of hospitalization of the patients.

2) Financing of Hospital Care The financing of German hospitals is regulated by the Hospital Financing Act of 1985 and the Hospital Care Rating Decree of 1985. These laws replaced and standardized former regulations, which were inadequate in various aspects.

The principal components of current arrangements for hospital financing are:

a) capital expenditures are totally financed by federal budget funds;
b) the hospital's current costs (that is operating costs) must be financed by *per diem payments;* and
c) *per diem* rates must be fixed in such a way that they enable the hospital to cover all current costs of management.

If the hospital realizes a profit (surplus) it may keep it. However, the *per diems* will be reduced the following year. The *per diem* rates are uniform for all patients in the same hospital but differ among hospitals. Capital expenditures are defined by law as the construction costs of a hospital plus the costs for durable equipment. A precondition to receiving federal budget funds is that the hospital meets certain standards and conforms to the Hospital Need Plan (*Krankenhausbedarfsplan*) as discussed below.

Per diem rates are negotiated between the sickness funds and the individual hospitals. Prior to this, each hospital calculates its average cost per bed-day in a form specified by the decree. Since 1986 the *per diems* are prospective payments, that is if the hospital has lower cost than the *per diems* it may keep these profits and if it realizes a loss this has to be covered by the hospital or its owners. The sickness funds and the hospitals also agree on certain quality standards, length-of-stay and occupancy rates. On the one hand, hospitals have a legal claim to receive cost-covering rates. On the other hand, the sickness funds refer to article 17.1 BPV, which demands economical hospital management. Therefore it is not unusual in Germany to find that sickness funds as well as hospitals sue to change the stated rates. This system of setting rates on the basis of historical costs leads to great discrepancies in the rates.

The hospital financing scheme described above has an inherent problem: clearly there is no economical incentive for hospitals to shorten the length-of-stay. Patients are frequently hospitalized on Fridays and discharged on Mondays, even though no specific medical care is provided at weekends. The hospital financing system offers no incentive to reduce costs and to use resources economically, because the *per diem* rates are calculated on the basis of past cost data. The higher the costs of hospital care in the past, the higher the present rates will be.

Other forms of financing hospitals, such as decreasing *per diem* rates or diagnostic-related-group type of financing (DRG), are being discussed in Germany but seem to be unacceptable to all concerned.

3) Planning for Hospital Needs The Hospital Financing Act restricts federal funds for capital expenditures to those hospitals which have received accreditation. Combining hospital accreditation and financing was intended to achieve three major goals:

a) a more equitable regional distribution of hospital facilities and available hospital beds;
b) a well-balanced regionalized structure of hospitals;

c)   a reduction in the number of hospital beds with a concomitant increase in occupancy rates.

German hospital need-planning contains some obvious problems. First, the act contains no clear criteria or standards for states' hospital planning, therefore the criteria underlying the Hospital Need Plans differ from state to state or are not indicated explicitly at all. Second, in practice, hospital need planning affects only construction of new hospitals or additions to already existing ones. A hospital, once listed in a Hospital Need Plan can hardly be expelled from the plan. This is the reason why hospital need planning can only hope to change the structure and distribution of hospital care in the long run. Finally, hospital need planning seems to have paralysed the private sector by making it very difficult for private hospitals to become accredited. In 1985 only fourteen per cent of hospital beds were under private ownership. However, private hospitals are normally relatively small, which is why about thirty point five per cent of all hospitals are privately owned. The future problem will be to reduce the excess capacities of hospitals and to cover the increased demand for nursing homes, due to the dramatic demographic change taking place in Germany.

2.2.9 Pharmaceutical Care

The sickness funds spend about nineteen per cent of their entire expenditure on drugs and medical appliances; this is more than for dental care or for ambulatory physician care. These extraordinary high expenditures are due to excessive consumption and high prices. Surveys indicate that German doctors prescribe on average about 11 medicines per person per year, almost three times more than their American colleagues. Also surprising is the discovery that about sixty per cent of all medicines prescribed in Germany are prescribed primarily at the request of the patients. One reason for this relatively large consumption of drugs by German patients may be the coverage of prescribed drugs by sickness funds and by most private health insurers.

The German legislature has attempted to lower drug expenditures by the passage of article 368 of the Social Insurance Act in 1977. This mandated the creation of a blacklist of drugs normally used in the treatment of minor illnesses. Drugs on this list have to be paid for out of pocket by the patient and are no longer covered by sickness funds, even when they are prescribed. In addition, the co-payments for prescribed drugs were increased several times since 1983 and are currently DM 3.00 per prescribed medicine.

In addition to the large *per capita* consumption of pharmaceuticals, high prices also play an important role in determining the global expenditures for drugs. A more analytical look reveals that the demand side of the drug market involves three distinct sets of players: physicians, who decide what should be consumed but bear no portion of the cost; patients, who consume the drugs but decide neither what to consume nor how much to pay; and the sickness funds, which foot the bills but exercise no control over what is consumed. This three-way partition in decision, consumption, and funding, creates a situation in which market forces can hardly determine drug prices in West Germany and other countries underscores this dilemma.[6]

During the last several years, the government took two steps to revitalize price competition in the drug market. First, parliament created a drug 'Transparency' Commission. Its task is to publish and distribute lists comparing prices of medical compounds with the same uses and/or ingredients. Second, the Medical Association and the sickness funds are compelled by law to negotiate yearly an overall ceiling on expenditures for prescribed drugs. The Medical Association must then influence its members by moral persuasion, prescription guidelines and other measures to implement the negotiated ceiling. In addition, the recent Health Insurance Structural Reform, which became effective on 1 January 1989, will bring a fifteen per cent co-payment on all prescribed drugs and indemnity benefits for all compounds where generics exist. The indemnity benefits will be higher than the prices for generic drugs but lower than the prices for the original brand drugs.

2.2.10 Solidarity and Cost Control

The major goal of the German health policy is to achieve equal access to medical care for all citizens. This is guaranteed by the comprehensive and generous coverage of the sickness funds and the financing scheme. A second goal is freedom of choice and a high quality standard of services. However, as it was demonstrated in the beginning solidarity and freedom of choice cause the problem of cost control. Germany was very successful in controlling costs in past years. All parties concerned are represented in the National Health Conference. This Conference has to recommend expenditure targets and give guidelines for the regional price and quantity negotiation. Cost control is then achieved by negotiations between medical, dental and other suppliers' associations and the sickness funds, and the outcome of those negotiations are binding for everyone. In those cases where the outcome of negotiations of the sickness funds associations and the providers are not binding, for example the negotiations between the pharmaceutical associations are not binding for pharmaceutical companies, co-payments and quantity controls were imposed to contain costs.[7] The Health Insurance Structural Reform Law which became effective from 1 January 1989 proscribes that expenditure of the sickness funds may not increase faster than salaries. By this, Germany is the first country which explicitly defines by law the fraction of income spent on medical care.

2.2.11 Demographic Change

The German health care system is confronted with three challenges: the increase in the number of physicians, the sharp separation of ambulatory and hospital care and the rapid demographic change. The first two challenges are solved or can be solved by reforms of the ambulatory care and hospital financing. The third challenge, rapid demographic change, is only partly compensated by refugees coming from East Germany and East European countries. This demographic change is caused by a drastic increase in life-expectancy and a constant decline of fertility. In 1964 the demographic net-reproduction-rate, that is the average number of daughters a woman has during her whole life, was 1.18. The net-reproduction-rate dropped to 0.61 in 1984. We estimate that the German population in West Germany will decrease from 57.1 million to 34.8 million in the year 2030, so the whole population will decline from 61.6 to 46.1 million. This development will also lead to a drastic change of the population structure.

The number of elderly will increase over the next 40 years which will increase the demand for health services and for nursing care and old people's homes. The number of people in the workforce will decline. Because social security is financed by pay-as-you-earn premiums of the employees and their employers, contribution rates are increasing and will increase due to the change of population structure. We estimate that under *status quo* benefit rules the contribution rates for pension funds will increase from eighteen point seven per cent to between thirty-six point four and forty point one per cent in the year 2030. The average contribution rate for statutory sickness funds is currently twelve point six per cent of wages. This will increase to about twenty-one point six per cent in 2030 if no major reform takes place.

It is clear that future generations will not be willing to finance this burden; those who have children in particular, will prefer an intra-family transfer to an inter-family transfer which covers old age pensions and health care for the growing number of DINKS (double-income-no-kids).[8] Newly industrialized countries should avoid this trap of social security systems by employing a fully funded system accumulating age reserves. Social security reduces the incentives to have children, less children lead to an unbalanced population structure in a transition period and this transition period is a threat for a pay-as-you-earn financed social security scheme.

2.2.12 Europe after 1992 and Medical Care in Germany

The crucial question is, do we expect that the European harmonization process will lead to a change in the German health care system. In Germany there are no visible forces demanding a major reform of the German system, for three reasons. First, all those who are living for and living from the health care system do live quite well, with the exception of nurses who are poorly paid in Germany, therefore nobody is calling for change. The pharmaceutical industry in particular fears that the EC-harmonization will lower the price levels for pharmaceutical products. Second, the German unification process demands a lot of attention and resources. East German hospitals are obsolete and many East German physicians are poorly trained because they have worked in administration. Third, the German health care system has shown the capability to provide high quality care and to contain cost. Why should it be changed in a more centralized and regulated or in a more market-orientated system?

However, I still see five forces which could lead to a major change and a convergence of social health insurance in the EC countries:

a)   increasing patient mobility;
b)   a deregulation of private health insurance;
c)   increasing border crossing of physicians, dentists and other health services personnel;
d)   a growing number of internationally-operating hospital chains; and the free trade of pharmaceutical products.

Differences in Europe will induce movements of patients, products and health care suppliers which in itself will speed up the harmonization of the different European social security schemes. As in former times the harmonization process is more enforced by the dynamics of international trade and the interaction of international product and labour markets than by political decisions made in Brussels.

1 See for a detailed description of the German health care system: Glaser, W.A. (1978), *Health insurance bargaining: foreign lessons for Americans.* New York, Gardner Press, 95-116; Landsberger, H.A. (1981), *The control of cost in the Federal Republic of Germany. Lessons for America?* Washington DC: Department of Health and Human Services, publication no. (HRA) 81-14003; Reinhardt, U.W. (1981), Health insurance and health policy in the Federal Republic of Germany. *Health Care Finance Rev,* 3, 1-14; Stone, D.A. (1979), Health care cost containment in West Germany, *Health Politics Policy Law,* 4, 176-99; Stone, D.A. (1980), *The limits of professional power: national health care in the Federal Republic of Germany,* University of Chicago Press, Chicago.
2 Geissler, H. (1973), *Krankenversicherungs-Budget,* Mainz, Regierung Rheinland Pfalz.
3 See OECD (1987), *Financing and Delivering Health Care, A Comparative Analysis of OECD-Countries,* Paris, 55.
4 *Sachverständigenrat für die Konzertierte Aktion im Gesundheitswesen,* Jahresgutachten 1989, Baden-Baden 1989.
5 Cf. Schulenburg, J.-M. Graf v.d. (1987), Die Ärzteschwemme und ihre Auswirkungen auf die ambulante Versorgung, in Brennecke, R., Schach, E. (eds), *Ambulante Versorgung: Nachfrage und Seuerung,* Berlin, 125-139. Kraft, K., Schulenburg, J.-M. Graf v.d. (1986), Co-Insurance and Supplier-Induced Demand in Medical Care, *Journal of Institutional and Theoretical Economics,* 142, 360-79.
6 Schulenburg, J.-M. Graf v.d. (1983), Report from Germany: Current conditions and controversies in the health care system. *Journal of Health Politics Policy and the Law,* 8, 320-51.
7 See for the forms and effects of co-payments Schulenburg, J.- M. Graf v.d. (1987), *Selbstbeteiligung,* Tübingen; Knappe, E., Leu, R., Schulenburg, J.-M. Graf v.d. (1988), *Der Indemnitätstarif,* Frankfurt.
8 See Breyer, F., Schulenburg, J.-M. Graf v.d., *Family Ties and Social Security in a Democracy, Public Choice* (forthcoming) and *Voting on Social Security: The Family as Decision-Making Unit,* Kyklos 1987, 40, 529-547.

2.3 Competition and the New Structure of the Health Care System in the Netherlands
F.P. Broere

2.3.1 Room for Competition in the Common Market

After 1992 the EC is thought to become one big market. There will be a fully liberalized movement of goods, services, labour and capital. Whether this will become reality remains to be seen, but if so, exceptions may still exist, a very likely one of which would seem to be health care. The main reason for this lies in the vast differences in organization of the health care systems of the Member States. As yet, the EC has not given incentives for harmonizing the health care systems.

Consumers may wish to buy health services in other countries than their own, suppliers of care may wish to set up establishments in other countries. Both groups will succeed only if Governments allow them to do so and if insurers are willing to pay. Governments tend to see health care as related to their welfare and social security policies and will try to retain autonomy in these fields.

However, European citizens are already seeking access to health care in other Member States when they feel the level of medical care is higher and/or service elements of the care supplied are better than in their native country. Also if regulations limit domestic options they will want to go abroad, thus some international competition is already developing.

To get an impression of how competition at a European level could take place, the new structure of the health care system in Holland will be used as a starting point for a discussion about the scope for competition and the shape that competition may take. The effects on the behaviour of the parties in the market of government policy will be analyzed.

2.3.2 Governments and Competition

As pointed out above, national Governments want to influence the way in which health care is provided and financed; they set the constraints for competition. They may choose to regulate the health care system thoroughly or may leave the outcome of supply and demand largely to market forces. Within the British National Health Service for example, there is no competition but next to this system a commercial health care exists. In the future Dutch system a form of competition, called administered competition, will be implemented. Dutch Government will no longer control the process but will try to steer the outcomes by the constraints it sets on the operations on the market.

An outline will be given of the proposed system for the Dutch health care.

2.3.3 Government Plan for Changes is the Structure and Finance of Health Care in the Netherlands

In the Netherlands over the last decades state regulation has been growing with the aim of keeping the costs of health care at an acceptable level. But despite its growth, regulation proved to be ineffective or even counterproductive. There are several reasons for altering the system:

a)   the inability of Government to control costs by controlling the system;
b)   the disadvantages of the current system which are in part related to state regulation;
c)   the general shift in society away from state influence towards market mechanism.

One of the political goals of Dutch Government (the Lubbers administration) is reaching a degree of deregulation. For health care this means that the Government should create conditions for the proper functioning of health care and should steer processes only globally. However, Government still aims at cost containment and high efficiency and will continue to maintain a high level of quality of health care. Also, health services should stay accessible for all citizens.

In August 1986 a committee was appointed by the Government, called the Committee on Structure and Financing of Health Care, which had as its chairman Professor Dr. W. Dekker, then president of the Supervisory Board of Philips Inc.

In March 1987 the Dekker Committee presented its report entitled 'Willingness to change'.[1] The committee designed a structure based in part on ideas that were already known by health economists.[2] In its proposals there is more room for competition and limited room for Government regulation. Government should give incentives and as few directives as possible. Through competition, via the market or price mechanism a continuous process of weighing costs against benefits takes place. Within health care this will give rise to more careful spending of scarcer funds, nevertheless competition will be curtailed by certain rules ('regulated' or 'administered' competition). A large measure of solidarity is guaranteed.

The Dekker Committee advocated more flexibility and a higher rate of efficiency through the introduction of the market mechanism. One way of reaching this goal is through a reform of the insurance system. Instead of the existing dual system (compulsory insurance for people within the lower income brackets and voluntary insurance for the higher income groups) all insurers would compete on an equal basis. All citizens would have a basic insurance covering about eighty-five per cent of the former compulsory package, as well as the state insurance for extraordinary health risks. They could extend their insurance with a voluntary supplementary package covering the 'remaining fifteen per cent'. Both the basic insurance and the supplementary package could be insured by the former sick funds as well as the insurance companies.

According to the proposals the insured are paying for the compulsory package partly by an income-related premium and partly by a fixed amount, the latter being dependent on the efficiency of the insurance company and of the health care the company has contracted. People buying supplementary insurances pay a premium reflecting the size of the package as well as the efficiency of the insurance company and of the contracted suppliers of health care.

Unlike the current situation, insurers do not have the obligation to contract all state-recognized health care. They can choose the more efficient suppliers of health services and/or the ones that deliver better quality. On the other hand, the insured will have the possibility of changing insurer, without losing their rights.

In a recent publication of the Department of Health Care, the outline of the earlier proposals remained intact.[3] However, the basic insurance will probably cover more than ninety-five per cent of the former compulsory and state packages (see above) leaving only some three to five per cent for voluntary supplementary packages. The idea underlying the shift towards a higher percentage may be the supposed growth of the voluntary package at the expense of the basic package after the new system is introduced.

2.3.4 Where to Choose from? (Is there a real choice available?)

The choice for the consumer of health care may not differ very much under the system the Dekker Committee and the Department of Health Care propose. As previously he may choose his doctor and the doctor will direct him to the second layer (hospitals and medical specialists). Although this in theory is the choice of the consumer, in practice he will follow the advice of his doctor, because the doctor has knowledge of the medical treatment of specialists and knows what type of specialized medical treatment the consumer/patients needs. In reality the consumer almost always has a preference for a hospital only, not being acquainted with specialists. Hospitals - as currently perceived by health consumers - don't differ very much, they tend to opt for a local hospital facility.

Insurance companies will be able to choose from suppliers of health care. According to the Dekker Committee they will choose the most efficient ones, because those suppliers are cheapest. This could restrict the freedom of choice of the insured, as insurers will not contract every supplier of care. However, consumers can move from one insurance to another. A reason for change may be that they like a local hospital better than a cheaper hospital that is not much different but farther away, and in this case they will not favour the lower cost insurer.

2.3.5 What sort of competition will take place?

In the vision of the Dekker Committee insurance companies will compete with each other to attract customers; price is the weapon used in the struggle for the customer. The same is true for the competition between suppliers of health care to obtain a contract with as many insurers as possible. Lower prices will occur only when both insurers and suppliers of health care tighten their costs and boost their efficiency. Insurance companies compete on the financing market. In addition, these suppliers compete on the care delivery market in which consumers receive services from institutions and physicians.[4]

Two forms of competition may occur: price competition and 'service' competition.

1) Price competition In the proposals of the Dekker Committee the only form of competition that may appear to take place will be price competition. This presupposes many parties of about the same size that are homogeneous in their services. However, in larger urban areas oligopolistic competition between hospitals exists. Outside these areas hospitals are regional monopolists, and general practitioners almost everywhere are monopolistic competitors. It is doubtful whether price competition as Dekker sees it will occur.

There are still many sickness funds (that will in future no longer differ from insurance companies), but in view of the changes to come, many of them are merging to form larger entities that will be able to compete with the private insurance companies. To avoid competition, (groups of) sickness funds may merge with non-profit or even for-profit insurance companies and what remains is perhaps less than 20 entities among which will be a few large ones.[5] The insurance market may become an oligopoly also.

In the Dekker proposals, competition is thought to take the form of price competition and seems to satisfy the outcomes of microeconomic models. This, however, is a very lean form of competition as the choice to consumers as well as to insurers is very limited. A richer form is possible in combination with an acceptable level of social justice.

2) 'Service' competition For the compulsory package, price competition is limited to the nominal premium (independent of income, dependent on efficiency). This may also, but not necessarily, be the case with the voluntary package.

The voluntary package will comprise special types of medical treatment not included in the compulsory package, but may also include more service elements: higher premiums will buy these packages. For the compulsory package higher (service) quality may be wanted also and may be paid for via the 'nominal' premium.

2.3.6 The Shape Competition may take

Health care is aimed at the well-being of people. There is no fundamental difference between people buying health care or any other service, but with health care, people may lack sufficient knowledge of the service they are considering. They can gain information by reading advertisements, test reports, articles about the experiences of others, or by consulting experts. In general there exists freedom of choice. The needs and wants of consumers differ from each other, but usual groups of consumers can be identified that have certain specific needs and wants in common.

Organizations that offer goods or services will be able to reach their goals better by researching the needs and wants of certain customer groups and offering such goods or services and in such a way as best matches those needs and wants. Serving different groups with different services can be both more efficient and more effective than serving everyone with one service.[6] In health care preferences also differ, although some systems offer only one type of service for all patients. People can perhaps live with a limited range of choices, nevertheless those who can afford it will look for alternatives to obtain the care that suits them, for example in other Member States of the EC.

If the outcome of the process of supplying and asking for health care is left to the market to a larger extent, competition will not be so homogeneous as the Dekker Committee expects and taking into account the needs and wants of patients need not be so homogeneous. This is not to say that enormous differences in care or overly luxurious care is advocated here. A few conditions should be set:

a)   to a certain degree health care should be accessible for every citizen;
b)   there should exist a certain (high) quality of medical care;
c)   to a certain extent there should be solidarity both in income and in health risk.

The Dekker Committee incorporates these conditions in its proposals. It has also tried to design a structure in which more market - more competition - and less government will be present. It suffers from myopia in that it looks at price competition only.

The second form of competition, non-price competition, will most probably occur. Health insurers will try to control costs. They can ask for lower premiums or provide their insured with better benefits. These benefits can take the form of better quality of service in a broad sense. More specifically, this could take the form of service elements such as faster treatment, shorter waiting lists for medical treatment for certain specialisms that are in short supply, and gimmicks such as using one's PC in a hospital room (useful for businessmen and scientists). Another type of benefit could be personal attention, for example good communication and information exchange with specialists, explanation of the types of therapies and treatments and more personal care.

The examples mentioned above can be elements of different packages specially designed for certain target groups; these groups are formed by segmenting the total population of potential patients. On the basis of demographic, geographic and psychographic characteristics, groups can be distinguished with homogeneous needs and wants. The marketing policy of suppliers of health services will be to offer each package to a specific target group. They can try and convince some insurance companies to offer such packages as a voluntary type of health insurance and together they can aim at selected target groups.

In this approach there is a benefit for many people. The conditions for the health system as a whole are unaffected; the compulsory package guarantees access to a high level of health care and there are incentives for efficient operations via price competition. At the same time a certain degree of non-price competition can exist because the quality of the care the insurers provide may differ. Consumers wanting more and different medical treatment and/or service elements will not be limited in their choice. They can choose from several types of (voluntary) packages, and as a consequence some rise in the level of expenditure will occur, but these are not the result of insufficient care in the compulsory package.

2.3.7 The Common Market

Both in the Netherlands and in the EC, on an aggregated level there are three parties in the market: insurers, suppliers of health services and patients. Suppliers of care and insurers will compete if circumstances make it attractive for them to do so. European and national authorities play an important part in creating room for competition.

To obtain a better understanding of these three parties, their conduct will be examined below.

1) Suppliers of health care Two levels of international competition seem possible and occasionally have already taken place.

a) Top-level clinical care may compete throughout the EC. Competition will be directed towards patients and insurers in supplying care. Wealthy patients can look for the best medical treatment, because they can afford it. Sometimes patients' organizations may utilize foreign hospitals for their members, because of a shortage of top quality care in their own country.

b) The other level will be competition within regions and between adjacent regions. Examples are areas on both sides of a border.

Competition on a European level already exists between hospitals, research institutes and universities, aimed at undertaking contract research and consultancy for the pharmaceutical industry and suppliers of medical hardware.

2) Insurers Already insurance companies can compete in other markets than their home market. Whether they will enter the market of an EC-Member State depends upon the possibility of reaching their goals, that is making profit of serving certain social purposes.

As a consequence of competition between suppliers of health care, patients could ask their insurer to compensate them for the consumption of care in other countries than their own. Whether insurers will be inclined to pay for health services from foreign suppliers depends upon the cost structure of health care in the home countries of the suppliers and upon the willingness of the insurers to seek this kind of competition. In this case top-level clinical care may be an object of competition. Insurers can look for top clinical care in other countries, because cost comparisons indicate to them that it is cheaper there (sometimes as a consequence of government subsidies, thus disguising the real costs).

3) Patients Apart from top-level clinical care, there is much uniformity among suppliers of care. If health care institutions are not willing or able to differentiate their services from other institutions by using distinguishable mixes of product, price, promotion, distribution and personnel, patients will not have anything to choose from. In that case competition is non-existent, with the possible exception of strong international differences. Even so, insurers may compete with each other to attract patients by selling policies that are more or less comprehensive.

2.3.8   Conclusions for Competition in Europe

In this paper an outline is given of the proposals for more market elements in Dutch health care of the Dekker Committee; also the two forms of competition that may take place are described in brief. It is unlikely that competition will be limited to pure price competition. A description of the conduct of the parties involved in health care made clear that a real freedom of choice for patients is a necessary condition for competition. It will come to pass only if patients can choose between suppliers as well as between insurers on the basis of differences in both price and quality.

The division of the health insurance into a compulsory element amounting to about ninety-five per cent of the current package of the Sick Funds and a voluntary element of only less than five per cent may frustrate competition. There is also a tendency among suppliers of health care, as well as among insurers, to reduce competition by merging into larger entities.

The proposals of the Dekker Committee offer a structure that can be used as a model for the development of a European policy for health care. It meets the need for competition on a European level. However, the European Commission should take several measures to create competition and keep it intact.

On social grounds a compulsory health insurance can be defended, although some incentives for cost conscious behaviour of consumers of health services should be part of this. Also, there should exist a relatively large voluntary element to stimulate mutual competition between suppliers of health care and between insurers of health care. Anti-trust legislation should avoid unacceptable concentration of power among suppliers of health services as well as among insurers. By doing so suppliers and insurers will compete on both price and quality; cost of health care may rise somewhat as a result of higher qualities, including better service, asked for by the patients, but there remains pressure on the costs of health care in general. Competition also prevents health care from becoming rigid and less innovative.

The possible alternatives are either separate health care systems for each of the Member States or a European Health System, EC owned or heavily regulated. Looking at the vast differences in the national health care structures, harmonization on an EC level still seems many years away. For health care after 1992 the frontiers will still exist. Nevertheless, Europe as an economic entity needs free movement of health care as well as a free movement of labour, capital and goods. International competition seems more in line with the policy aimed at Europe without economic frontiers than a structure heavily dominated and regulated by 'Brussels'.

2.3.9   Notes

1 Commissie Structuur en Financiering Gezondheidszorg, Bereidheid tot verandering, The Hague, 1987.
2 The ideas put forward by the Dekker Committee were inspired in part by Professor A.C. Enthoven of the Graduate School of Business at Stanford University. In his book called 'Health Plan, The only solution to the soaring cost of medical care' (Reading, MA, 1980), he pleads for a system in which providers are rewarded for finding ways to give better care at less costs.

3 Annex to "Working on renewal of care" (Werken aan zorgvernieuwing) entitled *Note regarding the change of the health system* (Notitie inzake de stelselwijziging zorgsector), The Hague, May 10th, 1990.
4 Schut, F.T. and W.P.M.M. van de Ven, (eds) (1987), *Proceedings of the conference on regulated competition in the Dutch health care system*, Lecture by J.F.G.M. de Beer, Rotterdam, 6.
5 In the recent publications of the department of Health Care (see note 4 above) it is suggested that a health insurance, being a social insurance, only can be executed by non-profit insurers. Commercial insurance companies need not cease trading; they can create a non-profit subsidiary to run this part of their business. Besides, it is not clear whether a health insurance must be seen as a social insurance as is an unemployment insurance.
6 Marketing theory has brought this insight. For a thorough description of marketing theory for health services see Ph. Kotler and R.N. Clarke (1987), *Marketing for health care organizations*, Englewood Cliffs, N.J.

2.4 A Competitive Strategy for the Efficient Organization of Out-patient Services
M. Campari

2.4.1 Introduction

At the beginning of the 1970s a working party of diverse businessmen and professionals examined the feasibility of introducing a completely new type of service into the Italian health system - a system whose organization at that time was almost totally devoted to in-patient care.

After a careful analysis of health services and their likely development in several countries, the group identified a number of fundamental trends, then in their initial states, that were likely to become increasingly evident as the years went by, for instance:

a) People would demand health services of ever higher quality and greater efficiency; no longer basing their judgement of those services solely on the skills of the doctor but on the entire package available.

b) Technological innovation would radically modify diagnostic techniques, which would become much quicker, non-invasive and highly sophisticated, leading to a major reduction in the length of time a patient remained in hospital for diagnosis.

c) The development of medical knowledge would result in modifications to many surgical and therapeutic procedures; this too would tend to expand the out-patient sector.

d) Early diagnosis and primary prevention would grow in importance in the eyes of the public and politicians; awareness of the relevance of such concepts as risk factors, environmental conditions, life style and early diagnosis in relation to disease would grow sharply.

These trends were evident in the context of a situation in Italy whereby its National Health Service, partly based on the British model, was, at the end of the 1970s, about to be officially inaugurated.

The ideology behind Italian health reform dates back to the 1960s and may be summarized by the principle of a complete range of health care being provided 'free' to all citizens. The service was to be largely provided and administered by a structure consisting of about 700 Local Health Units covering the whole of Italy. The private health care sector was to have an agreed role within the system: it would provide its services to citizens at the request of a general practitioner after approval by the Local Health Unit. Charges would be agreed nationally and payment would be made by the same Local Health Unit.

The payment mechanisms usually adopted differed according to whether out-patient services were provided or if the patient was admitted; in the former case payment depended on actual services provided, in the latter it depended only on the number of days spent in the private hospital. Assuming that the payment mechanisms always involved controls encouraging behaviour consistent with propriety and economy, it was unfortunately true that, while the payment methods operative in the out-patient sector encouraged productivity with respect to service provision, those operating in the in-patient sector encouraged long stays.

The payment mechanism provided no incentive to reduce the time spent by a patient in the nursing home, since if this were done it would have reduced bed utilization which was the most important measure of nursing home profitability. In the USA this problem had been recognized and strict monitoring of hospital 'residence' times in relation to different diseases was carried out. In Italy, the largest mutual health insurance organization, INAM (abolished with the introduction of the 'free' service) used to carry out similar controls. It was thought that, once the confusion due to the actual introduction of the reform had subsided, better mechanisms for remunerating private hospitals for treating in-patients, and for evaluating the productivity of public hospitals, would be identified.

Not least with regard to payment mechanisms, the out-patient sector was more modern and efficient and it was expected that the methods employed there would have been progressively extended to the other sectors of the Italian Health Service. The speed of this extension was, and continues to be, very slow; not just because of the complexities involved, but also because of the opposition and powerful negotiating positions of hospital trades unions and the private hospital associations.

Having analyzed the international trends on the one hand, the pattern of development of the Italian Health Service on the other, and various services reimbursement possibilities as well, the opportunities and dangers associated with a major new initiative in the provision of out-patient services were painstakingly identified:

2.4.2 Opportunities:

a) The demand for out-patient and early diagnosis services was growing and was likely to grow faster in the future.
b) The continuing development of medical knowledge and technology led to the expectation of significant expansion of the diagnostic techniques and therapies available for application in the out-patient sector.
c) The more traditional diagnostic services had also undergone major administrative reforms designed to allow the patient to receive several different types of examination at one centre and within a very brief period.

d)   The service, however, left much to be desired, based as it was on units that were too small and centred around freelance doctors; there was no awareness of the needs of the market.

e)   The out-patient sector could then, as a whole, be considered 'emergent': the rules of play had not yet been established, and would have a tendency to develop in the direction considered most convenient. In other words the sector was 'malleable'.

f)   The advance of new technology would have brought with it anyway an influx of capital into the out-patient sector, as had happened previously in the case of nursing homes.

2.4.3   Dangers:

a)   Politicians would have interpreted the initiative as a reaction of the private sector against the Italian Health Service, then about to be conceived; they would have opposed it, possibly killing the scheme entirely.

b)   The freelance doctors operating in the sector would have felt threatened by the new scheme and opposed it, instead of seeing the opportunities it presented to develop their businesses.

c)   The new out-patient centres envisaged would have required efficient management; the particular kind of health manager required was not available on the market, and training would have taken a long time.

d)   The innovations that were part and parcel of the scheme were wide-ranging and would all have to have been implemented more or less at the same time, otherwise there was a real danger that the scheme would have been a failure.

Having carefully weighed up these pros and cons, it was decided to go ahead and develop a large (10 000 sq.m) out-patient centre, fully equipped with all the latest diagnostic apparatus and so on, including computers, where the patient could, in the space of a single day, undergo all the tests and diagnostic procedures requested by his GP, in a comfortable ambience and in the care of attentive and efficient staff who treated him as an individual.

Five strategic factors were identified as essential to the success of the initiative and the consolidation of a material advantage over the competition; their correct implementation implied efficient and highly innovative management. They were:

a)   Identification of the best organizational procedures, using industrial and service industry experience as models, and implementing modifications appropriate to the out-patient sector; the modifications eventually required were rather unexpected.

b)   Major reliance on computers, whose use at that time was growing rapidly in the health sector.

c)   Implementation of the right kind of personnel structure, so that the relation between organizational hierarchy and function would be compatible with the freelance attitudes of the staff working in the centre.

d)   Requirement for training of staff. In view of their strong specialist bias, staff would have little awareness of the organizational and managerial aspects of their work, less so of the human relations skills essential for good client rapport.

e) Identification of the publicity techniques to best inform the public of the new Centre, taking account of the major restraints imposed in this area by the Italian Medical Associations ('Ordine dei Medici') at both national and regional levels.

2.4.4 First Factor: Organization

The primary requirement of an out-patient centre incorporating a full range of diagnostic techniques and not a few treatment services, is to be able to manage the comings and goings of large numbers of people (about 2 000 per day), each requiring a particular combination of examinations and tests, selected from among the thousands available.

The first problem to solve was to decide how much space would be needed, how many staff required and where they would be accommodated; to assist with this, traffic and transport control methods were used (queue theories, and so on) as well as the use of models simulating the workings of the various departments as a function of workload.

With the opening of the Centre, ideas for improving procedures and workplace arrangements were formulated, and additional medical equipment needs were identified. Experience was gained rapidly, and as the volume of work expanded major economies of scale were identified, particularly with respect to the laboratory analyses. It was discovered that the question of organization within the Italian Health Service had been completely neglected even though it constituted a fundamental issue.

It was also discovered by a careful study of the way people were 'processed' through the system (information, booking appointments, acceptance for tests, carrying out tests, provision of results) that processing could be divided into stages with the introduction of quality controls at each stage. Improved quality coincides with reduced costs in as much as the rooting out and correction of problems becomes more difficult and costly the longer the delay between emergence of that problem and its identification. Total commitment to quality was a strategic element of major importance.

2.4.5 Second Factor: Computerization

As procedures developed and experience of them was gained, so too were the best ways to computerize them sought, making maximum use of the most sophisticated and modern hardware and software technologies available.

From the beginning the Centre had been fully equipped with impressive data-processing capacity; the professionals working there were immediately exposed to computers and soon gained confidence in their use. There was a mainframe with its 'high priests' - the programmers - and a network of many terminals, which were dedicated or intended for general use in the departments. The idea that the computer was an instrument like any other, and was there to be used and exploited to the full, steadily took root among the staff. The medical staff too, quickly learned to use a computer and soon overcame, for example, their suspicions of computerized diagnostic protocols, realizing that these were only a codification of their own experience and knowledge, which put on computer allowed more efficient use of the same.

2.4.6 Third Factor: Personnel Structure

Within the out-patient sector in general (which was and remains considerably behind in terms of management techniques even in comparison with the poor state of affairs in in-patient care) the peculiar problem of how to tailor a managerial structure to the needs of freelance professionals had never been approached; it was therefore necessary to start from scratch. The first step was to appoint a managing director (Direttore Generale) in overall charge of both medical and non-medical personnel. The person appointed was not in this case a doctor, but an engineer, coming from a firm of Italian-American management consultants charged to carry out the original feasibility study for the Centre.

Once the go-ahead for the Centre had been given, the managing director's job was to set it up according to policy guidelines provided by a managing committee, and subsequently to manage it adopting a type of personnel structure which had been developed successfully in other countries. His most important decision was to link a young manager to the doctor in charge of a section. The manager was competent in organizational aspects and would soon develop an understanding of the operational problems and staff mentality associated with that area of the health sector. The doctor, obviously responsible for the quality of the services he and his colleagues provided, but not desirous of mastering management techniques, was happy to leave these to an expert. The only exception to this arrangement was in the laboratories, where the biological sciences graduates proved themselves both willing and able to adopt and improve the new procedures. Even today this is the only section where the organizational manager is not a trained manager but a trained scientist.

The limited size of the staff structure meant that the usual expedient was followed of allowing the testing technician to be responsible for the entire testing process: from patient reception to handing over the results. This arrangement was criticized within the organization since investigation had shown that the stages of this process could be grouped into two distinct 'cycles', each requiring different sets of skills on the part of the person performing them.

There was a 'patient cycle', concerned with provision of information, appointments, reception and conveyance of test results; and an 'examination cycle' involving either analysis of samples provided by the patient, or examination of the patient. The staff concerned with the 'patient cycle' did not necessarily have to be medical or paramedical professionals, but had to be competent in the management of client contact so that the client felt that he mattered, was important. It is during the 'patient cycle' that patients' expectations are very high: they hope to be treated with attentive courtesy and very much appreciate the presence of someone to listen to what they want and be sympathetic to their doubts and fears.

In the 'examination cycle' the client is more concerned with the technical skills and experience of the person carrying out the test and although, as always, courtesy is never amiss, here it is not essential.

Having thus subdivided the above process into two cycles, the post of 'patient cycle' manager was created, responsible to the sector or sector group manager. Integration of 'patient cycle' personnel with those carrying out tests and so on, was a rather delicate matter; the manager in charge of both these operating sectors having a very complex management task, a task of major strategic importance within the organization. That organization, that subdivision of function, in accordance with company policy, has to be clearly evident in the personnel structure, which in turn must accurately reflect strategy. It is from the personnel structure of the Italian Diagnostic Centre that the dual aspects of market orientation and good working organization based on advanced management techniques derive.

2.4.7 Fourth Factor: Training

Having clearly established the personnel structure, and hence the allocation of duties at various levels, the next necessary step was to ascertain to what extent managerial expertise could be purchased on the job market and what would have to be provided in-house via training programmes.

It quickly became apparent that trained health service managers were not to be had on the job market. This is a serious problem in Italy; there are no degree courses in health services management, only brief seminar courses which are not substantial enough to provide serious training. It has been only a few years, however, since the Italian NHS identified a need for people with real managerial skills to run its hospitals and Local Health Units. This discovery has not yet given rise to legislative changes which would allow hospital restructuring and give the necessary administrative powers to able managers; nor yet have any health management schools been inaugurated to train such managers.

Since it could not obtain its managers by recruitment, the Centre's policy from the outset had to be one of training its most able staff for managerial responsibility, knowing full well that it would also be training managers for their competitors.

With regard to the 'patient cycle', the requirement was for personnel who were very good with people; a health service background was not necessary. Staff were in fact selected from among candidates with excellent basic experience without family commitments. Courses were prepared for them, given by doctors, introducing medical terminology; there were also seminars which emphasized the importance of quality of service - particularly as to how this was perceived by the patient. Consciousness of patient/client needs and measurement of the extent to which they are satisfied (by means of patient questionnaires) is the method, even now, of identifying weak points within the organization: modifications and improvements result. Changes are also made following suggestions submitted by staff at fortnightly meetings aimed at service improvement. Additionally, all staff undergo personal development courses to improve interpersonal and client relationships.

The results allow the affirmation that, beyond all doubt, there is a strong positive sense of identification with the company and its aims among all employees, and this is the best guarantee that the success enjoyed today by the Centre will continue in the future.

2.4.8 Fifth Factor: Informing the User

The old Italian formula for success, *'Fare, Far bene, Far sapere'* rendered in English, with some loss of epigrammatic quality as, 'Do, Do well, Tell people what you're doing!' is valid for much of human enterprise. Its application to the Italian health sector becomes highly problematic, however, with respect to *'Far sapere'*. The debates over the regulation of health information and health advertising are ongoing and the legislation governing these areas is unsatisfactory - nor, even, is it uniform in all regions of the country.

The subject is an extremely complex and delicate one, since on the one hand advertising is an efficient means of disseminating information and on the other it conditions individual choice. Some would claim that the consumer must be informed before real choice is possible, even though publicity information may prompt him to make harmful choices. Others hold that the average citizen is poorly equipped to choose the best medicine for himself, and should take his doctor's advice. Health advertising, therefore, should be directed only at the doctor. The latter point of view is that of the Federation of Italian Medical Associations (La Federazione degli Ordini dei Medici); they have great difficulty, however, in checking and controlling the various forms of advertising, which anyway, should always be subject to approval by local medical associations.

The complexity of the work of control and the differing ways in which control is exercised have created serious inconsistencies between different areas of health publicity. Certainly the medical authorities pay a great deal of attention to the various forms of advertising that the large health organizations attempt to put out.

The situation is different for the medical specialist, who operates from his clinic, often part-time, and relies on his own medical expertise rather than heavy capital investment. It is he who, worried about loosing his patients, puts pressure on the Italian Medical Associations to restrict the publicity output of the large private establishments.

The corporate concerns are resisting this attitude as part of their policy of promoting new out-patient centres and developing the health sector in general. The accepted central importance of the doctor is often used in this debate to slow the progress which must come eventually. A similar situation was played out in England a number of years ago. In Italy too, a solution, a new equilibrium, will certainly be found: it will favour neither the doctor nor the large private centres, but the citizen.

2.4.9 Conclusion

The planning, realization and running of a large private out-patient health centre has demonstrated that the ability to clearly define strategic objectives and identify competitive pressures are what contribute to success even when operating in the health sector.

Experience gained on the Health Planning Committee under the Italian Ministry of Health and as Vice Director of the 'Ospedale Maggiore', Milan, leads one to affirm that the possibilities of collaboration between the private and public sectors in the health field are enormous. The private sector is in a position to experiment with new planning and management methods which, once proven, should be applied in the public sector as well.

If it is true that the Italian health system is there, not to make profits for business, but to provide a good service to the public, although the value of that service, unlike business profit, is not amenable to simple quantitative measure, it is also true that those profits will soon disappear when business fails to satisfy, or retain the confidence of, its clients. The mechanisms used to identify and establish organizational and management strategies in business, which are the *sine qua non* of profit, are also able to deliver a high level of client satisfaction; that level of satisfaction must also be the objective of the public sector.

3 Medical Ethics

Contents

3 Medical Ethics

3.0 Introduction
M.A. Verkerk

For the problematics of European integration, health care and ethics are one single question of the utmost importance, 'Are European ethical guidelines possible and necessary with reference to ethical questions in health care?'

For the necessity of European ethical guidelines one can point to the fact that many ethical questions on health care cannot be handled adequately without referring to the European context. Next, one has to consider that some ethical questions present themselves more urgently, if European integration becomes a more serious matter. When opening the congress, from which the present studies result, the secretary of state responsible for health care problems, mentions in this context, questions around patients' rights, organ transplants, AIDS, ...

Though the points just mentioned argue in favour of the relevance, of the question of European ethical guidelines, the question of their possibility should also be raised: 'Are European ethical guidelines at all possible?'

A positive answer to this question is not apparent immediately. In the first place one is confronted with the absence of a moral consensus in Europe; most scholars have noticed this lack of existence. Professor Riis, discussing 'informed consent' states that:

...differences in relation to informed consent exist within the European nations.

The main cause is the existence of different views on the common citizen's right to information and the right to influence professional decision-making. Attitudes that are deeply rooted and not restricted to medicine or research.

In the same vein Moerkerk pointed out differences with respect to the AIDS-problematics.

Secondly, there are differences as to which ethical questions have to be put on the agenda. Professor Doxiadis mentioned that some questions, thought to be relevant in some parts of Europe, are not seen as problems in south-european countries.

Taking into account the above considerations, doubts can be expressed as to the feasibility of European ethical guidelines. That does not mean however, that ethics and European integration have no mutual connections.

In the first place one has to distinguish between 'ethics' and 'morals'; as Berkesteyn put it:

Ethics as a systematic and scientific reflection on our morality. From this point of view, ethics and morality are not identical to each other but complimentary. Many still employ the word ethics when they mean morality and especially their personal morality.

If one cannot speak of any moral consensus, is there maybe a role for ethics? That role does not exist for Buise, 'ethical aspects play no important part in policy questions'. Berkesteyn however, was much more ambitious in his plea for the creation of a European Ethical Council which should advise European politics. Professor Doxiadis gives high priority to 'Teaching of Medical Ethics' in the whole of Europe.

Though European ethical guidelines are thought of as not immediately possible, there is a necessity for an open moral debate. Such a debate should be guided by the results of ethical analysis and reflection. Ethical reflection should extend to the meaning of 'illness' and 'health', and of 'solidarity and equal access to health care'. The latter concepts are not purely economic, but also have moral implications.

As an answer to the question of the possibility of European ethical guidelines, the thesis of Mrs Borst-Eilers is, in our opinion, correct when she states:

The value of medical ethics however lies more in the debate than in the establishment of guidelines. Discussing ethical issues in medicine on a European scale should therefore be encouraged, even if it will not lead to common European guidelines after 1992.

3.1 Harmonization of Medical Ethics; a Civil Servants View
R.V. Buise

3.1.1 Introduction

One of the tasks of the International Health Affairs Division is to represent the Netherlands in the various European organizations where health matters are on the agenda at the governmental level, that is mainly the Council of Europe and the EC.

The viewpoint of my contribution will be that of a person involved in the bureaucratic components of the process of policy-making on a European scale. My background in this respect is partly the medical and partly the legal profession, so it is obvious I cannot claim any specific ethical qualification or competence.

I feel comforted by the fact that I share this lack of knowledge with the vast majority of participants to any given debate on ethical matters and I would like to point out that in the course of my work I don't see too much reason to regret this deficiency overmuch.

The environment in which I have the opportunity to contribute to the gradual process of European integration, is a somewhat formal one. In the context of the EC and within the Council of Europe as well, contacts between the national representatives are of a fairly abstract nature, as communication is supposed to pass between nations and their administrators, rather than between individual experts on the various topics. This implies that all opinions and proposals brought forward by those around the table, have emerged from some national 'policy well' and have subsequently passed the various bureaucratic riddles and filters. The routes and procedures that have to be followed guarantee the firm embedding of any view presented in Brussels or Strasbourg in the political and civil reality of national policies in general, and health protection and promotion policies in particular. This evidently tends to reduce the freedom for each delegate to act or react, very much depending on the civil and political culture in his or her 'Base Camp'. Ethical matters, like any other business, will pass through those same filters.

In addition to this, each and every item on the agenda will have to be dealt with and will eventually lead to some form of conclusion, whether it is equally convenient to the political agenda of all Member States or not. The formal structure also implicates that it is hardly possible for a national delegation to do such 'emotional' things as withdraw from a meeting for reasons of, for example, the presence of a member or delegation that is known to hold certain views that are considered ethically unacceptable.

As a contrasting example I compare this situation to that of Dutch Professors Leenen and Hubben who recently decided to cancel their attendance at an international symposium on biotechnology, ethics and mental handicap, when they found out that one of the other invited experts had been banned for holding certain views. They balanced arguments as independent scientists and were in a position to prioritize accordingly.

3.1.2   Theme 1

The brief outline I have just sketched of international civil service, brings me to my first remark on the ethical aspects of European policy-making:

It is pointless to try and reach *'communis opinio'* (or should I say Community's opinio) on European scale concerning the current ethical issues in medicine and health care, as the various national attitudes on these themes are deeply rooted in their respective national cultural backgrounds and consequently are mutually exclusive. In other words: there is no willingness to conduct trade in these issues, as they are considered elements of national cultural identity.

One knows that national authorities represented in Brussels and Strasbourg, are almost completely autonomous in deciding which position they wish to take on each key factual issue, let alone on sensitive ethical issues. Their culturally-, religiously- or politically-based reservations on any proposal will be treated respectfully by all other members and so will all delicate specific national sensitivities that lay behind them.

From there it must follow that there is no positive contribution to European integration to be expected from explicit debate on ethical issues between governmental representatives of the Member States, in the course of their regular work. It may even be counterproductive to the process moving forward, to allow the same arbitrary mix of influences and arguments to steer the process at Community level, as seems to be the case in the national health field.

Let me quote an example of the latter.

A major Dutch business newspaper features the following editorial on 10 October 1989: 'Ban advocated on performing lung-transplants'. It quotes the Dutch Secretary of State for Health, Dees, as stating in a parliamentary debate on the boundaries of health care, 'he wanted a dialogue in Parliament on the subject, before the performance of such operations could be started'.

It also quotes the head of the medical advice board of the Sick Fund Council (the national body of medical social insurance), Dr S. Van der Kooij, who sums up his objections at the start of lung transplants in the Netherlands:

a) The council preferred to await developments abroad.
b) Because of the limited character of financial means available for health care, the council opposes experimental treatments as the growth-rate of the care delivered has to be kept down.
c) He questions whether this particular group of patients would benefit from the proposed prolongation of their lives, leaving aside the quality this extended life could have.

Here we see a most interesting example of the very confusing phenomenon of mixing ethically completely incomparable elements for the sake of argument. He expects the discrepancy between supply and demand to become gigantic. This induces the tendency to avoid starting this new type of treatment at all.

On 18 September 1989 the first lung transplant in the Netherlands was nevertheless performed successfully. For the financing of the treatment, the patient's family had called upon Municipal Welfare for the operation itself and upon the Medical Social Insurance Fund for the aftercare. Both institutions considered this to be within their line of duty, given the 'life-or-death' circumstances: the ultimate ethical implication of welfare, so to speak.

I present this story as an example of multi-incidental policy-making (or perhaps I should say multi-policy incident-making) on the national level, the way I would very much prefer not to see it happen on the European level.

3.1.3 Theme 2

The only effective way of bringing about a viable degree of harmonization between the various care systems (not applicable to the systems of cure), is dealing actually in Brussels or Strasbourg with each of the growing number of European-size health issues, in a business-like fashion, banning from the representatives debate the many aspects that must be supposed to have been carefully considered beforehand - the homework - such as the ethical aspects.

So, contrary to what Professor Riis says on the subject in this symposium, I believe that international cooperation within medical ethics, if at all possible, will not help to overcome actual differences between Member States' policies on a number of matters essential to high quality health care, like, for example, the issue of informed consent.

In order to achieve progress in this area, reaching agreement between experts on demarcated elements of the inter-European differences in clinical and experimental habits and procedures, including their ethical aspects, will have to be attempted. This on an element-to-element basis, with ethical issues serving only as an 'aide-memoire' and as background information for the benefit of those involved in the exchange of national health policy views.

As I see it, harmonization of medical ethics within the EC, is just as small a goal to be pursued, as is harmonization of the various actual cure facilities on that scale. This does not, however, interfere with continuation of the process of harmonizing within Europe certain ethically relevant features of various forms of practice in health care. Just like for example, harmonizing the criteria for assessing the quality of medical and paramedical diplomas is a useful contribution to the protection of consumers of health care within the EC, a similar story can be told for dealing with the procurement of organs and body substances, as Professor Roscam Abbing has pointed out.

Here again it will not be the harmonization of the ethics behind the issues that will make the European flag fly over these matters; it is a down-to-earth process of negotiating mutually acceptable agreements on practical matters among medical experts in EC Member States.

Although not unlimited, there is a respectable number of ethically relevant issues to be put on the agendas of the European Ministers of Health. Just recently, a renowned Professor of Health Law, in an opinion programme on Dutch television, called for Government action on the subject of the potential use of genetic information, made available by taking cells, with consent, for a specific purpose, for a different, not consented purpose, by, for example, insurance companies. The opening of the European borders to large, multi-national insurance companies, makes this an issue of European dimensions, with an important ethical impact, particularly in the field of life insurance. Here again, ethical debate as such will not help out.

In pragmatic terms however, exchange of policy views on the subject of classifying patients on the basis of genetic data, might simultaneously shed some light on the problems around the steadily increasing need to select patients for the available number of health facilities and services; that is, and will remain, a limited number. That is where the ethical implications of any chosen policy, become particularly poignant. I continue not to expect viable solutions from attempts to reach ethical consensus on these matters, but rather from creative efforts to take pragmatic and, if need be, legally binding measures.

On the subject of clinical trials with voluntary participants, a major step towards better protection of the volunteer was seemingly taken when GCP-procedures were introduced, in the USA at first, in response to FDA (Food and Drugs Administration)-formulated standards.

According to publicist Laurence Gerlis in The Lancet of 6 May 1989, American scientists have, on these grounds, come to feel quite superior to their European colleagues, who they expect to experience a 'culture shock' when confronted with the need to present a clinical trial participant with a four-page consent form that sets out all possible side-effects of a drug and even details of how to obtain compensation should anything go wrong.

Apart from whether or not freedom of information and the rights of the individual do indeed lag behind in Europe, I seriously doubt that simply putting things on paper will bring an airtight solution to the ethical requirement of optimal consumer protection, as is indicated in the next example:

> The same Dutch business newspaper features an editorial on October 13th under the heading 'Research for US on the effects on marijuana'. It tells of a Dutch institute for Medicine, Safety and Behaviour that is going to perform an experiment on the ability to drive a car under the influence for marijuana. The experiment, at the request of the US Department of Transportation, will have Dutch volunteers driving up and down a closed section of highway in the south of The Netherlands (that is thus indeed temporarily transformed into a 'Highway'). The article quotes an American official as saying that they had come to the Netherlands because an experiment like that would be practically impossible to insure in the United States. There are too many lawyers in the business of suing researchers, while proposing to split the proceeds. Moving the entire project across the Atlantic seemingly was the best 'solution', thereby willingly circumventing certain factors effectively protecting volunteers.

What I read in this message is the warning that standard solutions do not exist and that attaining a high level of legal patient protection in any given test situation, however ethically desirable this may be, is not achieved properly by simply formalizing this demand. Several other factors have to be taken into account as well, again leading to a rather complex process of weighing and balancing all aspects of the matter, with ethics as only one of the elements, albeit an important one.

Let me finally give you two quite different examples from my own recent experience in the European field, of how ethical considerations can in practice be moved to a less prominent place than they appear to deserve, simply as a consequence of the pragmatic requirements of decision-making.

> Some weeks ago I was invited to attend a working session for the *Eurobarometer*, an EC project that seeks to gather information periodically from European citizens in the form of an opinion poll. Instead of being able to formulate the questions that we considered most relevant and informative at the time to the consumer- and health-protection issues we were dealing with, we were warned, as delegates, about a host of practical limitations on the project, mainly of the nature of timing and financing.

This made me wonder whether the questions we finally agreed to put to the sample of Euro-citizens, could, after ample dilution, still be considered proper and acceptable to the Community standards and whether I had reason to look upon myself as working to substandard ethics, by accepting these pragmatic constrictions on the overriding principle of consumer protection.

And now to conclude, here is another question to be put at involvement in ethics, as well as at the ethics of involvement:

The October issue of the journal of the Dutch Motorist Associations features an interview with a trained male nurse, who is a crew member of an ambulance. He tells the readers of this 2.5 million copy journal what, quite frankly, most people in the medical and nursing professions have known for years: that each and every day nurses perform several manoeuvres that are in fact strictly limited in law to physicians only, such as intubations.

Knowing this, and knowing that more and more people in the general public have come to know this too, gives me an uneasy feeling about the ethical content of the agreement that was recently reached in my presence at a Council of Europe's Health Committee meeting on Emergency Medical Assistance Services and that re-emphasized the strict separation of the various levels of training required for health personnel involved, and of the manipulations allowed to them on that basis.

Here again the performance of ethics is easily confused with the ethics of the performers, nobody seriously having doubts about their good intentions.

This takes me back to what I hinted at earlier: don't expect any life-size contributions to the process of European integration in the complex and heterogenic field of health, from civil servants like myself becoming involved in explicit debate on the ethical aspects of the matters we deal with.

We have trouble enough doing the job as it is.

3.2 Toward European Guidelines on Ethical Issues in Medicine
Th.M.G. van Berkestijn

3.2.1 The Existing Code: Does it Work?

In January 1987, during the International Conference of the Medical Order and organizations placed on the same footing, a medical ethical code was decided on. This conference, founded by the French Medical Order, meets two to three times a year in order to discuss all kinds of subjects about the mutual co-operation and links in carrying out the medical profession in Europe. It is especially owing to the efforts of the Belgian physician, Dr Farber, that the European medical ethical code came into existence. In itself it is a laudable and important initiative; but what is the meaning of this code? Many years' negotiations and endless discussions preceded it. The authors co-operated in writing it without really having been granted the authority by their colleagues. Many important issues, such as euthanasia for example, were evaded through clever formulations, and the document lives and breathes the atmosphere of compromise in a number of other fields as well. In particular those issues are mentioned on which everybody can agree, and, of course, that is important.

However, the main issues of our time with their large number of ethical aspects have been left undiscussed: abortion, euthanasia, AIDS.

In another European context, the Standing Committee of Doctors in the European Community, discrepancies in these issues were expressed quite clearly and they have led to a deadlock. Even the World Medical Association, the world forum of old in which all doctors worldwide found one another after the Second World War (during which period some doctors were guided by Nazism), was incapable of living up to the ambitions on which it was based at the time: medical ethics based on the Hippocratic code and the generally accepted standards and principles of the western world.

In recent years politicians have also made themselves heard. Partly as a result of the jurisprudence realized in this field, laws have come into being in several countries trying to regulate medical actions from an ethical and medical legal point of view. In a motion, the European Parliament declared itself in favour of a more active participation of politics and authorities in these matters, and a restriction on the influence of medical associations. It is not only as regards content that there are differences of opinion, but apparently with respect to the question of who has the final word as well. Nevertheless, it is becoming more important than ever to reach a consensus of opinion in the field of medical ethics.

Borders are fading away, our society has become more multiform than ever before, culturally as well as socially speaking, due to the growing travel and migration possibilities and the problems are only increasing. In order to examine how uniformity in the field of medical ethics is to be reached, it is important to know how developments have been up to now.

3.2.2 From Unity to Division: How did it Happen?

Up to the Second World War there were hardly any problems at all. The development and application of medical science and learning were a concern of the western world. Abiding by the Hippocratic rules of conduct, physicians were able to manage quite well. 'The patient's welfare, the main rule'. All else followed from this. Fighting against death and fighting against suffering were practically identical. That had to be done at all costs. Fundamental changes were developed after the Second World War enforcing a new approach. I would like to divide these changes into four major groups:

In the first place, the possibilities of intervening by medical means in the lives and sufferings of people have increased enormously. So much so, that fighting for life and against suffering are no longer considered to be synonymous. The possibilities which have been created to intervene at the start of life affect existence itself in the depth of its being.

In the second place, the possibilities are well nigh limitless technically speaking; economically and financially, on the other hand, they are not unlimited. This is encroaching one of the basic principle of Hippocratic thinking: that everything has to give way to the interest of the patient. The moral: 'the patient's welfare, the main rule' no longer holds true.

In the third place, our whole society has not become multiform simply in a cultural and social sense, but also in moral and religious aspects. Up to now, sophisticated medical science was monopolized by the mono-cultural western world. This has changed in two ways. Western medical science has expanded all over the world. In addition, cultures from elsewhere have pervaded ours.

In the fourth place, others besides doctors, politicians and authorities in accordance with policy-makers, ethicists and lawyers, have started involving themselves with what is called medical ethics, and rightly so.

I would like to look more closely at these four factors in order to consider subsequently whether it is to be discovered from this analysis how one should proceed for the future and give the unification of Europe a good chance in the field of medical ethics as well.

As I have said, the medical technological possibilities have increased so greatly that fighting for the extension of life is not always identical any more with fighting against suffering. On the contrary: sometimes extension or even just starting a treatment causes so much distress that in doing so, medical science is overshooting one of its main purposes. The developments in neonatology, for example, have resulted in keeping alive small individuals who did not stand a chance until recently. With the aid of a lot of medical technology we can now keep them alive, but at the cost of the quality of their lives which hardly meets the basic requirements called for. For some people the extension of their suffering is experienced as being so severe that they ask for a merciful release. Because of this, heated discussions have arisen about what to do once this point has been reached. An example hereof is the discussion about euthanasia. In these discussions attention has not shifted enough yet to avoid such situations. 'Look before you leap' as a modern variant on *in dubio abstine* is hard to learn for physicians who are used to proceeding actively. Most technological developments, luckily, did involve undisputed advantages for medicine, and yet, many of these improvements cost so much money that limitations will have to be imposed. Consequently choices will have to be made. By whom and for whom? The *Salus aegroti suprema lex* still holds true for physicians: they will not sell 'no' to a patient. But who will? It is the politicians who will have to set the financial limits, but what are their responsibilities towards that one patient who sees all hope lost?

3.2.3   From Division back to Unity: how can that be reached?

The answers to these questions are not easily given. These are new problems which apparently cannot be solved with the Hippocratic ethics and moral principles generally accepted in our western culture. As I have said, our society is rapidly becoming a multiform one. Who would have thought twenty years ago that mosques would be springing up in almost all Western European cities! Besides, the interpretation of values and principles, even within our Christian culture, is strongly dependent on the times we live in. That which was once reprehensible in view of those principles, is now permitted and vice versa with those same basic principles as a background. Personal rights have changed. Not everybody has a right to everything any more now that economic lines have been drawn.

Other basic rights may yet change as well. Will the individual right of procreation, now generally approved of, still be inviolable if, in the future, it may turn out that the environmental problem is in fact a problem of overpopulation and that we are no longer able to cope with the life-threatening issue of pollution?

In order to answer these questions we can no longer simply consult our own personal consciences. It is true, basic principles such as respect for life remain intact in a multiform society but applying these principles to a new situation is not easy and it may give the insecure something to hold on to, but it does not offer a real solution. That is why systematic reflection and a methodologically sound approach to these problems are needed. It is in this sense that I want to interpret the meaning of ethics: as a systematic and scientific reflection on our morality. From this point of view ethics and morality are not identical to each other but complimentary. However, many still employ the word ethics when they mean morality, and especially their personal morality.

3.2.4 A Systematic Approach: Analysis first, and then Solutions

It will be quite clear that such a scientific and systematic approach will require its own discipline. Doctors, politicians and jurists have not been equipped for this kind of work during their training. Professional ethicists will have to show us the way via systematic analyses to teach us how to tackle an ethical problem. In doing this, other disciplines, such as behavioural sciences and comparative studies of the world's main cultural and moral trends, will also have to proffer a helping hand. As a result some ethicists and other people with important positions in the field of medical ethics in the Netherlands have developed the idea of founding an international European council of professional people in the field of medical ethics to advise the ministers and politicians in Europe about the ethical implications of the progress in medical science. Only then will we be able to start fruitful discussions which will probably lead to even more questions. Whatever the case, let us hope that they will not lead to closed attitudes where contents and positions are concerned.

However, ethicists should not only be called upon for help in analyzing the problems and contributions to reach solutions. If ethicists and those who are concerned with medical-ethical issues in practice are to understand one another, then the latter will also have to be taught the methods of ethics right from the start. For this reason medical ethics ought to be a basic discipline in medical schooling, just as it should be one for the law student. In the future it will be just as important a condition for the functioning of politicians as their understanding of financial-economic questions is now.

If all concerned can be convinced of this, detailed negotiations about a medical ethical code will not be necessary, at least not as a first step. For the present, politicians, universities and the medical world will have to make out a case for a considerable contribution of the ethical discipline as a basic subject in medical training and research. Only then will the problems become clear through good analyses. This will not lead to one code full of compromises reached by way of negotiations on firm standpoints, but to sympathy for different ideas, plain and clear as regards the patient, who, after all, is the one that matters. He will then be offered practical options, as is befitting a multiform society.

3.3 Ethical Issues in Health Promotion
S.A. Doxiadis

The attempt to investigate 'Ethical Issues in Health Promotion', as is the title of my contribution, requires an agreement among scientists and decision-makers in the various European countries on the meaning of health. In spite of the universal acceptance of the World Health Organization (WHO) definition of health which '... is a state of complete physical, mental and social well being and not merely the absence of disease or infirmity', most people still centre their thoughts and acts around the concept of 'negative health'. This means concern for the absence of 'ill health' which is again a vague notion comprising illness, disease, injury, handicap.

The WHO definition uses the word 'well being' first, therefore it gives priority to 'positive health'. However if we ask ourselves what is 'physical, mental and social well being', here again it is most likely that there will not be general agreement, and the lack of agreement becomes increasingly stronger when we move from physical to mental and from mental to social well being.

So, one of the targets of our Congress 'Health Care after 1992' was to start from first principles and try to agree on the meaning of health in its various aspects; negative, positive, well being, and to this we add fitness.

The above is not an academic exercise. It has practical significance because clear definition of the above terms is a prerequisite in order to distinguish between 'health needs' and 'health wants' of a population. Again this distinction is important as even now, but increasingly so after 1992, citizens of all countries will be asking their governments to cover all they desire in the field of health. Governments and other social agencies on the other hand, working under the inevitable budgetary restrictions, would like from the scientific community a more clear definition of the real health needs of the population.

This is no easy task. If we aim at some sort of European chart for health care, we have to define in a realistic way what are the needs and not the demands of our citizens. To cover the **needs** in an adequate way would then be the duty of the state or of any state-controlled agency.

You may now ask what this has got to do with ethics. To illustrate the relationship I mention some of the ethical problems in **preventive medicine** which constitutes a large part of health promotion.

Almost all authors writing on the ethical problems of medicine describe situations of a one-to-one relationship, doctor to patient or healthy subject, or at the most the relationship of a small group, the health team, to an equally small group, the patient and his or her family. However, little attention is paid to ethical problems, equally or more important, in the fields of preventive medicine and health promotion.

There are six reasons why I consider the ethical issues in these two fields equally worthy of attention as those in therapeutic medicine.

First, in therapeutic medicine, one person or a small number of people present the health problem. In preventive medicine much larger numbers are involved. An unethical decision would, therefore, affect many more people.

Second, in therapeutic medicine, the person or persons are ill when they present the problem. However, particularly in primary prevention, the subjects are usually healthy. Unethical decisions will therefore affect people who have been previously entirely or apparently healthy.

Third, the responsibility in therapeutic medicine is usually vested in one doctor or a small number of doctors or other health professionals. In this context, the responsibility of the state for ethical matters as distinct from legal responsibility is very remote. In preventive medicine, on the other hand, the direct responsibility of the state is often considerable, but the community physician or health planner is rarely in individual contact with the subject of his work and may therefore feel less responsible for his decisions. The problem of abortion, of euthanasia, of the mentally defective newborn presented in a clinical situation with an individual patient will appear very different from a consideration of similar problems in a large anonymous population. Furthermore there can be great danger when 'systems' make decisions.

Fourth, in therapeutic medicine, the results of a decision are usually assessed within a few days, weeks or months of consultation. The results of decisions in preventive medicine frequently take a much longer time to evaluate. Again the responsibility is remote, and it may, therefore, tend to be forgotten.

Fifth, in therapeutic medicine, the criteria of success or failure are easily defined - death or life, an additional life or not, interruption of pregnancy or not, transplantation or not. In preventive medicine, the criteria of success or failure are defined much less easily or clearly because there are so many factors involved. Here again, this complexity of aetiological or contributing factors may tend to lessen the feeling of responsibility in those making the decisions.

Last, while decisions in therapeutic medicine are usually independent of the cultural, social and economic background of the subject, many decisions in preventive medicine affect disadvantaged groups with inadequate knowledge of their own rights and of the consequences of possible courses of action. Our responsibility to protect the rights of such groups is great. In an undernourished population, for example, the manifestion causing most concern among parents is blindness of their children caused by vitamin A deficiency. This can be prevented by administration of some vitamin drops, a relatively easy and cheap measure which will satisfy the parents, but this result may blunt their sensitivity to the more difficult and equally serious problem of under nutrition and may also provoke, among the administrators or other groups able to help, a feeling of false satisfaction and therefore lead to inertia.

The ethical dilemmas are even less well known, have been less discussed when we examine other aspects of health promotion such as health education and environmental or economic issues.

This brings me to the last part of my lecture. Since important aspects of medical ethics are little known, even among doctors and much less among politicians or the wider public, what should one of our main targets be for the last decade of the twentieth century? For 'Health Care after 1992'?

I put to you that all of us should give high priority to the teaching of Medical Ethics. Let me finish with a brief mention of what teaching Medical Ethics should achieve and what would be the benefits.

The programme of education in Medical ethics should make students and doctors:

a) aware that medical practice is repeatedly facing 'value judgements' and not only technical problems;
b) able to take decisions based on logical arguments and not on intuition or compassion;
c) recognize that in cases of uncertainty the answer is seldom the only correct one, but also to accept that there are answers which are undoubtedly better than others;
d) accept that the validity of a decision may not be related to the sincerity or honesty of the person taking it: even the most 'moral' of doctors may make wrong decisions;

e) acquire such a breadth in their thoughts as to accepts that all persons engaged in health care may have a very wide spectrum of values, concepts and attitudes;
f) realise that patients and the public should participate in decisions, because doctors alone should not solve moral dilemmas.

With emphasis on the teaching of Medical Ethics we may hope that greater knowledge, more awareness, increased sensitivity of the medical profession (and other health professionals) in this field will spread to other sections of society and will be the best protection, and the best health promotion measure of individuals, communities and whole countries.

3.3.1 References

For further reading on Ethics of Health Promotion, see:

Boyd, K. (Ed.) (1987), Report of a Working Party on the Teaching of Medical Ethics (Chairman Sir Desmond Pond), Institute of Medical Ethics, London.
Doxiadis, S.A. (Ed.) (1987), *Ethical Dilemmas in Health Promotion*, John Wiley and Sons, Chichester.
Doxiadis, S.A. (Ed.) (1990), *Ethics in Health Education*, John Wiley and Sons, Chichester.

3.4 Informed Consent in Research and Non-Research Situations
Povl Riis

Fundamental human rights in a European and North American perspective are related to such famous years as 1776, 1789 and 1948. The declarations from these years express the citizens' right to life, to personal safety, to freedom in general, to never be subjected to torture or cruelty, inhuman or degrading treatment, and to freedom of speech. Equity is a fundamental principle underlying these fundamental rights.

3.4.1 Human Integrity

The term human integrity is often used in ethical contexts, and consequently often when describing patients' overall rights in health systems and as participants in biomedical research.
    The term usually creates an awesome impression among users. It has, however, strong elements of defence and self-protection, and thus merely expresses the last stage in citizens' reactions to coercion. Such a last line of defence is certainly important, but health systems and research communities in open democratic societies ought to respect citizens' fundamental human rights long before the stage of defending human integrity.

3.4.2 Personal Norms

Both patients' and health professionals' personal norms interact strongly with the patient-physician-, the patient-nurse- and the patient-researcher-relationships. In more homogenous societies a substantial core of personal norms constitutes the normative part of the national culture. However, with increasing personal freedom in European and North American societies (an important progress in itself) the amount of normative pluralism has increased considerably. This means that even fundamental human rights on a citizen level can be modified, especially if they are not repeatedly evaluated in the light of basic human rights.

Even in several of the ethical dilemmas created within the frame of a patient-doctor-relationship or a patient-researcher-relationship the ethical problems will be influenced strongly by the patients', the citizens', the doctors' or the researchers' personal norms. Consider for instance the difference in patients' attitudes to participating in biomedical research, whether they wish to help other patients by their participation, that is behaving altruistically, or they consider such participation only to be evaluated from an angle of personal benefit or not. Another example is an elderly patient's reaction to the possible respirator treatment of his or her chronic bronchitis, varying with the patients' personal norm being based either on self-interest or altruism.

3.4.3 Equity and Freedom

When fundamental human rights in health and biomedical research communities are made operational, that is applicable in daily professional situations, the key words are *equity* and *freedom*. These key terms further lead to the ultimate operational term of a patient's meeting the health professional or the researcher: **the right to autonomy**.

3.4.4 The Complementarity of Right and Duties

The societal developments during the latest decennia have strongly emphasized citizens' rights and authorities' and institutions' duties. What is sometimes forgotten is the logical interaction between the two terms. The linkage is obvious, that no-one can possess rights without others having duties and vice-versa.

Probably even more critical in applying these terms is their societal interaction. In an open democratic society no person or group can possess only rights and others only duties. With the exception of very small groups of multi-handicapped with severe mental retardation, all citizens, in their contact with fellow citizens, institutions, agencies, health systems and so on, have both rights and duties.

3.4.5 Citizens as Patients and Research Subjects

The era of paternalism has lasted until recently in Europe. One might even still find small resistance groups considering their professional work as justifying residual elements of paternalism.

In the 1960s and 1970s a strong movement in Europe had forwarded the era of autonomy, now dominating, when citizens meet institutions and professionals. The dominance of autonomy has sometimes been so strong, that both citizens and professionals have considered being *pro*-autonomy and *contra*-paternalism a solution to all ethical problems in the health sector.

We must, however, face the need for accepting a future, more complex era, in which the right to autonomy is accepted as fundamental, but at the same time being able to disclose situations where the patient does **not** wish to apply this right, but instead expresses a need for 'loving paternalism', from the nurse, the doctor and so on. 'Loving paternalism', means that the health professional, after having emphasized the right to autonomy, is willing to take upon her- or himself the burden of being the ultimate decision-maker on behalf of the patient. In this perspective, vigorous pointing to autonomy can sometimes be rather cruel, and the willingness to accept paternalism in selected cases can, on the contrary, sometimes be very benevolent.

Patients in clinical, non-research situations will as a rule have the right to information and consent. According to the above emphasis laid on the complementarity of rights and duties, patients also have duties towards health personnel and fellow patients, in the last case in accepting for instance fellow patients' fair share of scarce health resources.

In addition, patients joining investigations as research subjects have of course a right to information and autonomy, but again they also have duties in a historic and future perspective. Patients of our time benefit in many ways from controlled trials and other systematized clinical experiences from patients of earlier generations. In this way patients of our time have a moral obligation to pay their contribution to contemporary and future patients. Patients of our time further benefit from research in other countries, consequently they have moral duties to contribute to the global sum of reliable clinical information.

3.4.6 Conclusion

Without losing any rights from the era of autonomy, future patients will find themselves in the post-autonomy era, in which they must combine their rights to autonomy, security, equity and so on with duties contributing to the global sum of clinical knowledge and experience. They will still have the right to autonomy, and to say no to such an obligation. They should, however, also consider the serious consequences, if all citizens and patients chose to apply their right to autonomy in such a restricted and selfish way.

3.5 Implication of a European AIDS Policy
H. Moerkerk

While opinions differ on many of the scientific, medical and social issues associated with HIV infection and AIDS, on one thing experts and politicians seem to agree: prevention was, is and for the next few years will be, the most important means by which we can respond to the challenge of a viral infection with often devastating consequences.

In this short article I will try to make clear that although the statement that prevention is our only weapon in the fight against AIDS, the chance for a joint European approach for this objective is limited because politically linked and ethical questions are creating numerous barriers between European countries. When we speak of Europe, we should not have in mind a single united continent, since within it there are considerable differences in political structure, cultural background and social development. In some countries such as the republic of Ireland, sex between men is still illegal, while in others such as the Netherlands the advent of AIDS has in some respects provided further impetus for gay-emancipation. It is crucial not to view Europe as a single entity but as the sum of many different cultures and political structures which have responded inconsistently and unevenly to the advent of AIDS. All this needs to be borne in mind when considering the ways in which different countries have responded. Western and northern European countries are characterized by the fact that the majority of reported cases of HIV infection and AIDS consist of men who have sex with men. On average, this comprises about seventy per cent of reported cases in this part of Europe, although this proportion is decreasing with the growth of infection amongst injecting drug users. Heterosexuals acquired infections that are not linked to injecting drug use are still relatively rare in these parts of Europe.

In southern Europe on the other hand, there are higher proportions of injecting drug users amongst people with HIV infection and AIDS. This is particularly the case in Italy and Spain. However, it is important to recognize that less efficient reporting in southern European countries may mean that the numbers of gay and bisexual men who are affected are under-reported at present. In southern European countries too, there has been a more rapid increase in reported cases of HIV infection amongst children and amongst heterosexuals.

In eastern Europe, HIV and AIDS have only recently been identified as potential problems, and governments are now beginning to move beyond an initial response which suggested that AIDS was a sickness confined to African students or Capitalist gays. Nevertheless, the impression continues to be given that HIV is a virus which can and should be stopped at the border. A good example is Bulgaria which intends to introduce mandatory screening of the entire population between 16 and 65 and requirs antibody-negative certificates for foreigners who stay longer than one month. Even inside the kingdom of the Netherlands, on the island of Aruba, prostitutes applying for a working permit need to be tested compulsorily and sero-positive individuals are refused entrance to the island, to keep Aruba AIDS-free. At this moment Europe can count approximately 30 000 diagnosed cases of AIDS registered on a cumulative basis since 1982. The number of HIV-infected people is unknown, but can be estimated between 300 000 and 500 000. Aids will lay a heavy burden on the European health system in the next decades!

Examining the different ways European countries have tried to organize their AIDS activities, first of all it is necessary to recognize the fact that many NGOs (National Government Organizations) have played a key role and have sometimes been the initiators of activities on a national scale. However, considering the political implications of AIDS, for the moment I want to limit myself by looking at 'official' policies developed by government bodies charged with AIDS control.

I should like to make a distinction between four groups of countries which show different types of official responses:

Type 1 - pragmatic responses
Type 2 - 'political' responses
Type 3 - biomedical responses

Type 4 - emergent responses

The first type of countries have put the emphasis of their activities on planning, evaluation, pragmatisms and consensus and do not rely on prohibition and other coercive forms of control. Norway, Denmark, Switzerland and the Netherlands seem to be good examples. The second group of countries have developed an AIDS policy in accordance with what is politically possible or politically desirable. The UK, the Federal Republic of Germany (FRG) and Sweden are good examples. Because such a politically-influenced policy can have enormous repercussions on ethical and legal questions, I shall discuss the Swedish example in more detail. The government there has developed a comprehensive and committed AIDS policy as part of a pre-existing system of social and public health. For many years, and in accordance with reformist and neo-pluralist principles, efforts have been made to socially engineer 'desirable' solutions to a wide range of health problems. As a consequence, substantial resources have been made available for public education and health care. This kind of state involvement in health issues generally has had important consequences with respect to ethical issues.

Overall, Swedish policy takes the view that the state should regulate and set clear boundaries on human behaviour, and legislation is seen as an important instrument in the attainment of this politically-formulated objective. It is not surprising, therefore, that HIV antibody testing has become one of the most important components of prevention programmes, with current legislation requiring anyone suspecting that they might have been infected by HIV to undergo examination by a doctor. The so-called 'treating doctor' has the responsibility of prescribing how the patient should behave. Together with a well-developed system of contact tracing, these measures constitute an important part of Swedish AIDS prevention policy. By overstressing the 'general interest' and making individual rights and responsibilities of a second order, I think that the Swedes introduced an example of ignoring ethical elements in public health policy.

I still owe a short explanation of the other two groups of countries which I mentioned.

The third type I called 'the biomedical' response, where AIDS is regarded primarily as a problem which is amenable to biomedical solutions. In these countries, like Belgium, France, Spain and Italy, governments have displayed only short-term interest in the issues; they have established medical institutions charged with determining official policies and interventions. Finally there are those countries in which HIV disease has only recent been identified as a serious concern; most east European countries, dealing at the same time with 'glasnost', fall within this category and have in the interim resorted to the use of existing legislation as a means of AIDS control.

It cannot be denied that health legislation plays an important role in AIDS control in a good and also in a bad way. The Australian Judge Kirby, member of the Global Commission on AIDS, once described law as 'marching with medicine, but in the rear and limping a little'; as countries develop and refine their legal responses to AIDS, there is a growing realization of the limits to what can be achieved by the law in epidemic control. At the same time societies are confronted with ethical questions as to what extent prevention activities have been complicated by the passing into law of section 28 of the 1988 Local Government Act which prohibits local authorities from (what is called) 'promoting homosexuality'.

AIDS has raised a number of complex legal and ethical issues which cut across the fields of public health law, criminal law, human rights and standard ethical procedures in medicine. If national and local legislatures have been slow to legislate along the same lines it may be partly because in most countries there is no tradition of public health law being subjected to close scrutiny from a human rights perspective. For instance the importance of confidentiality means that anti-discrimination legislation must be accompanied by legal guarantees of strict confidentiality of information relating to a person's HIV sero-status. It must be obvious to all that the conditions for such a development are very different in Europe and that the question arises whether a European AIDS policy can help us.

It will be useful to see to what extent international organizations constitute an active and perhaps effective instrument. We will begin by briefly saying something about the context within which this kind of co-operation would take place. It should be clear from what has been said so far that AIDS control strategies vary considerably between countries. This raises important questions about the extent to which a common approach is possible, or even desirable. In this kind of situation, it may be better to aim for what can be described as condition-creating activities concerned with AIDS prevention than to seek to develop uniform (and possibly monolithic) programmes. These might include the setting up of information services that cross national boundaries as well as the establishment of a common set of ethical and legal principles relating to the rights of people with HIV infection and AIDS. It also would seem important that international co-operation is facilitative rather than restrictive in its effects. This is made all the more complicated by the diversity of organizations that already exist. The European Community, the Council of European regions of the World Health Organization all have their own aims and objectives. Efforts will need to be made to clarify the roles and responsibilities of each of these bodies if a clear and unambiguous set of priorities is to be established.

3.5.1 The European Community

The European Community occupies an important position when it comes to decision-making in respect of political and social issues. This is true insofar as non-member countries are concerned also that the actions of the European Community are central in climate building throughout the continent. Already declarations about HIV/AIDS have been made by European Government leaders (1987) and the Council of Ministers of Health (1987, 1988). The important factor now is to turn these statements of principle into deeds. This is where problems are likely to arise, particularly in a body in which the main lines of policy are largely shaped by political considerations. This is certainly true of public health which is not mentioned explicitly in the Treaty of Rome, and in which strong nationally-oriented traditions exist. On the other hand, there have been sustained efforts to develop a European Community stance on health protection and environmental issues. The major question now is in what respect and to what extent is AIDS policy a matter which falls within the competence of the European Commission? Besides, the commission itself violated all partial declaration, by testing all new applicants for jobs at the beginning of 1988.

3.5.2   The Council of Europe

Twenty-three northern, western and southern European countries are currently active in this organization, particularly with respect to cultural, educational and ethical matters.   In 1986, this organization also designated AIDS as one of the areas in which it would become active, and in November 1987 detailed plans for prevention programmes were announced along with a series of statements concerning the legal position of people with HIV infection and AIDS.   In 1988, further recommendations were made concerning AIDS and prisoners, and AIDS and work, and in the autumn of 1989 statements on the social and ethical implications were published.   The emphasis so far, though, has been whether these will be followed by legislation requiring the development of consistent approaches.

3.5.3   The World Health Organization

The World Health Organization's role in the development of AIDS control activities across Europe has so far been relatively low key, being confined to the facilitation of expert meetings and consultations, and the support of limited programmes of research and development.   In many ways it would seem quite inappropriate for a European equivalent of WHO's Global Programme on AIDS to be developed, since this would run the risk of duplicating existing patterns of provision.   Nevertheless, there is important work to be done in facilitating better communication between eastern and western European countries, and European nations themselves have an obligation to continue to support WHO's activities with respect to AIDS prevention in the third world.   The European Region of WHO also took the initiative to publish an important number of recommendations on legal and ethical issues on HIV infection as a result of a conference held in Oslo in 1988.

In the months and years ahead, a more consistent and coordinated approach to AIDS prevention in Europe will need to be developed, whilst recognizing that different groups may have different needs.   If prevention activities are to have long-term success, they will need to offer people positive and acceptable options. Desirable changes in behaviour can not be brought about by coercive and legalistic interventions; rather, they must be taught, encouraged and supported.   Insights will come from a wide range of social research into sexual motivations and behaviour. Only by doing this will it be possible to deal effectively with the complex biomedical and social challenges that HIV and AIDS present.   It is clear that ethical implications have to play an important role in this challenge.

4 Quality of Health Care and Position of the Patient

Contents

4 Quality of Health Care and Position of the Patient

4.0 Introduction
A.F. Casparie

In recent years in many countries much emphasis is placed on quality assurance in health care. Furthermore, in 1985 the European Member States of WHO formulated as target 31: 'by 1990 all Member States should have built effective mechanisms for ensuring quality of patient care within their health care systems'. However, quality of health care and quality assurance are not items on the agenda in Brussels in preparation for the European Community. This is all the more remarkable because after 1992 more competition between the health care systems in the European Member States can be expected, and besides costs, quality of care could be the issue on which competition will be carried out. Quality assessment could be the mechanism to assure that after the unification, health care provided in the various Member States will remain at a high standard. Even more striking is the fact that in the area of changing health care provision, still no attention is being paid to the position of the individual patient and of patient organizations.

Therefore in the Congress on Health Care in Europe after 1992, a separate session was devoted to the quality of care and the position of the patient. Four papers, based on oral presentations during the congress, were included. In the first paper, the concept of quality and the potential role of the patient in quality assurance is described. Based on an enquiry in eight countries it can be concluded that consumers' and patients' influences on health care, at macro-, meso- as well as micro-level, differ from country to country but seem to be rather limited. However, there is a trend toward more patient rights in the respective countries and this could lead, after 1992, to even more juridicalization and commercialization of health care if we look to the developments in the USA. The next paper looks at the possibilities and the problems of collaboration between patient organizations in the EC countries in order to obtain more influence on health care systems after 1992. The third paper deals with the problem of measuring consumer opinion and patient satisfaction with regard to quality of care. In the last paper the legislation regarding quality assurance in the various countries, or rather the absence of legislation, except for medical-technical equipment and application of X-rays is mentioned. A plan is drawn up for a framework legislation.

In conclusion: After the discussions at the Congress it was not clear whether quality would play a central role in the realization of a more uniform care system and to what extent patient organization will influence this system after 1992.

4.1 Quality of Care and the Involvement of the Patient
N.S. Klazinga

4.1.1 Introduction

In this article, first presented at the Congress 'Health Care in Europe after 1992', quality of care and involvement of the patient in quality assurance will be discussed. First, the concept of quality will be explained and from there the different functions that patient involvement can fulfil will be described. The situation with regard to patient involvement in quality assurance in the European Community will be discussed via the results of an inventory that has been held among experts from various countries who attended the preliminary meetings of this congress. Apart from an overview of patient involvement in quality assurance the agenda of patient rights in Europe will be discussed. This will be based upon a report of a WHO-Working Group on Patients' rights in Europe, presented in 1986. After discussion of the concepts of quality, involvement of the patient, and the factual situation at this time, trends towards 1992 will be discussed. The dangers that accompany the present developments will be emphasized and the presentation will end with a discussion of the various opportunities that more patient involvement in quality assurance would create for health care after 1992.

4.1.2 The Concept of Quality

In literature various definitions of quality can be found. For this presentation a definition is used that comes from quality assurance in industry. It runs as follows: *'quality is the degree in which the whole of characteristics of a product, process or service meet the requirements that spring from the goal of use'*. This phrase verbalizes the following elements of the concept of quality:

a) Health care is considered as a process with certain goals and objectives. This is a relatively new way of looking at health care and makes it necessary to formulate the objectives of care and consider quality assurance as a form of process management.

b) Within the concept of quality one can discern different aspects. The most well-known are effectiveness (if objectives are reached) and efficiency (how objectives are reached). However, other aspects of quality are also relevant, depending on the branch of health care you focus on. For instance accessibility, availability, safety, accountability and equity.

c)   Quality assurance implies the formulation of requirements, standards and criteria. According to the theory of Donabedian we can recognize three kinds of criteria. The criteria of the **structure**, the **process** and the **outcome** of health care. A structural criteria for instance, is the person, performing an operation, being a registered surgeon. Process criteria within the hospital setting are for instance waiting times, or outside the hospital, the time it takes for an ambulance to arrive for a patient with a cardiac arrest. Outcome criteria in the health care setting are for instance: mortality rates, complication rates and re-admission rates to hospitals.

d)   The concept of quality also implies comparing and adding value judgements. Apart from the formulation of criteria one should register what is actually happening and by comparing the ideal with the actual situation one should place a value judgement on the difference and decide upon necessary risks. Therefore, quality assurance has a lot in common with evaluation, but it goes one step further; it really tries to implement change. Given this concept of quality, what is the function of the patient?

4.1.3   Functions of Patient Involvement in Quality Assurance

According to Hannu Vuori, a quality assurance expert of WHO, patient involvement in quality assurance has different functions:

a)   Patient satisfaction is an outcome of care itself and therefore an objective of health care. This is all the more true when we consider the definition of WHO on health; the total well-being of an individual.

b)   Patient involvement is a prerequisite for compliance and with that an essential part to reach the main objective of health care, medical effectiveness. For instance a patient who doesn't take the antibiotics that are rightly prescribed to him will contribute to less effective health care.

c)   Patient experience can be used as an information source about the process of care. Patient experiences can be used as feedback to the process and add valuable information for the improvement of health care.

d)   Apart from an internal function towards quality assurance, patient opinions also have an external function towards quality assurance. Patient opinions can be used as a (valid) indicator of quality. This is certainly true for the interpersonal and organizational aspects of quality, but as Davies and Ware described in their studies in the United States, patient opinions also seem to be a valid indicator for some of the technical aspects of health care delivery.

4.1.4   Patient Involvement in Quality Assurance in Europe

To obtain a rough idea of the involvement of patients' and consumers' organizations in quality assurance in Europe we made an inquiry among the experts that attended the preliminary meeting to this congress. The sample of this inquiry is very small (eight countries, ten persons) and the results are only to a limited extent representative, and neither randomized nor controlled. However, they help to provide a framework for this presentation. The first question asked in the survey was: *'to what extent can patients' and consumers' organizations influence the national health policy?'* The results are presented in Figure 4.1.

1   Luxembourg
2   United Kingdom, Italy, Bundesrepublik Deutschland (BRD), Greece, the Netherlands
3   Ireland
4   Denmark

Figure 4.1 Influence on health policy

As you can see in the majority of countries of the European Community, the influence of patients on health policy is considered rather low. Somehow it seems to make no difference whether you live in a country with a national health system or in a system which is more market-oriented. In all cases the normal democratic representation of people through politics somehow is not considered as sufficient consumer and patient influence on the decision-making process about health care. We also asked: *'what formal and informal instruments were used by the patients' and consumers' organizations?'* The experts mentioned political lobbying, participation in advisory bodies (as for instance in the community health councils in the UK), media work and petitions and even some funding of targeted research by patients' organizations. Only one country, Luxembourg, in an expert's opinion, has not got a patient organization. The next question we asked was: *'to what extent has there been patient influence on institutions such as hospitals and long-term care facilities, sickness funds or insurance companies?'* The results are presented in Figure 4.2.

hospitals
1 Luxembourg, Greece
2 United Kingdom, Ireland
3 the Netherlands, Denmark, BRD
4 Italy

sick funds
1 Luxembourg
2 Italy
3 Ireland, BRD, Greece, the Netherlands

Figure 4.2 Patient/consumers influence on hospitals and sick funds

Again you can see that the relative influence of patients and consumers is considered low, although in hospital boards and boards of trustees as well as in the boards of trustees of sick funds there are often, by tradition, places for representatives of the community that these institutions serve. However, the influence of the real consumers on hospitals and sick funds is not considered very large.

The next question in the inquiry was: *'do these institutions (hospitals) use patient surveys and if so, what is done with the results?'* The answers are presented in Figure 4.3.

As you can see, in only four countries are surveys used to some extent and it seems that the UK is the most experienced in using patients' and consumers' opinions for their quality assurance programmes.

The last question we asked was: *'to what extent are patient organizations involved in establishing guidelines for health care and medical care, for example by means of conferences to develop a consensus on a certain problem?'* The answers showed that in only three countries consensus conferences are held: Denmark, the UK and the Netherlands. In Denmark and the UK there was some consumer involvement: in the Netherlands, only in two of the 25 conferences. Furthermore, in most countries specific patient organizations exist (chronic renal failure, diabetes) and they seem, to a limited extent, to be involved in guideline formulation.

Greece	no
Ireland, Luxembourg, BRD	not known
Italy	+
Denmark, the Netherlands	+ +
United Kingdom	+ + +

Figure 4.3 Use of patients surveys

Overall, consumer influence on health care seems to be very limited. However, in most countries we can see a trend towards more and more patient organizations and growing pressure for patient organizations to become involved in the actual decision making process about health care. Another point that is interesting in this respect is to see what happens with regard to patient rights in the European Community.

4.1.5 The Agenda for Patient Rights in Europe

In 1986 a working group of WHO chaired by Professor Leenen made an inventory of the different initiatives in the field of patient rights in Europe. From the results of the study one can derive the agenda for patient rights in Europe for the next decade. On the agenda one finds the following items: the right to privacy, the right to information (getting access to medical records), a general tendency to transform laws from a doctor's duties point of view towards a patient rights point of view, complaint handling procedures, experiments with human beings, legislation about compulsorily admitted psychiatric patients and legislation towards voluntary sterilization/abortion and euthanasia. The discussions during the session on ethics show that, especially with these last items, we are far from creating a uniform legislation within the European Community.

4.1.6 Trends of Patient Involvement in Quality Assurance

What is the overall picture one can derive from the present situation? The first trend that can be noticed is that in most countries there seem to be initiatives for legislation although most of these activities are either focused on patient rights or quality assurance. In none of the countries are the two combined. A second trend is that participation of patient organizations and consumer organizations in the decision-making process is growing. A third trend is that, on a small scale, more and more countries try to use consumer information for the evaluation of their health care. Last but not least, there seems to be more interest in the actual communication between patients and doctors. That's where the key to success lies, because communication between doctors and patients is the central element in producing quality. Just like an industry, quality should be built into the product, therefore improvement of communication between doctor and patient, discussion of their mutual expectations and the creation of mutual trust is an essential component for quality assurance.

Let me conclude by pointing out two dangers of the present situation. One danger is a polarization through juridicalization. This means that by making laws too quickly and too detailed the actual communication between patient and doctor will not be promoted but will be influenced in a negative way, because the law will promote that patients demand their rights whilst doctors will try to defend their positions. Therefore I propose a way of legislation that gives positive incentives to improvement of communication and not one that only adds more polarization to the doctor-patient relationship. Another danger lies in de-commercialization of health care. If patient information is used solely for marketing reasons one will probably only promote new demands and a thorough evaluation of actual needs, and feedback of patient information for quality assurance will play a less important role. The fact that in the United States the publication of mortality rates of hospitals in 1986 on the front page of the New York Times did not have any significant influence on consumer behaviour towards selecting hospitals (the reverse seemed to be the case, patients kept on selecting the hospital where the mortality rates were the highest) shows that consumers' preferences might lead us away from quality assurance in terms of medical effectiveness. However, the trends with regard to patient involvement in quality assurance also create new opportunities. One opportunity lies in cooperation between health care providers and consumers. A good example of this cooperation can be found in the Netherlands where in April, 1989 during a national conference, the different organizations in the health care field decided that the development of quality assurance systems is a common responsibility of providers, consumers and third party payers, and should be a concerted action. One result of this attitude is the agreement between the Dutch Patient Consumers Platform (LPCP) and the Royal Dutch Medical Association (KNMG) about a paper that describes the physician-patient relationship in terms of mutual duties and rights. The final opportunity lies, however, in the improvement of doctor-patient communication as a key factor to quality of care. In this respect patients and doctors try to achieve a common goal. To demonstrate that differences between the position of the patient and the physician towards quality assurance will always exist, a quote from Hannu Vuori: *'the difference between the physician and the patient in quality assurance resembles that of the hen and pig in the preparation of eggs and bacon: the hen is involved, but the pig is committed.'*

4.1.7 References

Davies, A.R., Ware, J.E., Brook, R.H., Peterson, J.R., Newhouse, J.P. (1986), Consumer acceptance of prepaid and fee-for-service medical care: results from a randomized controlled trial, *Health Services Research*, **21**, (3), 429-52.

Davies, A.R., Ware, J.E. (1988), Involving consumers in quality of care assessment, *Health Affairs*, spring, 33-48.

Gevers, J.K.M. (1987), Tien jaar op weg naar een rechtspositie van de patiënt. *Tijdschrift voor Gezondheidsrecht*, Jan/Feb, 7-11.

Intentieverklaring betreffende een te ontwikkelen kwaliteitsbeleid. Medisch Contact 1989; **44**, 605.

Kistemaker, J.W.G. (1988), De beleving van patiënten en de kwaliteit van het medisch en verpleegkundig handelen, in *Onderzoek naar de tevredenheid van ziekenhuispatiënten*, A.Ph. Visser (red.), De Tijdstroom, Lochem.

Leenen, H.J.J.(1987), Patients' rights in Europe, *Health Policy*, **8**, 33-8.

Legge, D. (1988), Quality assurance: what is the consumers' role?, *Australian Clinical Review*, December, 190-6.

Modelregeling arts-patiënt, in *Rapportenboekje 198ste Algemene Vergadering Koninklijke Nederlandsche Maatschappij tot bevordering der Geneeskunst*, 27 October 27, 1989.

Matthews, D.A., Feinstein, A.R. (1988), A review of systems for the personal aspects of patient care., *American Journal of the Medical Sciences*, **31**, 159-71.

Nationale Raad voor de Volksgezondheid. Concept-advies klachtenopvang in de gezondheidszorg, 1989.

Visser, A.Ph. (1984), *De beleving van het verblijf in het algemene ziekenhuis*, Van Gorcum, Assen.

Vladeck, B.C., Goodwin, E.J., Myers, L.P., Sinisi, M. (1988), Consumers and hospital use: the HCFA "death list", *Health Affairs*, spring, 122-5.

Vuori, H. (1988), Patient satisfaction: an attribute or indicator of quality care?, *International Journal of Health Care Quality Assurance*, 1,(2), 29-32.

Wendte, J.F. (1984), Patiënten in het ziekenhuis. De betekenis van medische gegevens voor de meningen van patiënten over hun verblijf in het ziekenhuis, Proefschrift, Leiden.

4.2 Possible Contributions towards Quality Assessment and Quality Regulations by Patient Organizations
M.G.E. Welle Donker

As with so many things in life, words often seem to mean something different from what one might think at first sight. Language after all, is an organic growth, while at the same time it is 'unorganic' in that it has no material body, and often defies definition. Yet once a concept has formed, it guides our thinking. In addition we have to agree with other people on a word's meaning, in order to communicate. Still, in spite of our efforts, meaning can be so diffuse and dependent on cultural overtones, that communication breakdowns threaten continually. This, however, is not a modern phenomenon. The eighteenth-century English writer Sterne, for instance, left a blank page in one of his novels, because he despaired of his readers' ability to understand his intentions. Don't be afraid I'll follow his example. Even though communication between professionals and patients is never a simple process, and communication between different nationalities has its own pitfalls, I believe in discussion to clarify ideas.

Quality is an excellent example of a concept that needs clarification. In itself a neutral word, it means different things to different people even in everyday life. Usually however, it has a positive connotation, in that it means 'good quality'. But 'good' differs from individual to individual, depending on time, place and situation.

Quality is not a novel concept either, but it has certainly been used in a novel way over the past few years, and definitions abound. Usually those definitions concern the quality of professional standards, or the quality of isolated institutions or services. The new emphasis on quality moreover, has led to a host of novel concepts that sprang up in its wake: Quality of life, quality of health, quality of health services, quality assurance, quality assessment are just some of the new terms.

Granting the importance of the quality concept in relation to health care, this means we have not only a problem of definition, and hence a problem of communication, but also three other key problems: what is to be measured, by whom and by what instrument.

It is not surprising that health care, which has been influenced to a large extent by technology, has turned to an industrial model of quality assurance. This may seem natural, but entails the risk that aspects in which health care as a product differs from other commercial services remain out of focus, if not out of sight. The effect of the services - the 'health' of the patient - is not produced by the professional only, but is the result of a joint effort by professional and patient. Equating a 'patient' with a 'consumer' is therefore only part of the picture and sadly incomplete.

A second difference is that patients, especially chronic patients, people with handicaps, or patients in an acute stage of illness, are not as free in deciding whether they want to use certain services or not, as in the case of eating out, selecting leisure activities, further education, or even deciding whether to have a yearly health checkup or not.

A third difference is that many services, like specialist care, hospital care or medicines are not freely obtainable.

Quality in health care, therefore, has many different aspects and will probably have a somewhat different impact compared to a free consumer market.

There is therefore some merit in the most current (Donabedian's) description of aspects of quality, in that it is so general. Structure, process and result can be applied to nearly anything. While this description does not say anything about content, about constituting parts, or the viewing angle, it is evident that the perception of quality changes according to whatever constituting parts are taken into account, by the person who looks and by the weight that is attached to certain constituent parts. This means that quality can only be properly assessed and assured by joint action of all concerned. Government, professionals, financing bodies and last but not least, the patients.

Though the quality of healthcare is ultimately actualized on the micro-level, in professional-patient interaction, it can only exist by virtue of an overall structure. I will therefore concentrate on the meso- and macro-levels, although the aggregated experience-base patients bring to bear in the quality debate, typically flows 'bottom-up'.

Patients in the Netherlands have only recently focused on quality as a separate concept in health care, though of course, many of their organizations stem directly from movements to improve certain health services. This means that implicitly, concerns about quality have been core activities from the very beginning. Although they were at first seen only as groups clamouring for their own narrow interests based on demands and not on needs, and dabbling in self-help, making fellow-patients sicker than they already were, this picture has changed.

The post-war years gave Holland not only a 'baby boom', but also an 'organization boom'. Globally speaking there were three rallying points:

a)   Patients and their direct relations have, of old, organized themselves round certain illnesses or dysfunctions, like blindness, deafness, diabetes mellitus, cara, cerebral palsy, psychiatric illness or mental retardation. Their membership typically ranges from a few hundred to tens of thousands; many of them organize nationally and/or regionally. These vastly different individual organizations formed three main national umberella organizations (to unit them into one seems to be just one bridge too far): one for psychiatric patients, one for mental retardation and one for people with physical handicaps. The last mentioned is the Dutch Council of the Disabled, which comprises around sixty specific organizations of the handicapped, with an advisory status for professional organizations.

118

b)   The 'democratic reform movement' of the sixties, which gave rise to groups organized round health care centres, groups interested in the organization of health care, in furthering patients' interests, or centred around thematic concepts such as 'health and law', 'christian fundamentalism', 'alternative cures', 'child and hospital' and the like. Some were active at a local level only, others regionally and nationally as well.

c)   A third movement was formed by the consumer organizations.

Towards the eighties these three movements were fully established and influential, and they forged a national platform, the LPCP, (National Patient and Consumer Platform) in order to be able to cover the total field of health from the patient perspective. At provincial and regional levels, more or less identical organizations are coming into existence at this very moment. Although (like all its participants) hampered by lack of funds, it has set itself the enormous task of finding consensus among so many diverse organizations, finding volunteers among the organizations' members to serve on committees and represent the movement in government or private institutions. Though not yet always impeccable in its internal coordination, it works, and has the potential to put forward the patients' perspective at national and provincial/regional levels.

As far as I know, this set-up is unique, not just in Europe, but even in the world. Whether it will prove a blueprint for new developments, or be discarded by other countries as just another 'Dutch Disease', I do not know. Internationally it is not so easy to copy the Dutch experience. First of all, organizations in the other European countries, with the exception of the consumer organizations, are very dissimilar. Very often organizations for the handicapped are charities governed by leading residents or professionals, or more or less professionally rendered services with varying input from handicapped people, such as RADAR in the UK. Only the situation in Scandinavia and Portugal is comparable to the Dutch situation as far as the physically handicapped are concerned.

Worldwide (but with European chapters), there are two organizations that have brought together organizations of the handicapped (Disabled People's International), or organizations of both the handicapped and the care-givers (Rehabilitation International). The Dutch Council of the Disabled is affiliated to both. Disabled People's International can barely survive through lack of funds, which makes even personal contact of board members a matter of personal expense.

Like it's worldwide organization, the European chapter of Rehabilitation International is, unlike the Dutch chapter, dominated by care-givers and shows little inclination to change. Another initiative 'Action Europeenne des Handicapes' (AEH) is limited to membership from two individual Dutch organizations of handicapped persons and some of their EEC counterparts and is ineffective.

The specific organizations, like those of the blind or the deaf, usually have stronger international ties. International cooperation, however, does not seem to be a priority, judging from the different positions they take in meetings of the non-Governmental organizations. Add to this the very limited, or non-existent interest of the European Community, its Parliament and its committees, the decrease in funding for handicapped people through the Helios programme, and the future is bleak. As a consequence, quality assurance so far has not appeared on the agenda of any of the international organizations mentioned above. Quality of life is the only sense in which the word quality is encountered throughout Europe among the organizations of the handicapped, usually in relation only to the beginning and end of life and genetic research.

Maybe the European consumer organizations can take the initiative towards European cooperation. They seem to have become sensitive to the needs and the potential of a unified European patient movement.

It is high time patients know of the strengths and weaknesses of health care in other countries; know of differences in ethical notions, differences in legal rights, before we start shuffling professionals and patients around. That patient's perspective can be made to count; can be seen from the Dutch experience.

Nationally patients have participated in a conference that is laying the foundations for the development of a coherent system of quality assurance by government, health care professionals, funding agencies/health insurance companies and patients. Regionally, the platforms are discussing the way in which they could best implement their role *vis-à-vis* national regulation, the care-givers and the financing institutions. Consensus-meetings to establish consumer standards are one idea; establishing independent 'experience centres' is an other. The pros and cons of co-contractorship are debated. Specific organizations have embarked with specialist institutions on the improvement of the quality of care by making patient experience available to professionals and patients through the initiation of, and participation in, experiments, visiting teams, and so on.

So far the aspect of quality that has received most attention has been the so-called 'process'. It certainly is the easiest to measure; it is also the aspect that lends itself most easily to patient judgement. Information, consent, respect, complaint procedures are easily identified. Important though those aspects of the process are, they should never be viewed in isolation. If it is at all possible for the professional to dissect structure, process and result, the essence of quality for the patient lies in the totality.

Deciding for services on process quality alone may even jeopardize the patient's health. A hospital that has the friendliest nurses might have the worst mortality rate, which again would not necessarily make that hospital's care worse than another hospital with a lower death rate.

Whereas strict protocols may ensure minimal professional standards at minimal cost and equality to both (highly prized qualities by governments and insurance companies perhaps), those are detrimental to an individual's option. Quality, or again, a qualitatively good service, like for instance, outreaching nursing care to an elementary school student with myelingomyecele, is available at his home, but not at school, thanks to certain regulations. As children of a certain age have to attend school during the greater part of the day, the available and needed service is unattainable for them, the needed services are accessible in a special school setting. Whatever the quality of the special school setting, seen from the point of view of those students and their parents, the quality of the services rendered is poor and even wasteful (being not what they seek, and more expensive).

Hence, not only the health services in isolation constitute quality for a given patient, but the way those services support and/or allow or hinder his functioning in all areas of life. To a patient, health services are a means, never an end in themselves. Quality, as seen from the patient's point of view, can only exist if the patient's inherent human worth and his autonomy are respected. Flexibility and individualized care merit quality ratings from his point of view. Measurability presses in another direction however: protocols and standardization.

If the structure and the process are not quite as easily measured as we might have thought at first sight, the measurement of the result is no less ambiguous. Expectations vary, and hence the perceived quality of the result. Adverse effects are weighed differently. The client is the only one who experiences the result and has to live with it. It may be important to investigate perceived quality, and a perceived cost-effect ratio as seen by the patient alongside professional measures to arrive at a balanced quality concept. Patient surveys may be a welcome instrument. It might be wise to consult ex-patients for topics to be covered, and ideas to implement.

If health is looked upon as a 'product', this implies there is a producer. In a narrow sense that is true. The professional produces (delivers) a service. This service in itself is already rather complex, but the result is even more so, as it is most certainly influenced by patient variables; not in the least by professional-patient interaction and by the patients' efforts to get well. Those two aspects, the professional's expertise and the patient's experience and knowledge-base must be brought into balance. The magic word 'trust' is insufficient in itself to bring about that just balance. There must be two-way traffic, as it were. From micro to macro - that is the way to improve quality.

Then there are prerequisites for good professional service delivery, related to the professional's expertise and skills. In this field the client can only monitor curricula, the procedures to maintain standards, safety procedures, and so on. The maintaining of and/or increase in professional expertise and skill is predominantly the professionals' responsibility, though consumers might hire expertise for this purpose. The English have a nice proverb. In all its simplicity it comprises the essence of quality assessment: *'The proof of the pudding is in the eating'*. True enough, but the problem with health services is that sometimes there is no second chance if the selected pudding did not look appetizing, or if the cook did not take into account the special peculiarities of the individual tastes or digestive tracks of the designated consumers. Let's write a wholesome recipe:

Possible quality assurance.
A possible construction might be:

International Consumer Standards:	EEC legislation
General Consumer Standards:	national; LPCP (including LODEP)
General Consumer Standards:	regional Platforms; Consumer bureaux
MESO-standards:	peer group assessment (including patients)
Professional standards:	professionals plus contribution from patients towards formulation of criteria, procedural assessment
Government:	minimum standards

4.3 Measurement of Patient Opinions
S. McIver

4.3.1 Introduction

The National Health Service Management Inquiry led by Sir Roy Griffiths in 1983 placed particular emphasis upon the customer voice in health service provision. It questioned whether the NHS was meeting the needs of the patient and of the community, and could prove that it was doing so.

The Government White Paper 'Working for Patients' produced in 1989, similarly drew attention to the experience of the customer as a vital aspect of health service provision.

This has meant that over the last few years health authorities in Britain have been required to examine their practices and procedures from the viewpoint of the service user, in order to develop a more customer-oriented service.

Research on consumer feedback activities in UK health authorities has shown that many managers are unsure about how to obtain feedback from their users, how to utilize the information obtained and how to make services more sensitive to the needs of users. The most frequent method used is market research, in the form of 'patient satisfaction surveys', but unfortunately there are many problems associated with this method.

4.3.2 The Patient Satisfaction Survey

Surveys of patient opinions are popular with health service managers for a number of reasons:

a) They have a limited, but respectable history of use in the NHS, through the work of Winifred Raphael of the King's Fund, and also indirectly through the work of many Community Health Councils.
b) Surveys were legitimized by the Griffiths Report in 1983, which made comparisons between health authorities and the private sector where market research is an important part of the development and selling of products.
c) The survey has credibility with other staff (particularly clinicians) because it can be summarized statistically. Highly technical procedures involving computer calculations are often equated with scientific procedures even though there is no necessary connection.
d) The survey is a tangible, finite and structured piece of work with a clear beginning and end. It *seems* to offer a quick and uncomplicated solution to the perceived problem of 'getting the patients' views'.

Patient satisfaction surveys may be attractive to health service managers, but there are serious limitations associated with this method of obtaining feedback from customers. Some of these are:

a) Agenda Setting: The agenda is usually set by health service providers who construct questions around the areas they consider to be important for patients. Often these are copied by one health authority from another under the assumption that because certain questions are usually asked, they must be crucial ones. The service user rarely has any input into decisions about which areas are to be covered by the questions.

b) Sensitivity: The survey method is not sensitive to complex issues where an explanation from the service user may be necessary in order to make a response understandable.

c) Type of Question: Satisfaction with services is far too general a question area to obtain any meaningful response. In addition many surveys use categories such as 'very satisfied' 'quite satisfied' and 'satisfied' and then conflate them to make a percentage of 'patients satisfied' statement, which makes it difficult to see why they bothered to have these responses in the first place. In addition, many questions rely on memory and/or a person's ability to be aware of what is happening to them during what is often a traumatic event.

d) Usability: Self-completion questionnaires are generally used in surveys for ease of administration and speed, but they will not record the views of those who are illiterate, who do not read English, who cannot use their hands, or who are blind or short-sighted and have forgotten their glasses (many elderly people are in this category). A number of people also find questionnaires off-putting and will refuse to complete them.

e) Implications for action: Health service managers frequently underestimate the cost and complexity of surveys. They find there is little time or money left for analysis and report writing, and so many end up gathering dust on shelves. Even when they are written into reports, either the time for action has passed, or the gap between results and what these mean in terms of 'action to improve services for patients' is so great that nothing changes.

There are two processes currently under way in the UK aimed at improving the current position relating to the measurement of patient opinions:

a) Improving the survey method so that it provides a better tool for use in health services.

b) Encouraging the development of other methods of obtaining feedback from health service users.

4.3.3 Improving the Survey Method

The survey method can be improved for health service use in four main ways:

a) Making sure that all questions relate to an agenda set by the patient. That is, establishing areas of importance for service users through interviews, discussion groups and critical incident technique before questionnaires are constructed.

b) Using specific questions about issues, rather than general ones about satisfaction. That is, questions such as 'Did the doctor answer your questions in a way you could understand?' rather than 'Were you satisfied with the way you were treated by the doctor?'

c) Constructing a number of short questionnaires on various topics rather than one long one covering many topics, as is usually the case in Britain. Short questionnaires are likely to be more acceptable to the patient, and of more use to managers as they provide a quicker turnover of information than one long one, more specific information which has a higher use value, and they can be rotated on a regular basis in order to monitor service provision.

d) Conducting surveys only in those areas and with those users for whom this method is appropriate. Other methods should be used in conjunction with surveys in order to obtain comprehensive feedback from service users.

4.3.4 Other Methods of Obtaining Feedback

There are a number of other methods currently being used in a small number of health authorities in Britain to obtain feedback from service users and it is hoped that these will become more widely used in the near future. Some of these are:

a) Observation
b) Participant observation
c) Patient flow analysis/timecards (for example, for waiting times)
d) Interviews and critical incident technique
e) Discussion groups
f) User advisory panels and forums
g) Patient advocates and liaison officers
h) User participation in planning and service development

4.3.5 Conclusion

The measurement of patient opinions is currently at a relatively unsophisticated level in Britain, but this picture is beginning to change. A number of people working in the area, both academics and health service managers, are beginning to question the survey method and call for the development and increased use of other methods of obtaining feedback from users.

They are also improving the survey method by developing a number of short standard questionnaires on different areas of service delivery. These questionnaires are being constructed so that they both relate to the patients' agenda and are designed to be of maximum use to the health service manager, by obtaining information which can be directly related to service change.

4.3.6 References

Carr-Hill, R., McIver, S. and Dixon, P. (1989), *The NHS and its Customers*, Centre for Health Economics, University of York.

4.4 Is Legislation about Quality Assessment and Quality Assurance Compulsory after 1992?
W.G. Fack

In 1984 the European Regional Committee of the World Health Organization adopted 38 targets to reach the organization's overriding policy goal of Health for All by the Year 2000. Target 31 reads:

'By 1990, all Member States could have built effective mechanisms for ensuring quality of patient care within their health care systems.'

The target document suggests that this could be achieved by establishing methods and procedures for systematically monitoring the quality of care given to patients, by making assessment and regulation a permanent component of health professionals' regular activities, and by providing all health personnel with training in quality assurance. The document emphasizes the need for clear national policies to state which procedures are to be assessed; how this should be organized; how health providers, politicians, and consumers should coordinate their efforts. These policies would involve provider groups, researchers, public health authorities and consumers. The WHO Regional Office for Europe had already launched a programme on quality assurance in 1980 to implement specific activities towards this target. As part of the programme, basic concepts and methods of quality assurance have been defined, principles of quality assurance identified, and an approach to develop a curriculum on quality assurance suggested 1982 to 1986. In 1986 another report defined practical steps in the organization of quality assurance, especially in hospitals and health centres, among Member States.[1]

Quality of patient care within the health care system is not only the case for health care providers, such as physicians and hospitals on the one side and for politicians on the other side, but also for the consumer, the patient. In recent years the public has become a better informed consumer of services which expects assurance that services within their health care system are good. In cases of malpractice, more and more patients do not accept the consequences but take their grievances to consumer organizations, ombudsmen, or in the last resort, to court.

The development of the organization for quality assurance in the different European countries differs. Even the position of the patient, especially the possibilities of safeguarding his rights, is very different in the European countries. In the following this state of affairs will be considered.

First, it is a fact that there does not exist at this time a representative or official overview about legislation on quality assurance and patient rights in the European countries, therefore the following opinions are based on unofficial information and cannot guarantee completeness and accuracy. Incidentally, the main emphasis of these considerations is based on regulations which are valid for hospitals.

In Belgium there is no special legislation for the area of quality assurance. There are only few patient organization activities in the field of health care. Hospitals and their personnel, especially the physicians, are insured against malpractice.

In Denmark at present, a bill is prepared on the settlement of malpractices. Since 1 October 1989, it is obligatory by law to have an ombudsman. Hospitals and their personnel are insured against malpractice; above that physicians are also personally insured.

France, too, has special acts for the areas of medicine, laboratories, medical equipment, and so on. Above that, internal quality assurance in hospitals has been required by law since 1986/87, and has to cover the areas of nursing and hygiene. For this purpose special commissions have to be created. Local consumer councils are active in the protection of patients, and for the geriatric area there are also special commissions.

Ireland has no special law concerning quality assurance. However, cases of malpractice are recorded by the physicians' organizations. The doctors have to be personally insured. The patient has comprehensive rights, for example the right of seeing his patient file, and, moreover, he can consult an ombudsman.

The Netherlands, too, have no special law on quality assurance. However, there are quality assurance institutions working on a voluntary basis in the hospital sector, for example, the CBO (Centraal Begeleidings Orgaan). Each patient has the right to see his patient file. Furthermore there are special organizations who speak up for certain patient groups such as those suffering from a heart condition or a kidney disease, or psychiatric patients).

No special legislation exists in Portugal, except for the control of stored blood. Hospitals, however, participate in voluntary quality assurance measures, for instance in the area of neonatology, obstetrics, and so on. Hospitals have appropriate insurances, including provision for malpractice by their personnel. This is not relevant for the doctors, however, who have to insure themselves personally.

Spain also does not have special legislation on the field of quality assurance. Hospital personnel are not insured against professional errors. In the case of damage the patient therefore has to enforce his rights directly against the causer or against the causer's private insurance. There is, however, the possibility of consulting an arbitration council.

Great Britain, too - as most other European countries - has no special legislation on the sector of quality assurance. However, there are organizations on a voluntary basis, such as the 'College of Health', who are engaged in quality assurance measures. Moreover, there exist advisory bodies as well as the institution of the ombudsman. The hospital personnel are in principle insured with respect to their professional activities. This does not apply for physicians, who have to insure themselves. Patients' rights are safeguarded by commissions, such as the 'Mental Welfare Commission', or local consumer councils. There is an arbitration board for medical malpractice, the so-called 'Blue Commission', which every patient can consult.

Luxembourg as well has no special legislation for quality assurance, except for the laboratory area of hospitals. The total hospital personnel is in principle insured against malpractice; physicians are in addition also personally insured. Consumer councils so far are only to a very small extent occupied in health care.

In Switzerland also, only general laws exist, such as technical instructions for medical-technical equipment. All hospitals have an insurance against malpractice, which in case of event has to stand for the patient. There are appropriate consumer councils and in some cantons there exists the institution of an ombudsman.

The Federal Republic of Germany is so far the only member of the European Community, that has enacted special laws for quality assurance. Within the bounds of the new Health Care Reform Act, being in force since 1 January 1989, the legislator lays down quality assurance measures for out-patient as well as for in-patient care. However this is only a general outline of the law. Exactly which measures in detail the doctors in private practice and the hospitals have to implement, are subject to contracts between the self-governing organizations of physicians, the health insurances and the hospitals. The standards for quality control in hospitals are to be fixed in special contracts also. Hospitals as such are insured against malpractice of their personnel. Doctors regularly have a supplementary private liability insurance, and some provincial Hospital Acts determine that hospitals have to appoint an ombudsman. Victim patients can consult a medical arbitration council at the provincial General Medical Council. The advantage of this procedure is that it is free of charge. Above that patients are of course free to take legal action. Furthermore there exist patient protection organizations and groups representing the interests of patients with special diseases (for example heart diseases, cancer, and so on).

As for the other European countries, only Norway and Sweden have a special act for quality assurance in the health care area.

In the USA, who have a comprehensive institutional quality assurance on a voluntary basis, there exists since 1986 a special act on quality assurance in health care (Health Care Quality Improvement Act of 1986). This Act created a public clearing authority which especially collects data of those physicians who have been proven of malpractice-behaviour. This is supposed to prevent a physician, who has attracted attention because of malpractice in one US state, from moving to another state and practising there.

In Sweden as well as in the United States there exists to a greater extent consumer councils which attend to patients' rights. Furthermore the ombudsman is a regular institution in Scandinavia.

Summing up, one can say that except for general Acts, as, for example, those on the security of medical-technical equipment, the application of X-rays, building constructions and so on, there is no special legislation on the quality assurance sector in most of the European countries. Representation of patients' rights are therefore dealt with respectively in extremely different ways. What are the consequences of this for 1990 with respect to 1992?

Considering the complex subject matter and in particular the problem of defining by law what quality assurance is, it is hardly advisable to demand a detailed legislation for the quality assurance sector in the different countries. On the other hand, it seems desirable that by means of a framework legislation the involved parties are principally committed to the undertaking of quality assurance measures and the control of same. The organization of those measures in detail should, however, really be left to the parties involved, because this is the only way to reach a high level of acceptance and, with that, also quality of the quality assurance. In the different countries the legislator should support all attempts to establish institutions for quality assurance on the voluntary basis of the parties involved. In the patients' interests it seems desirable that all countries establish the institution of an ombudsman. Furthermore it seems to be necessary that, by means of according regulations, the legislator works towards a sufficient insurance for the deliverer of health services in the case of claims for compensation. Moreover it has to be ascertained by relevant measures that patients' rights are realized as quickly and unbureaucratically as possible. Damage suits, which can go on for several years, are unreasonable for victim patients.

Last but not least, a still more intensive exchange of knowledge and data on quality assurance in the different countries has to take place, especially about successes and failures. This is the only way to guarantee the European citizen in all countries a relatively equal quality standard in 1990 with respect to 1992.

4.4.1 Notes

1 Shaw, Charles (1989), Organization for Quality Assurance, in: *Hospital Management International '89*, London, 174.

5 Pharmaceuticals

Contents

5   Pharmaceuticals

5.0   Introduction
B. Leijnse and P. de Wolf

After listening to the speakers and the discussion about pharmaceuticals, we have to admit that William Comanor was right in choosing the title of his famous survey article, *The Political Economy of Pharmaceuticals*, in the Journal of Economic Literature some years ago. By this we mean the important role of the different organizations in the European circus with their conflicting interests, coalitions and positions in the network.

We have seen the schemes on registration procedures, centralized and decentralized. We have heard the problems of harmonizing criteria on quality control, product information and the division between prescription drugs and OTC-drugs. The entrance of Spain, Portugal and Greece formed a new challenge for these issues, and the Mediterranean Challenge seems to add even more weight to the questions of patent protection, price levels and regulation.

After Mr. Sauer presented a comparative survey of EC price-levels in combination with a comparison of consumption per capita, we were almost inclined to think 'The fault of the Dutch is in swallowing too little and paying too much'.

We now know that the reliance of the European Commission on parallel imports to decrease the enormous price differences between EC countries has not been justified. The guideline on price transparency also seems a very modest step to solving this problem, as Mrs. Hancher criticised this guideline as being preoccupied with *administrative* criteria instead of using *substantive* criteria, based on a clear analysis and a clear vision of the goals of the **internal market**.

What economic effects do we expect of European economic integration in the market for pharmaceuticals? As far as the manufacturers are concerned, the estimated effects in terms of increased efficiency, leading to cost savings in production figures of maximum 0.6 per cent are mentioned by both the Economists Advisory Group and the Cecchini Report. We do not expect large economies of scale in an industry which is already of an international character, so the cost reductions are expected to come from harmonized registration procedures in the EC.

As long as distribution and marketing activities will be decentralized and based on special demands in national markets, economies of scale will *not* be reached for these costs. The high levels of marketing expenditures demonstrate the existence of competition in the form of all P's in the marketing mix, including a high degree of product differentiation and promotional costs, but excluding price competition, say in those countries where wholesalers have considerable market power, producers lose a part of their profit margin to wholesalers and sometimes to pharmacists. That is the well-known problem of the differences between list prices and transaction prices and the hidden discounts.

We hope that the databank on drugs that will be built up by Mr. Sauer will shed some light on all financial flows in the channels of the pharmaceutical sector. It also should reveal eventual hidden forms of national protection, that are certainly against the philosophy of economic integration.

Another important issue in the pharmaceutical industry is the continuity of the research-based firms and their production of real innovations seen as the background competition from firms of American and Japanese origin. The plea for restoration of the effective patent protection term must also be seen in international perspective and deserves serious investigation, but producers' associations always forget the first part of the so-called *Drug Price Competition and Patent Restoration Act of the US*, namely drug price competition that has taken the form of fierce generic competition in the United States, where nowadays the market share of generics has risen to twenty-five per cent.

It is obvious that real innovation has to be renumerated, but the absence of innovation, and that is the case in many European firms (also in West Germany despite its highest price level), means that generic substitution must not be hindered because this can lead to tremendous cost savings in the countries with higher price levels.

Representatives of producer's associations also plea for a situation of free price setting for pharmaceuticals. However, we have to remember that in economic theory the main conditions under which free pricing is said to be optimal in terms of efficient allocation of scarce resources are the presence of price competition amongst suppliers, the absence of oligopolistic markets and high barriers to entry, the absence of concerted actions or cartels between firms and last but not least, the presence of well-informed consumers who may decide whether they will buy or will not buy a product when confronted with the consumer prices.

It is obvious that the above-mentioned conditions do not prevail in the pharmaceutical industry and when we speak of the supply side of the industry we include all market levels in this branch, wholesalers and pharmacists. However, whereas many branches can be compared in terms of elements of market structure of the supply side (we mention the level of concentration, entry barriers and so on), the specific characteristics of the demand side of pharmaceuticals are obvious to anyone. Consumers are not well informed, they *do not* make decisions concerning price, quantity, brand name and so on of prescription medicines and we do not accept that some sick persons would not be able to buy medicines in the case of free pricing. That is why the insurance character is an element in this sector, and that is why governments feel justified to take measures that go beyond the scope of competition policy which can be applied to all industries.

5.1 The European Community's Pharmaceutical Policy
F. Sauer

5.1.1 EEC Pharmaceutical Regulations

The criteria and procedures for approval of human and veterinary medicines have been progressively harmonized in the European Community. By 1992 the EC pharmaceutical legislation will cover all industrially produced medicines, including vaccines, blood products and radiopharmaceuticals.

The criteria for the quality, safety and efficacy of medical products have been harmonized, as have certain aspects of procedures for marketing authorization (time-limits, giving of reasons, publication) or for manufacture (quality control, inspections). The analytical and pharmacotoxicological tests and clinical trials, performed in accordance with the Community rules, need no longer be repeated within the Community. The tests on manufacturing batches carried out in the producing country are accepted by the other Member States.

The Council has delegated to the Commission the power to update the technical requirements governing the testing of human and veterinary medicines in accordance with the so-called Regulatory Committee procedure, which involves the participation of governmental experts.

Table 5.1
The rules governing medicinal products in the European Community

Volume I	The rules governing medicinal products for human use in the European Community Catalogue number CB - 55 - 89 - 706 - EN - C
Volume II	Notice to applicants for marketing authorizations for medical products for human use in the Member States of the European Community Catalogue number CB - 55 - 89 - 293 - EN - C
Volume III	Guidelines on the quality, safety and efficacy of medicinal products for human use Catalogue number CB - 55 - 89 - 843 - EN - C
Volume IV	Guide to good manufacturing practice for the manufacture of medicinal products Catalogue number CB - 55 - 89 - 722 - EN - C
Volume V	The rules governing medicinal products for veterinary use in the European Community Catalogue number CB - 55 - 89 - 972 - EN - C

The recent so-called 'extension directives' covering GMP (directive 89/341/EEC), vaccines (directive 89/342/EEC), radiopharmaceuticals (directive 89/343/EEC) were published in the Official Journal Nr. L 142 of 25.5.89, and the directive on blood products (89/381/EEC) in O.J. L 181 of 28.6.89.

Note: These tests are on sale at the:
Office for Official Publications of the European Communities, 2, rue Mercier, L-2985 Luxembourg Tel. (352) 499281, Telex PUBOF LU 1324 b

The complete texts of the EC legislation presently applicable to medicinal products, comprising binding directives, test guidelines, notice to applicants, GMP guide and so on, have been published in a series of five volumes entitled 'The rules governing medicinal products in the European Community (Table 5.1).

5.1.2 EEC Coordination of Marketing Authorization

In spite of the scope of this harmonization, differences in the decisions taken by the national competent authorities are apparent. In order to reduce these differences, two committees, consisting of representatives both of the Member States and of the Commission, have been set up, one in 1977, the Committee for Proprietary Medicinal Products (CPMP), responsible for medicines for human use and the other in 1983, the Committee for Veterinary Medicinal Products (CVMP) (Table 5.2). Member States or the Commission can apply to these Committees to obtain advisory opinions on particular medicinal products, in particular in order to monitor the adverse effects of medicinal products (pharmacovigilance).

Table 5.2

In addition to purely national registration procedures, pharmaceutical companies may use two types of Community procedures which are intended to facilitate the adoption of a common position by the Member States on applications for authorization for medicinal products. The biotechnology/high technology procedure, which is governed by directive 87/22/EEC, is reserved for high technology medicinal products, in particular those derived from biotechnology. The competent authorities are obliged to systematically consult with each other, within the CPMP or the CVMP, before deciding to authorize, refuse or withdraw a product from the market. High technology medicinal products for human use, which have followed this procedure, benefit from a certain form of market exclusivity for a period of ten years running from the date of authorization to market the product within the Community.

The other procedure, known as the multi-state procedure, enables a company which has previously obtained authorization from one Member State in accordance with the Community directives to request the extension of the authorization to two or more of the other Member States. The Member States who receive an application are obliged to take the original authorization into due consideration and should normally grant a marketing authorization valid for their territories within 120 days of the receipt of the application.

The two Community procedures, whether centralized (high tech) or decentralized (multi-state) are based upon an evaluation undertaken by a national authority acting as rapporteur. The CPMP or the CVMP are simply responsible for coordinating the evaluations; they have no capacity to undertake an independent scientific evaluation at Community level (Table 5.3).

Table 5.3
Outcome of Community Procedures

Type of Procedure	Former CPMP (75/319/EEC)	Multi-State (83/570/EEC)	High/Biotech (87/22/EEC)
Period	1978 - 1986	1986 - Sept. '90	1987 - Sept. '90
Number of Dossiers	41	124	31
Number of Applications	253	625	372
Total Number (opinions)	41	90	10
- Favourable	28	81	10
- Unfavourable	13	9	0
Subsequent National Decisions			
Authorizations	175	273	66
Refusals	63	50	0
Outstanding	15	137	43

5.1.3 The Future EEC System for Drug Authorization

In order to prepare the proposals on the future system for the authorization of medicinal products for human or veterinary use within the Community, the services of the Commission have undertaken two rounds of consultation with the competent authorities of the Member States, the pharmaceutical industry and representatives of other interested European organizations. As a result of these consultations, it is possible to identify certain orientations for the proposals which the Commission will present shortly to the Council (COM (90) 283).

After 1992 there should be three authorization procedures:

a) a centralized Community procedure, reserved for certain new medicinal products and valid for all 12 Member States;
b) a decentralized procedure, which will cover a substantial majority of medicinal products, based upon the principle of mutual recognition, and concerning a variable number of Member States;
c) national procedures, limited in principle to applications concerning a single Member State.

Use of the centralized procedure will be compulsory for medicinal products derived from biotechnology, and available on an optional basis for other high-technology medicinal products and new active substances. Applications for authorization will be submitted directly to a European Medicines Agency, consisting primarily of the reinforced Committee for Proprietary Medicinal Products (CPMP) and the Committee for Veterinary Medicinal Products (CVMP), supported by an administrative and technical secretariat with appropriate logistical support and benefiting from substantial scientific support provided by the competent authorities of the Member States. The opinions of the CPMP and the CVMP will subsequently be transformed into decisions valid throughout the territory of the Community.

The objective of the decentralized procedure is to permit the extension of a marketing authorization granted by one Member State to one or more of the other Member States by means of the recognition of the original authorization. In the case of serious objections, and after the exhaustion of all possibilities for a bilateral resolution of the problem, the CPMP/CVMP will arbitrate. At the conclusion of these procedures, the opinions of the CPMP/CVMP will be transmitted to the applicant, the Commission and the Member States. In the absence of serious objections within 30 days of transmission, the Commission will adopt a decision to implement the opinion of the Committee. If objections are received, the Commission will reach a decision in consultation with a regulatory committee.

The Agency will also be responsible for the coordination of national activities in respect of pharmacovigilance, inspection and laboratory controls, in order to ensure the safety of medicinal products circulating within the Community.

5.1.4 Pricing of Medical Products

In order to control pharmaceutical expenditure, the majority of the Member States have adopted rules governing the pricing of medicinal products or limiting the range of medicinal products eligible for coverage by their national health insurance systems. On 21 December 1988, the Council adopted directive 89/105/EEC on the transparency of national measures regulating the control of prices of medicinal products for human use and their inclusion within the scope of the national health insurance systems. The directive entered into force in January 1990. The main purpose of the directive is to ensure that national decisions on the pricing and reimbursement of medicinal products are adopted in a fair and transparent manner in accordance with objective and verifiable criteria. The directive lays down a series of procedural provisions relating to the time limits for decisions, the giving of reasons, rights of appeal and publication of decisions which take account of the different types of measures adopted by the Member States.

The directive also lays down a framework for future Community cooperation in this complex field. A new Advisory Committee has been established in November 1989. The

Member States are required to provide the Commission with detailed information about the operation of their national systems. In the light of experience, the Commission will be required to present, before 1 January 1992, any necessary further proposals to eliminate the disruptive effects which the existence of national controls may have on the operation of the internal market.

In addition, the European Parliament requested that more action be taken to increase the actual transparency of the pharmaceutical market. With the support of the Council, the Commission has therefore undertaken to establish a database on pharmaceuticals which will include approved product information together with information about prices. This database will be progressively established by 1993.

Finally the Commission has proposed a further means to increase the protection of pharmaceutical innovation, and to restore patent protection, in particular by creating an appropriate extension certificate (O.J. n° C 114 of 08.05.1990).

5.1.5 New Activities

1) Extension Directives In May and June 1989, the Council adopted four directives extending the EEC pharmaceutical legislation to areas not yet covered, such as immunologicals, radiopharmaceuticals, blood products and exports to the Third World. These extension directives will be supplemented by five detailed Commission technical directives currently under preparation.

2) European pharmacopoeia The convention relating to the elaboration of a European Pharmacopoeia was signed in 1964 within the framework of the Council of Europe. Currently 19 European countries are parties to the Convention. A protocol for the accession of the EEC to the European pharmacopoeia was signed in November 1989.

3) Veterinary proposals In January 1989, the Commission presented to the Council a package of three proposals on veterinary medicinal products (O.J. n° C 61, 10.03.89) which cover:

a)   a Regulation for the institution of a centralized Community system for determining acceptable levels for residues of veterinary medicinal products in foodstuffs of animal origin;
b)   a directive improving the multi-state procedure and updating the detailed provisions of directive 81/851/EEC and 81/852/EEC, in the light of experience;
c)   a directive for the extension of the veterinary medicines directives to cover immunological veterinary medicinal products.

Following the debate in Parliament, the Commission has submitted to Council several amendments to these proposals (COM(90)135 of 26.04.1990). Regulation (EEC) n° 2377/90 was subsequently adopted by Council on 26 June 1990 (O.J. n° L 224 of 18.8.90, p.1). The two proposals for a directive were finalized at the beginning of 1991.

4) Rational Use of Drugs The existing Community directives already contain a number of provisions concerning information to doctors and patients about medicinal products. The summary of product characteristics introduced by directive 83/570/EC provides a standardized basis for checking the accuracy of information. The Commission has convened an *ad hoc* group consisting of representatives of consumer groups, doctors, pharmacists and the pharmaceutical industry to discuss the type of information which should systematically be provided to patients and the manner in which it should be presented in order to promote a better use of medicinal products.

The three outstanding proposals in the pharmaceutical sector under the White Paper programme for the completion of the Internal Market were transmitted to the Council on 26 January 1990. Their common objective is a more rational use of drugs (O.J. n° C 58 of 08.03.1990).

The first proposal aims at eliminating obstacles to the free circulation of pharmaceuticals through the control of the wholesale channel of distribution of medicinal products, including the recall of defective medicinal products.

The second proposal tends to harmonize the legal status for the supply of medicinal products, in particular of those available on prescription only.

The third proposal deals with patient information and tends to harmonize the content of the labelling and package leaflets accompanying medicinal products.

5) Pharmaceutical Advertising The Commission has also submitted to Council a proposal for a directive concerning advertising of medicinal products for human use (O.J. n° C 163 of 4.7.90, p. 10). The proposal provides for separate rules for, on the one hand advertising to the general public and, on the other, advertising to health professionals. Advertising to the general public is authorized only with respect to self-medication; furthermore, it is subject in this case to certain conditions, positive and negative. Advertising to health professionals is subject to a more complete system of rules which covers in particular: medical sales representatives, financial inducements, and the distribution of free samples. Finally, provisions are made for the monitoring of advertising of medicinal products, with a special provision for self-regulation.

6) Homeopathic Medicines After more than two years of consultations with interested parties, the Commission has submitted two proposals to the Council to guarantee the quality and the safety of homeopathic medicinal products for human and veterinary use (O.J. n° C 108 of 01.05.1990).

5.1.6 The Need for International Harmonization of Drug Testing

The substantial progress made by European harmonization enables the Community to exercise international responsibilities in the pharmaceutical sector. Regular contacts with non-EEC regulatory authorities, in particular through the international Conference of Drug Regulatory Authorities (ICDRA), the World Health Organization (WHO) and the Codex Alimentarius. The Commission has conducted sectorial discussions on pharmaceuticals with Japan, which produced very positive results. Fruitful discussions have started with the European countries belonging to EFTA and with the US Food and Drugs Administration. These multilateral contacts could lead to better international harmonization of pharmaceutical regulatory requirements, preventing unnecessary repetition of tests in humans and animals and thus significantly reducing R and D costs. The efforts are fully supported by the pharmaceutical industry represented in Europe by the European Federation of Pharmaceutical Industry Associations (EFPIA) and worldwide by the International Federation of Pharmaceutical Medicinal Associations (IFPMA), who will jointly organize an international symposium on the subject in Brussels in November 1991; this symposium will be co-sponsored by the European Community, the Japanese Ministry of Health and Welfare and the US Food and Drugs Administration (FDA).

5.2 Uniformity versus Diversity: Opportunities and Risks for the Pharmaceutical Industry from the Different EC Health Care Systems
J.C. Matthews

5.2.1 Introduction

As an Englishman invited by this University named after Erasmus, I am put in mind of Erasmus's contacts with scholars in England and in particular of Thomas More, lawyer, statesman and Lord Chancellor of England who first met Erasmus around the year 1515 while on a diplomatic mission to Flanders.

More's famous book 'Utopia' published in 1516 was actually a kind of social and political satire, though the word 'Utopia' has come in our day to mean some unattainable, idealized, objective - rather like the public expectations or our national health care systems!

In More's Utopia the 'hospitals are so well run and so well supplied with all types of medical equipment, the nurses are so sympathetic and conscientious, and there are so many experienced doctors constantly available, that, though nobody's forced to go there, practically everyone would rather be ill in hospitals than at home.' - not a bad statement of objectives for today's health care system, though in the sixteenth-century there were few medicines and medical care consisted of trying to help the body's own recovery processes. With modern medicines and surgery, our expectations can be so much broader.

5.2.2 Need for New Medicines

But whatever one's views about the range of treatments available in Europe today, there is the inescapable fact that there are whole areas of disease for which there is no treatment at all or no really effective treatment. This proposition was put the opposite way by the President of our Royal Society of Medicine, Sir Christopher Booth, in a recent lecture[1]:

'It is not so much that there are lacunae in our present therapeutic armamentarium. Rather the world of the clinic should be regarded as a vast desert of uncertainty within which there are only oases of rational treatment.'

Many problems will require the greater understanding brought about only by research. We urgently require new antiviral agents, as well as new substances that can counter resistance in either bacteria such as staphylococci or parasites like malaria. Our treatment of many forms of cancer remains inadequate. We are making a start in the prevention of genetic conditions but so much more remains to be done. The list of 'holes in therapy' includes AIDS, Alzheimer's disease, and virtually all forms of cancer. While much has been achieved in treating cardiovascular disease, the major killer in the western world, we are still far from effective prevention.

And I could go on ....

Most of the medicines made available in the past forty years have been discovered and developed in the research laboratories of the pharmaceutical industry. The track record of the European research-based industry in developing new 'world-class' products is very good - as Table 5.4, based on an analysis by Barral of 12 years of research shows. There is a great difference between discovering a new medicinal substance (or New Chemical Entity) and achieving its acceptance on world markets, so can I direct your attention to the second column of this table showing NCE's marketed in all of seven leading markets. No less than thirty-seven per cent of these were discovered in the UK, Germany, Switzerland and France combined, although only one in ten of new substances achieved worldwide marketing.

Table 5.4
Per cent of New Chemical Entities marketed, by country of origin

Country of Origin	% of total	
	All NCEs	'Worldwide' NCEs
United States	25	42
Japan	19	5
Germany	13	7
France	12	5
Switzerland	6	7
United Kingdom	5	18
Italy	10	0
All others	10	16
Total	100	100
Number of NCEs	610	60

Source: Barral, 1985 and update 1987[2]

However, there is a worrying trend that Europe is losing its position for the future, shown if we look at expenditure on research and development. If in Table 5.5 we compare average expenditure in 1980 - 1983, with 1987, and express all the figures at 1987 exchange rate, then we see that the European share has fallen by seven percentage points, while the US and Japanese shares have increased. The absolute level of spending by American companies will probably overtake that of the whole of western Europe put together by 1990.

Table 5.5
Estimated Percentage Shares of World Pharmaceutical R and D Expenditure

	Average 1980 - '83*	1987
Companies		
American	30	36
Japanese	18	20
West European	48	41
Others	4	3
	100	100
* at 1987 exchange rates		

Source: Redwood (3)

Figure 5.1 taken from Redwood's recent publication illustrates the interaction between the scientific and financial parameters in drug discovery, development, marketing, and eventually reinvestment of profit in research.[3] The area of high-risk spending is shaded and covers about two-thirds or more of the total time cycle of more than 20 years. The phases of highest risk are development and international marketing. The main decision on revenue spending is whether to begin clinical and other expensive forms of development of a new compound, and whether to maintain it until launch or abandon the project somewhere along the way.

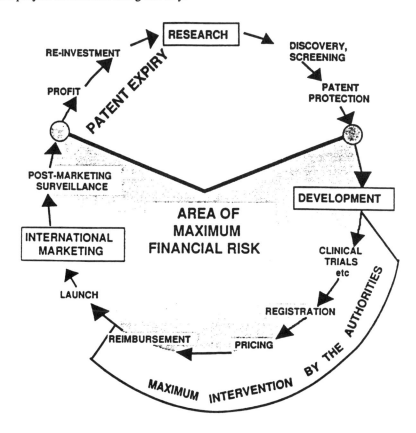

Figure 5.1 The 'science-finance' cycle pharmaceutical industry
Source: Redwood, 'The Price of Health'[3]

Development absorbs on average about two-thirds of the 12-13 years of R and D from discovery to launch, as well as two-thirds or more of total R and D expenditure. It is only when all three stages; product development, pricing/reimbursement *and* international marketing with an adequate period of patent protection are successful that a financial return can be achieved from R and D.

So, to put the issue very simply, if the European industry is to deliver its contribution to society in the discovery and development of new medicines, then we have to maintain, and preferably improve, the climate and opportunities for companies to invest their funds in research for the future.

This is a crucial standard against which to judge the value in the pharmaceutical sector of the process of completing the European internal market.

5.2.3 Opportunities

Measures in hand or proposed should offer opportunities to reduce the industry's costs and improve efficiency.

At the moment, when a manufacturer wishes to market his product in all EC Member States, he has to obtain a separate marketing approval in each state. During the past 20 years the requirements of the national regulatory authorities have converged as a result of progressive EC directives.

In practice, however, there are still substantial differences between one country and another. Methods of evaluation vary, as do perceptions of the weight to be put on particular kinds of evidence.

The Commission has just completed an extensive consultation on the form of a future system for a single marketing authorization valid in all Member States. The pharmaceutical industry's objectives are a Community-wide authorization of consistent character, granted on a single assessment of a single dossier, on the sole basis of quality, safety and efficacy. The method must be transparent, predictable, practicable and *rapid*.

Suffice it to say that the industry favours what we call a Harmonized System, providing for two procedures:

a)   a centralized 'common assessment procedure' with direct access
b)   a decentralized 'acceptance procedure' based on confirmation of existing national procedures

with freedom for the applicant to choose the most suitable of these options.

What would be the benefits? Frankly, they will be few unless the new system achieves much more rapid approval than the two years or more currently being taken by some national authorities and the three years or more needed to achieve approvals across the Community.

In a report to the Commission in 1988, the Economists Advisory Group estimated that delays in the marketing approval process, additional administrative costs and the time lost imposed a total cost of 160-260 million Ecus, or 0.4 to 0.6 per cent of industry costs within the Community.[4]

The single market also provides the possibility of cost savings in production. The industry is international and many companies have plants for formulation of dosage forms in all the important markets. There are good reasons for this: local medical practices influence the preferred form of administration of a medicine, the labelling and product information has to be in the local language, and there is value in being seen as an investor in the local economy - not to mention government pressure, often expressed in the course of price negotiations. Increasingly, however, companies will be rationalizing their production on a pan-European basis, such as producing several markets' requirements of a given product in one plant. It is difficult to put a figure on the savings which could result from better usage of the installed production capacity, since companies will not engage in widespread plant closures - that would be politically and commercially damaging. An admittedly high estimate by the Economists Advisory Group suggested saving in the range 260 to 530 million Ecus, or 0.8 to 1.6 per cent of unit production costs.

Finally, the most important and very positive measure relates to restoring the period of patent protection lost due to the ten years or so of the patent life which is used in the testing of a new medicine and obtaining marketing approval. An effective patent system is a crucial incentive for continuing investment in research.

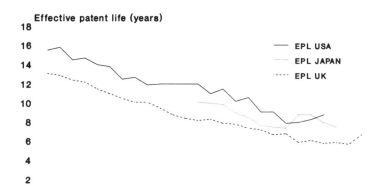

Figure 5.2 Internal Erosion of Effective Patent Life
Source: Centre for Medicines Research

As Figure 5.2 illustrates, the period of the nominally 20 years' patent protection which is left by the time a product is granted marketing approval has fallen to only eight to ten years.

The Commission has been persuaded of the need to take an initiative on this question, to avoid Europe being disadvantaged against the USA and Japan, which have already acted, and the industry welcomes the proposals about a 'complementary certificate of protection'.

Having reviewed these potential benefits from the completion of the internal market, their value of the first two in the short term is comparatively modest - less than two per cent of costs - and could be easily outweighed by the economic risks.

5.2.4 Risks

Central to any discussion of the economic position of the European pharmaceutical industry is the question of prices.

All Member countries of the Community control pharmaceutical expenditure by one means or another. The methods used are summarized in Table 5.6.

Table 5.6
General Outline of National Reimbursement Systems in EC Countries

	B	D	F	G	Gr	Ir	It	NL	P	S	UK
Nature of controls											
1 Price profits control	□	□	□		□	□	□		□	□	□
2 Official price approval required before any marketing	□						□		□	□	
3 Prior price approval for health service listing or reimbursement	□	□	□		□		□		□	□	
4 Positive reimbursement list	□		□	□	□		□		□	□	
5 Some types of products excluded but all others allowed				□		□		□			□
Contribution by the patient (products covered by social security)											
6 Fixed fee per item			□					□			□
7 Fixed fee plus variable element							□				
8 Percentage of controlled public price	□	□	□		□				□	□	
9 No charge						□					
Percentage of insurance or state spending of total spending on medicines (inc. non-prescription products)	52	53	65	56	n/a	48	64	64	67	67	76

Source: ABPI/EFPIA (Association of the British Pharmaceutical Industry, European Federation of Pharmaceutical Industry Associations).

The majority of Member nations of the Community regulate the prices of individual products. The methods used may be summarized as cost-plus, internal comparison and external comparison. Cost-plus bases the permitted price on the costs of production, allowance being made for marketing and R and D expenditure. Internal comparison fixes prices by reference to comparable products already on the national market, concessions being made to innovative products with therapeutic advantages. In external comparison, the price of the particular medicine in other countries is the key factor.

Several Member nations, however, do not fix the prices of individual medicines. The Netherlands nominally operates a free market, relying on other means such as voluntary agreements to control total pharmaceutical expenditure. Denmark in effect does the same. West Germany, formerly the great European example of free pricing, now restricts reimbursement under the national health insurance system to a fixed sum for multi-source products with identical active ingredients.

The United Kingdom is unique in controlling the profitability of companies rather than the price of their products. Each year firms negotiate with the UK Department of Health a global return on capital based on their sales to the National Health Service in the previous year. The rate of return is fixed company-by-company 'having regard to the scale and nature of the company's long-term risks'. Provided that this rate is not systematically exceeded, firms are then free to set the prices of new products as they see fit.

Such major differences in the ways in which pharmaceutical prices are controlled - or not controlled - would be expected to lead to corresponding variations between European countries in price levels, and they do. They are accentuated by the fact that price increases to compensate for, say, rising costs usually require official permission, which may well not be forthcoming. Price freezes are common. Companies aim for a pan-European price for a new product only to see it disappear amid national differences in exchange rates, the progress of inflation and official responses to these factors. To add to the problem, rates of VAT and wholesale and retail mark-up vary markedly between countries.

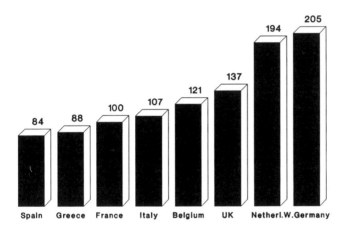

Figure 5.3 Price Index for Pharmaceutical Specialities, 1987 (France = 100)
Source: Syndicat National de l'Industrie Pharmaceutique

The outcome is clear. As Figure 5.3 shows, the ratio of average prices between the cheapest and the most expensive Member nations of the Community is of the order of 1 to 2.5. Medicines are relatively expensive in Denmark, West Germany, Ireland, the Netherlands and the UK and relatively cheap in France, Italy, Spain and Portugal.

The fact of finding variations between countries is not, of itself surprising or confined to medicines. Some product categories have even wider spreads but these are a response to market conditions, differing distribution margins, and so on. In the case of pharmaceuticals the cause is price control by Member States. The low prices in France, Spain, Italy, Portugal and Greece do not provide an adequate margin to fund future research and if it was not for the contribution to research funding which companies can achieve from the German, UK, Danish and Dutch markets, as well as from exports, then those countries would not have the benefit of new European-discovered medicines. To put it another way, consumers in some EC Member States are riding on the back of research paid for by consumers in other Member States.

Is this fair or equitable? Can the industry continue to sustain this imbalance in a Single European Market? The answer is that the imbalance must be expected to even out. The crucial question is - at what new level? Will it be at a level which allows prices which can continue to support a research spend of the order of fifteen per cent of sales income, or will it be at a lower level which risks undermining an industry which is a European social and industrial asset?

A clue to the future scenario is provided by the level of parallel trading in medicines which is already going on and growing, under existing Commission guidance in the light of various interpretations by the European Court of Article 30 of the EC Treaty. Already parallel imports into the United Kingdom account for an estimated eight per cent of the market, encouraged by government action to make an arbitrary deduction form the reimbursement of retail pharmacists on the theory that they are all profiting from parallel imports. The extent of parallel trading here in the Netherlands is, I understand, similar, and that in Germany is less but still significant.

One can, evidently, do various estimates of the loss of overall income to the European pharmaceutical industry if such pressures cause the effective prices in those countries which do adequately recognize research costs to fall to the levels of those countries which do not. One estimate by the independent London financial analysts of Shearson Lehman Hutton is that if all prices fell to the Belgian level, then the industry would lose the equivalent of six billion dollars, or a twenty per cent reduction in the market.[5] Allowing, however, for those products which would not be attractive to parallel trade suggested to the analysts that 'a realistic estimate of the potential of the market to shrink should parallel trade increase markedly is around ten per cent (£1.7 billion)'. Other independent observers have published similar estimates.

Since costs would not fall, then this loss would go right through the account to reduce the industry's profitability, by an amount which is comparable to the funds needed for investment in research.

Compare this ten per cent cut in income and profits with the possible two per cent reduction in costs from the positive 'single market' market-measures, and you have the dimension of how the risks outweigh the opportunities.

5.2.5 Reducing the Risks

So, what can be done to reduce this risk of undermining the industry's innovative potential? Let me at this point emphasize that the question has to be directed to national health authorities as much as to the European Commission.

The new directive 89/105 on the transparency of pricing and reimbursement systems, which came into force from 1 January 1990, should help to disclose price control practices which are discriminatory between different companies, such as between those which do or do not have manufacturing or research investment in the country. Its provisions should also help to speed up the decisions of pricing and reimbursement authorities, which currently can add a further one or two years' delay even after a marketing authorization is received.

However, while requiring more disclosure of the criteria of national pricing decisions, the directive leaves untouched the question of the validity, equity or acceptability of those criteria. A complete re-evaluation is needed of the way in which new products are priced in order to allow a more competitive market after 1992.

Pharmaceutical manufacturers seek the same opportunities as other manufacturing sectors in the Community to choose their ex-factory prices in accordance with the competitive market conditions for their products. National health care authorities would continue to decide what proportion of the cost of prescription medicines they will contribute to the patient and by what mechanism.

The increasing competition between companies and the heightened pressure on health budgets means that the case for artificial price control has become weaker.

The market for medicines is increasingly price sensitive. This is mainly because of the growing pressure on health care budgets everywhere. Within each therapeutic area, a range of products compete in terms of price and performance.

The attitudes of doctors and patients to the medicines they use are changing. Doctors can no longer be regarded as insensitive to price as pressures to prescribe cost-effectively are increasing. Patients are increasingly well-informed and vocal in expressing their wishes about their treatment.

With very rare exceptions, no medicine is free from competition. Usually several more or less similar products compete directly. Where this is not the case, a choice exists between different classes of medicine or between different forms of treatment. Experience in the United Kingdom and the other countries where companies are free to set their own launch price clearly shows the impact of both price and product competition. Equally, if an innovative new medicine commands a premium at the outset, competitors entering the market subsequently will aim to compete on prices as well as performance.

Because of the complex interaction between price control, reimbursement, industry cash flow and research investment conditions, some of the distortions must be removed before the single market aggravates them:

a) for new products (that is, new chemical or biological entities) manufacturers should be free to establish their own competitive prices throughout the European Community immediately on receipt of a Community based marketing authorization;

b) for other products (that is, existing entities which cannot immediately be integrated into the Single Market) manufacturers should be allowed to adjust existing prices annually to compensate for inflation and exchange rate movements over an appropriate interim period;

c) 'modulation' or adjustment of prices within the product range without affecting total revenue by the manufacturer within each Member State should be allowed, in order to minimize cross-border disparities. This could be done without leading to any consequent increase of costs within the Member State.

As for any transitional arrangements, the impact of free pricing for new products would be very gradual as only a small number of significant new chemical entities (less than 30) come on to the market each year.

The industry looks to the Member States and the Commission to consider a scenario along these lines.

5.2.6 Diversity of Markets

While we believe that the diversity of national price control systems has risks for the Community if it is combined with frontier-free trading of medicines, this is not to suggest that diversity between Member States should or could disappear after 1992.

After all, we are not, nor will we be, dealing with some amorphous 'Euro-medicine' but with real people - patients, doctors, pharmacists - who are the products of the various national cultures around the European Community.

Quite apart from differences of language there are clear differences in the way in which doctors from different EC countries are trained to approach a given disease or condition, and in our various national attitudes to our bodies and disease. I could instance the French pre-occupation with the liver, but also their concern for the integrity of the whole body and use of less invasive techniques than, say, in England or the USA. Then one asks how it is that German doctors use seven times as much of cardiac glycosides per head then the French, and six times more than the English, and at the widespread diagnosis of low blood pressure, which would be considered a non-diagnosis in England. Why do the Germans and French prescribe about twice the number of medicines per person per year than the British?

There are national differences in the preferences for modes of administration of medicines - for example, a greater use of injections in pharmacies for antibiotics in Italy or Spain compared with Britain - or the French preference for rectal administration of certain products.

Pharmaceutical manufacturers have to recognize these national differences in their communications with the medical profession, which is why company marketing activities will continue to be organized on a national basis, though there is likely to be a greater degree of pan-European management and control to reflect the needs of the single market.

This national diversity will also have to be taken into account as we move to implement the directive requiring provision of written information for patients about their prescribed medicines. The industry is in favour of this move - indeed, in Britain the industry went on record as advocating patient information leaflets even before the Community directive was proposed. However, coming as we do from a situation where there are no package leaflets, and many prescriptions are dispensed by pharmacists out of bulk containers, we want to be sure that the leaflets are understandable by patients and provide enough information to enable them to take their medicines correctly, rather than just repeating the prescribing information as provided to doctors. There should be a core of information on the product which is common across the Community, but manufacturers have to work within the reality that there can be differences between Member States in the terms of the marketing authorizations granted to a given product.

It is clear that the successful pharmaceutical companies will be those which can achieve more efficient operations in a pan-European system yet be sensitive to local differences and customer needs.

5.2.7 Conclusions

I have briefly examined the opportunities and the risks for the pharmaceutical industry after 1992 arising from the different health care systems in EC Member States.

The main opportunities arise from harnessing those systems together towards achieving a single Community-wide marketing authorization and from improved opportunities for manufacturers to rationalize their production capacity around the Community.

Separately, but most importantly, there are the proposals to significantly improve the protection for innovation in the industry.

In looking for a positive climate for innovation we do not expect a haven for risk-free enterprise. We recognize the need to maintain efficient management of innovation and to produce evidence of the cost-effectiveness and health care benefits of new medicines. We also recognise the reality of generic competition after patent expiry.

Europeans, as patients and as contributors to health care systems, need assurance that the European Community will at best maintain and preferably enhance its capacity to discover and develop new medicines. Measured against that social objective, the negative economic risks from free circulation of those price control systems which do not allow for research investment will outweigh the positive benefits unless, in their diverse health care systems, Member States are willing to act in ways which recognize the value to them and their patients of maintaining the pharmaceutical industry as a European asset.

5.2.8 Notes

1 Booth, C. (May 1989), *'Holes in Therapy'*, lecture to European Federation of Pharmaceutical Industry Associations, Paris.
2 Barral, E. (1985), *'Dix ans de resultats de la recherche pharmaceutique dans le monde'*, Perspective et Santé Publique, Paris (update 1987).
3 Redwood, H. (1989), *'The Price of Health'*, Adam Smith Institute, London.
4 Burstall, M.C. and Reuben, B.G. (1988), 'The Cost of "Non-Europe" in the Pharmaceutical Industry', *Basic Findings, Volume 15*, Commission of the European Communities.
5 Walton, J. *et al.* (1989), 'A Controversial Vision of the Future: Challenges Posed by Pharmaceutical Deregulation', Shearson Lehman Hutton, London.

5.3 The 'Gesundheits-Reformgesetz' and the Realization of the Common-internal (EC) Market in 1993
H.R. Vogel

The pharmaceutical industry in Germany sees its position and perspective strongly influenced by two important incidents: the coming into force of the 'Gesundheits-Reformgesetz' at the beginning of this year and the realization of the common-internal (EC) market in 1993.

I would like to put forward my opinion on these two fixed points which will substantially influence the mid-term developments of the pharmaceutical sector in Germany.

The 'Gesundheits-Reformgesetz' (the health care reform act) already gives us reason to expect far reaching consequences for the German pharmaceutical market in the near future. To start with there is the 'Festbetragsregelung' (a fixed reimbursement price-system) which creates for the sickness funds the possibility of price-fixing for pharmaceuticals. Though this 'Festbetragsregelung' is a completely new and until now without any precedent elsewhere, let alone proven, instrument to economize on costs of pharmaceutical aid, it was tough - not to say insensitive - put into practice. The first fixed prices have already been executed. Since then it has become clear that at least the 'Festbeträge' will lead to price limiting, if not a total fixing of a maximum price by the sickness funds holding a demand-monopoly. These fixed prices have led to significant price-cuts; for the specialities often in a range of about thirty per cent. If this constitutes a signal for the future I would not dare to predict the outcome.

On the one hand, it will not be possible for pharmaceutical enterprises, simply for industrial managerial reasons, to cut prices with the thirty per cent mentioned across a broad range of their product-mix; with individual products it could be realized, under strong pressure, but on the total product-mix it is untenable. On the other hand, in view of the hugely positive results for the sickness funds it is to be feared that the latter will enjoy a kind of power-hungry attitude and try to impose on the pharmaceutical manufacturers even lower fixed prices.

It is a rather shocking fact that the social sickness fund, by establishing fixed pricing, is only recognizing the possibilities of obtaining the best economic prospects. Social political viewpoints are fully dominating these aspects. Meanwhile industrial- and research-policy aspects are ignored. The consequences of industrial- and research-policies as to the fixed amounts can be predicted.

For research-based companies they mean the end of the so-called generation-contract for pharmaceuticals: older products which ran out of patent from now on cannot contribute to the research and development of new pharmaceuticals. The presently used mixed-financing of pharmaceutical research will come to an end. When the financial means for research are diminishing, it is necessary to make significant cutbacks. When it is not possible to invest in research, it is clear that in the long run little will come out of that research. The research-successes - both medical and economical - of successful pharmaceuticals will decline. This again will negatively influence the international competitiveness of the research-based German pharmaceutical industry which can hold its position on the world-market only with competitive modern products.

In addition, the generic manufacturers suffer from fixed pricing policies. When the original products have to be brought down in price according to the fixed amounts, they begin to approach the price of generics. When the original products and the generics approach each other in price or maybe even reach the same price, the generics will lose the most important competition-instrument, namely the price-advantage. In that case the medical practitioner does not see any sense based on economical grounds in prescribing generics and will prescribe specialities instead.

However, it is not only the fixed amounts that cause great worry to the German pharmaceutical manufacturers. They are very anxious about a foreseeable fixed quantity-system. Quite arbitrarily the Healthcare Reform Act orders that both organizations of medial practitioners connected with sickness funds and the regional organizations of the sickness funds have to decide on fixed standards for the quantity of prescribed performance, especially for pharmaceuticals and therapeuticals. As to the set-up and consequences of the fixed quantities' system we remain in the dark, so until now it has not been recognizable whether the fixed quantities have to cut the prescription value or quantity. For both possibilities reasons can be found. However, no reasonable ground is to be found, in the minds of many representatives of the sickness funds, for fixed quantities to bring about a detailed control of the medical prescription pattern.

The Healthcare Reform Act with the above mentioned fixed amounts and fixed quantities is not the only concern for the German pharmaceutical manufacturing and dispensing. A number of further problems will arise. Simply as an example I refer to the application jam at the registration authority, while more than 10 000 applications lie untouched, dumped in containers at the BGA. A manufacturer who today applies for his product may hope to get market-permission for it in the middle of the nineties. I only mention this for completeness sake because the endless time required for the application procedure reduces more and more the effective patent term. The application misery has been well-known for years, and complained about everywhere: a solution to the problems is not yet expected.

Furthermore the continuing discussion on animal tests causes problems. The enemies of animals tests continue to question the necessity of animal testing and would like to abolish all pharmaceutical research involving animals. They have considerable public support, which in its turn influences politics. A parallel to animal-testing is to be found in gentechnology. Some activists commit themselves against gentechnology; they stir up basic fears and therefore draw a substantial number of people to their side. Finally politicians focus on that concept. The pharmaceutical industry is not able to stop this trend alone. In Germany, it is not allowed to produce pharmaceuticals by means of gentechnology, whilst abroad this is approved. As a result, pharmaceutical companies will be forced more and more to leave Germany as their home-base. These are only a couple of issues. We cannot, however, content ourselves with simply looking at events happening in Germany. We have to look more to the creating process of the EC internal market.

The tension between the harmonizing process on the one hand and the diversity on the other is the prime challenge of the EEC with regard to the pharmaceutical industry. In the pharmaceutical field, this diversity generally shows - in the different social security systems - in the strongly divergent price- and reimbursement regulations. There is an important role in this framework to be played by the transparency directive and by this directive constituted evaluation committee.

It is in this very directive that the European Commission clearly stated that there should be a balance between the need for the national governments to keep the costs for national health care under control but at the same time the need for a strong European research-based pharmaceutical industry.

The divergence shows itself not only in the systems but in the different medical schools and traditions as well. Moreover there is a diversity of margins and assessment rates for pharmaceuticals. Convergence of prices has to be expected within the EC internal market, to mention only the effect of an internationally-operating wholesale activity. The question remains at what level will the prices convert? The subsequent question is whether this levelling of pharmaceutical prices will lead to changes in the level of health care in the individual EC Member States. One thing we can take for granted: a high level of care at the lowest prices cannot be realized.

When no active and offensive industry- and research-policy is formulated, but only social policy is imposed, the EC will lose every connection with the USA and Japan with respect to pharmaceuticals. It is necessary to create long term secured pre-requisites to enable successful (and substantial) research. The process of pricing should be left to the market and market forces. Directly or indirectly price regulations have to be rejected in principle.

With regard to market authorization, one should not be too hasty in choosing certain solutions. In principle the possibility of choice between a supra-national and national system of market authorization should be preserved.

Notwithstanding the internal troubles with the German registration authority mentioned before, there should be an opportunity for an evolution, and not a revolution, of the registration system. There is a need for adaptation time towards harmonization. A strong pressure for a centralized system within a short time might, for example, lead to the same congestion at European level as on certain national levels at the present time.

Besides, one should avoid the creation of a supra-national European bureaucracy in matters of application and admission to the market of pharmaceuticals. Once again, they seem to be excepted from the general free movement of goods by their special status at national level due to the divergency of price- and reimbursement systems.

Which way and what procedures will be the right and acceptable ones we will see in the coming years.

5.4 A New Directive Relative to Medicines: The Transparency Directive
D. Bégué-Aboulker, F. Courcelle, G. Duru

The establishment of the European Economic Community (EEC) by the Treaty of Rome goes back to 1957. The sought-after and time and again reaffirmed objective is an economic one; it is, in effect, to ensure that within the community itself there is free circulation of good, people, services and capital. Health itself was not mentioned specifically by the Treaty which simply gave the Commission of the European Communities the very general mission of 'promoting tight collaboration between States in the social field'. Social and health problems constitute no less of a priority where they are at the source of severe distortions of competition linked to disparities in social security contributions endured by different national industries.

To carry out an exhaustive evaluation of European policy on medicinal products constituted a very heavy task, so great were the facts in 1989. We also voluntarily limited ourselves to the analysis of one of the most recent directives to have appeared on the subject, directive 85/105/EEC of 21 December 1988, 'concerning the transparency of measures regulating the fixing of prices of medicinal products for human use and their inclusion in the field of national health insurance systems'. This directive entered into effect on 1 January 1990.

Our work is based around three ideas:

a) the relatively fast adoption of the directive - the first proposal dates from December 1986 - could not mask the difficulties of its conception nor belittle its originality;
b) the analysis of the text should not be a simple commentary of the measures adopted but must permit us to differentiate between that which was truly the subject of a consensus and that which is nothing but a compromise, liable to be changed in the future;
c) the range of the directive will depend upon the effective use which is made of it.

5.4.1 The Position of the Transparency Directive

The transparency directive represents the first legislative initiative taken by the community authorities that is aimed directly at the economic and social dimension of medicinal products.

Table 5.7
Principle directives, recommendations and decisions of the council
governing medicines for human use in the European Community

65/65/EEC	First directive; Definition of the general framework
75/318/EEC	Analytical, pharmaceutical and clinical norms and protocols to control trials of pharmaceutical products.
75/319/EEC	Second directive, specifying the general framework and establishing the Committee for Proprietary Medicinal Products and the procedure for partial mutual recognition.
75/320/EEC	Decision to set up a pharmaceutical Committee.
78/420/EEC	Directive amending the procedure of the CPMP instituted by directive 75/319/EEC (now replaced)
83/570/EEC	Directive amending 65/65/EEC, 75/318/EEC and 75/319/EEC in the procedures and requirements of applications.
83/571/EEC	Recommendations to the Council introducing explanatory notes relative to pre-clinical and clinical trials.
78/25/EEC	Colouring agents.
81/464/EEC	Directive amending directive 78/25/EEC on colouring agents.
87/19/EEC	Directive amending directive 75/318/EEC on the norms and protocols, and establishing a committee for the adaptation to technical progress of directives aimed at the elimination of technical barriers to trade in the proprietary medicinal products sector.
87/21/EEC	Directive amending directive 65/65/EEC as to protection with respect to a second applicant.
87/22/EEC	Directive concerning high technology products, in particular those from biotechnology and the instituting of a planning procedure.
89/176/EEC	Recommendation from the Council proposing new explanatory notes.
89/342/EEC	Directive enlarging the scope of directives 65/65/EEC and 75/319/EEC and foreseeing complementary dispositions for immunological medicines consisting of vaccines, toxins and serums.
89/343/EEC	Directive enlarging the scope of directives 65/65/EEC and 75/319/EEC and foreseeing complementary dispositions for radiopharmaceutical medicines.
89/381/EEC	Directive enlarging the scope of directives 65/65/EEC and 75/319/EEC concerning the harmonization of legislative, regulatory and administrative positions relative to proprietary medicinal products, and foreseeing special arrangements for medicines derived from human blood or plasma.

1) Until now the aspect of technical regulation had almost been exclusively privileged This can be explained by a matter of principle: it is natural that when concerning medicines the question of public health is a duty and favours reflection on the conditions of marketing authorization; things were made easier in practice by the fact that disparities exposed in marketing authorizations never went to the core - there was an identical philosophical base, always with the same requirements of harmlessness, safety and effectiveness of remedy - and only revealed differences as to the treatment of applications, relatively easy to iron out. Thus a whole series of directives has been adopted since 1965, as Table 5.7 shows.

2) On the other hand the economic, social and fiscal implications of medicinal products were long neglected This backwardness can be explained by the extraordinary range of solutions retained within the EEC regarding the price of medicines and the control of this by the health insurance systems. Certainly, the health needs expressed in the different European states are tending to come closer together and the same necessity to achieve better control over spending is emerging forcefully everywhere. However this is not enough; the heterogeneity of national regulations remains wide (Table 5.6) and the price levels for medicinal products are very disparate from one country to another (see Figure 5.3).

Other factors accentuate the gaps, such as the existence or not of a system of third-payer for medical consultations and visits, for example. These conditions, which reflect habits, mentalities and cultures, all at once very deep and very different from one another, render the harmonization of economic and social legislation on medicinal products totally unrealistic, at least for the time being. They also stand in the way of the setting up of a uniform European system, which would combine elements which have each proved their worth on a national level.

3) In the face of such great obstacles, the European Commission could have been tempted to give up. Despite appearances, it has not

a) A very apprehensive start If one refers to the multitude of decisions taken in the field of technical regulation it is probable that the balance on the side of anything to do with economic, social and fiscal aspects of medicinal production is small. Apart from the elimination of tariff barriers between the diverse countries of the EEC, not limited only to pharmaceutical products, and the presentation of a proposition for a directive on the harmonization of Value Added Tax (VAT) rates, the only provision having had a noticeable economic effect on medicinal products comes from directive 87/21/EEC which foresees, in particular for high technology products and in the absence of protection by patent, the possibility of a period of ten years exclusivity over the entire EEC running from the date of delivery of the first marketing authorization of the original medicine.

b) A long wait The Commission did in fact carry out a long drawn-out study of which the transparency directive was the outcome. Very early on, the Commission, guardian of the Treaty of Rome, saw itself posed with the problem of properly respecting the principle of free circulation of pharmaceutical products. As a general rule these are subject to article 30 of the Treaty of Rome which forbids the setting up of any measures equivalent to quantitative restrictions on trade, as these are explained by directive 70/50/EEC of 22 December 1969. Thus the question of compatibility between community law and national regulations on the price of a medicine and the control of that price by the national health insurance system had to be raised. The Commission obviously leant on the judgement given by the European Court of Justice who have had several occasions to pronounce themselves on this subject [1] and little by little establish a position of principle: it allows Member States, because of the specific nature of the market for medicinal products, the possibility 'to fight against inflation and to take measures destined to check the rise in the price of medicines, from whatever origin' and allows them 'to rearrange their social security system ... in particular to take dispositions destined to regulate the consumption of pharmaceutical products, in the interest of the financial stability of their health care insurance regime'. However in corollary and very strictly, it establishes three rules that the states must observe absolutely: non discrimination, objectivity and proportionality of decisions taken. To the Court of Luxembourg, it is clear that the circulation of a medicine between the countries in which it has obtained a marketing authorization must be total. Just as in the past however, certain Member States did not take this case-law sufficiently into account, thus falling under the blow of article 169 of the EEC-Treaty. Following several such cases the Commission announced its intentions very clearly in the White Paper on the completion of the single internal market which came out in 1985. Paragraphs 153, 154 and 155 of this document describe this most eloquently:

Paragraph 153: Of the total number of complaints received by the Commission, around sixty per cent, that is on average 255 complaints per year, are about articles 30 to 36 of the Treaty, but due to a lack of resources, they can only resolve about 100 cases per year. The delays and dossiers held up which result, are to the advantage of the offending states, prevent systematic action, create political and economic disequilibriums in the infringement procedures and a loss of confidence from industry as well as from the man in the street. Measures to remedy this situation are imperative.

Paragraph 154: In addition, the Commission will pursue its general action of improving and rationalizing its internal procedures so as to eliminate offences rapidly and efficiently. It will closely combine its preventative and penalizing actions, will examine the possibility of establishing sanctions and will consider all provisional measures which can be taken in order to halt the introduction of national dispositions which go blatantly against community law.

Paragraph 155: The elimination of unjustified barriers to exchange is traditionally done case by case by individual infringement procedures. Considering the practical inconveniences of these step-by-step procedures, the Commission will have to undertake more systematic action in publishing general communications which give the precise legal position which results notably from articles 30 to 36 for a whole economic sector or with regard to a determined type of barrier to trade.

It is the same in paragraph 156, where the Commission commits itself to 'give priority to publishing communications on ... pharmaceutical products'. This promise was kept in 1986 with the apparition of 'A communication from the Commission concerning the compatibility with article 30 of the EEC Treaty of measures taken by Member States as to the control of prices and reimbursements of medicines (86/C 310/08)' which summed up the state of positive law on the subject and stated the procedural rules to follow. Parallel to this is a proposition for a directive on price transparency of pharmaceutical products and the system of payments for medicines. After discussion, the directive itself was adopted by the Council on 21 December 1988. The timetable initially envisaged by the White Paper was thus scrupulously respected.

5.4.2 The Contents of the Directive

The analysis of the text can appear simple to non-forewarned readers. In fact, one must read between the lines and know the interests of the parties concerned well to be able to sort out what is definitively marked down and met with a consensus *grosso modo*, from what is likely to evolve further under various pressures.

1) The different protagonists

a) The Commission and the Member States It was the Commission which deemed it necessary to elaborate a directive aimed at transparency.

The directive is aimed at the Member State of the EEC (article 12); the operations foreseen, however, are not the same in every case. Thus it is that an exception is made for those who, like West Germany have adopted a policy which 'is founded principally on free competition to determine the price of medicines'. For the others, the demands vary according to the type of regulations in force (direct or indirect control on the price of the medicine, the existence of positive or negative lists ...), but with all the states having to conform to the directive by 31 December 1989 (article 11). However, nothing has changed deep down since 'these demands do not affect... the national policies in the matter of price fixing and the establishment of social security systems' and they put forward principles recognized by everybody since they emanate from Community legislation and of the judgement of the Court of Luxembourg. The independence of the states remains intact, as does their sovereignty.

b) The Industries and the Consumers The Commission and the Member States are not, however, the only players and in the wings the medicinal products industry and the European consumers stand out. One common worry moves them: to be associated as much as possible in the discussions to do with the directive so as to be able to present arguments and counter-arguments and thus best defend their interests. The stakes are high since in the system instituted by the EEC, Community regulations prevail over national regulations, and all directives, if they impose new constraints, equally constitute the pledge of a certain security by making the basic principles, the retained solutions and the procedures instituted, precise in the directive's field of action. Thus, the two groups show the same desire to participate, but - and this will not surprise anyone - each pursue their own objectives.

The European pharmaceutical industries have known for a long time of the need to be present at every strategic level. This is why, whilst continuing to develop individual strategies, they have for the most part re-grouped themselves around local associations, the latter all being adherents to the European Federation of Pharmaceutical Industry Associations (EFPIA), which serves as a privileged relay to the community institutions. Their hope of being associated, directly or indirectly, in negotiations has been all the better taken into consideration because they represent an economic force to be reckoned with: 2 000 firms, responsible for around thirty per cent of world production in medicinal products and generators of a positive trade balance of around 3.7 billion Ecus. Their immediate reaction when faced with the directive was negative, as it was against everything perpetuating controls hindering the freedom of prices. In their view, a product-by-product system of controls levels prices down, compromises companies' efforts in research and development and in the medium to long term damages their international competitivity. This evident hostility from business circles ran into the stoicism of the European Commission which judges this type of stand very unrealistic as long as the national authorities take on board an important part of the costs in medicines. Thus the industries made the best of the directive as a last resource from which they would force themselves to squeeze the maximum profit.

According to the European consumers, they themselves hold diametrically opposed arguments; in their view, in a situation where competition plays little or no part, the maintenance of prices at a reasonable level passes through a policy of price control. On this point, they are pleased with the judgement of the European Community Court of Justice but not with the directive and thus through this the Commission, because a lack of ambition in its past will play into the hands of the industries: 'The notion of transparency must not be exclusively for regulations but must apply equally to prices, the market and to research policy'. In particular, the directive as it is understood, 'does not aim for price transparency, but only for the transparency of price regulations'.[2] Their main fear, as expressed by the European Bureau of Consumer Unions (BEUC) is of seeing prices for medicines in Europe rise substantially, estimated at up to a hundred per cent in Spain, eighty per cent in Portugal and in France, seventy per cent in Italy and fifty per cent in Belgium.

The European consumers also regret not having been consulted as were the industries, and they denounce the lack of communication given out by the community authorities. This phenomena is not new, since in a decision of 28 October 1980, the Consumers Consultative Committee on the harmonization of European legislation of medicinal products stressed already the necessity for the Commission to 'not only submit its preliminary propositions to the industry but also to the consumers'.

In nine years, then, the consumers do not seem to have succeeded in enlarging their audience, despite the weight of 320 million European citizens for whom they wish to be the mouthpiece. Conscious of their setback they adapted themselves to the situation and, for want of being heard directly, they circulated their points of view by means of regular publications and they met a certain number of useful contacts such as, for example, members of the European Parliament, who on this occasion made themselves defenders of the consumer cause (note the case of Mr. Metten, socialist, the Netherlands, during the debate on the transparency directive).

2) The text itself   The provisions put to work by the directive call for comparison in their analysis. In effect the multiplicity of interested parties, the diversity of interests at stake, the differences in degrees of involvement at the time of discussion, have rendered the emergence of a true consensus very difficult and if certain provisions did not bring up major problems when they were adopted, some on the other hand, were keenly debated.

a) The elements of a certain consensus
The general philosophy of the text   This emphasizes the notions of transparency and competition, which could not fail to harvest the approval of all the parties.

In one of its first preambles, the directive recalls that 'the Member States adopted measures of an economic nature relative to the commercialization of medicinal products with a view to mastering spending on Public Health'. It then defines the pursued goals 'promoting public health by assuring a sufficient supply of medicinal products as a reasonable cost', and this whilst also bringing to the European pharmaceutical industry in a market which suffers unfortunately from 'insufficiency or absence of competition', the means of increasing its scope: 'such measures should also be destined to increasing the returns on production of medicines and to encourage research and the development of new medicinal products'.

The points of disaccord The consensus is broken when action must be taken and a directive must be elaborated upon. For the Commission, favouring transparency is

obtaining a view as a whole of the national agreements on price fixing including the way in which they apply to individual cases and all the criteria on which they are based, and to supply public access to all people concerned with the market for pharmaceutical products within the Member States.

But, as we have already underlined, neither the consumers nor the industries want to subcribe to this analysis. The consumers reject a text which only concerns transparency in pricing procedure and not price transparency itself. They cannot accept that a country such as West Germany should be excluded from the field of application of the directive, where price freedom at production goes hand in hand with high prices for medicines and they defend the idea that if a really effective intervention had to be carried out concerning transparency, then adequate measures have not yet been taken. The industry, for its part, continues to preach the abandonment of all controls and would like to see the directive being utilized as just a necessary but transitory stage on the road to price freedom for medicines.

The progress nevertheless realized Despite these disaccords on the surface, it is incontestable that the application of the directive will allow a greater transparency. Some of its provisions in effect encompass the national procedures for the price control of medicinal products, putting them in a common framework which appears more constraining for the authorities than in the past; others carry out the same exercise in the matter of the payment for pharmaceutical products by the Member States of the EEC. These procedures are shown in detail in Tables 3 and 4. From the evidence, the industries seem to be doing well: as the direct beneficiaries of new measures they are alleviated of most of the obligations decreed by the directive (time limits, justifications) which are incumbent and deplored by the BEUC upon the Member States.

b) A hard fought compromise The principal difficulties were concerned with the therapeutic classification of the medicines, with the eventual harmonizing of the transfer prices of pharmaceutical products between the 12 countries of the Community and with the setting up of the new Consultative Committee on Pharmaceutical Pricing (articles 8 and 10). The setting up of a databank was also the object of very serious controversy.[3]

The problem of therapeutic classification Arranging all the medicines existing in a given country by therapeutic class and sub-class constitutes a very difficult exercise on a scientific level if only for the reason of the possibility of multiple uses for the same medicine, and of the diversity of patients to which it can be prescribed. The comparison of different international systems has shown, furthermore, that extrapolation on a European scale of a national system is without value, given the persistence, even today, of deep differences in medical culture between neighbouring countries. The interest of

158

a classification is evident when considering that this system permits both the choice of products with adequate reference when the price of a new medicine is fixed and the almost automatic attribution of a rate of reimbursement to the products in question. Was it not necessary, then, to reply fully to the objectives of transparency in the directive and hence improve the functioning of the Common Market, to agree to the wishes that the Commission had formulated in the first version of its directive project and let it adopt, if it judged it necessary, 'a directive on the harmonization of national dispositions relative to the classification of medicines for the use of the Social Security systems'?

Only the consumers showed themselves favourable towards this idea; for their part, manufacturing circles, the European Parliament and the Council judged this rapprochement premature and declared themselves hostile to any delegation of power over the subject to the Commission. Prudence prevailed and the directive is content to impose on Member States, the communication before 31 December 1989 of the 'criteria concerning the therapeutic classification of medicines...used by the competent authorities to the end of applying to the national system of Social Security'.

The problem of transfer prices In this area too, the Commission allowed itself the possibility of adopting, after consulting the Consultative Committee, 'a directive for formulating guiding principles relative to the harmonization of national criteria concerning the verification of the fair nature of the transfer prices'. The Parliament and the Council reacted in the same manner as before in condemning the slightest inclination towards delegating to the Commission. However, the case is not exactly the same as in that of therapeutic classification and the bargaining was more complex. From the beginning, the pharmaceutical industry strongly affirmed its suspicions with regard to all efforts to bring national criteria on transfer prices into line with each other - illusory whilst there are such great differences between the Twelve in rate of inflation, exchange rates and fiscal policies.... The industry has always underlined the horizontal nature of the problem, common to all industrial producers from multinational companies and recalled that the OCDE had already defined basic principles, recognized and applied by fiscal as well as customs authorities. As to Parliament, divided on the question, some of its members recommended the setting up of more ample measures, notably obliging the multinational pharmaceutical companies to transmit all the necessary information on the transparency of transfer prices to the authorities. Facing such divergent points of view, the Council played the role of referee and came up with the following compromise: certain disputed dispositions concerning transfer prices in particular would disappear from the directive; instead a databank would be created.

The databank The birth of this databank brought out some very animated debates. First of all it became the object of one of the 21 amendments adopted in the first reading by the European Parliament in March 1988, the objective sought being to improve competition even more in the pharmaceutical sector and to promote a more rational use of medicines. Such an amendment adopted by a very large majority (299 votes for, seven against), did not impede the Commission from the moment where it did not involve the publication of confidential information and where it remained compatible with the decreed rules on competition, it was also incorporated without discussion, into the revised directive project. But certain delegations expressed their reservations on the way the databank was to be drawn up and opposed the insertion of such a measure in the body of the directive. However, it appeared impossible to drop this idea and for two reasons: first, the insistence of parliament and second, the symbolic value attached to the databank, considered as a favourable aid to abandoning certain stray impulses concerning therapeutic classification and transfer prices. Thus a compromise solution was found, the Council choosing to record its interest in the question in a supplementary political declaration and upholding the databank's constitution under the aegis of the Commission with a set budget and subject to parliamentary control. The databank should have been set up from December 1988 with the joint aid of the Member States, the industry and the importers. Its content is fixed by statute; in particular for each product will appear the summary of its principal characteristics as mentioned in directive 65/65/EEC; pharmaceutical form, its pharmacological and clinical properties, its pharmaceutical peculiarities, its ex-factory price, its retail price, the cost of usual daily treatment and the dispensary characteristics (hospital, chemist, self-medication or prescription).

The Consultative Committee The chance to create a Consultative Committee which would make a pair with the Committee for proprietary medicinal products of a more scientific vocation was never contested. The tasks that it might be set, on the other hand, have greatly evolved over time. It was proposed:

a) that it discuss and supply a judgement on questions that the Commission could bring up about therapeutic classifications of medicines or about the criteria used by competent national authorities to verify the fair nature of transfer prices;
b) that it encourage the development of a European policy on medicine;
c) that it examine all questions relative to the application of the directive, whether asked by a Member State, the President of the Committee or whether it has come from the Committee's own initiative.

Finally, only the last of these tasks was retained with, however, one restriction, since the Committee no longer possesses the power of self-initiative and thus is totally reliant in its function on the good patronage of the Commission and the Member States. It still represents no less of an important organ of reflection and recommendation. It remains to be seen what its true audience will be and in what measure the Commission will take it into account.

5.4.3 What Future for the Transparency Directive

The problem which poses itself is, what real impact will the directive have? If any certainties do exist, numerous hypotheses still remain.

1) A certain number of guarantees exist
a) Some are linked to the principles of Community law
The possibility of the transparency directive being applied directly In the vast majority, dispositions of European law are immediately applicable from the moment they are clear, precise, unconditional and need no intervention of any subsequent act. The Treaty of Rome only expressly foresees transparency for regulations; on the other hand, in principle, the directives cannot display their full potential until they have been transposed into internal national law.

In fact, this last demand was considerably softened, thanks to the judgement of the European Community Court of Justice, concerned above all with maintaining the rights of those justifiable in the case of incorrect or non-transposition of a directive (Van Duyn judgement, 1979): so long as the time period allowed for the transposition has not run out, no steps are possible; on the other hand, after the expiry of the time period and if the decreed dispositions are sufficiently clear and precise (as in the case concerning transparency), any national of the EEC can appeal for the directive in front of the law courts of his country.

It must be stated that there is a characteristic of the transparency directive which reinforces its potential effectiveness; this detail is that the date on which the fixed time limit for the transposition to internal law expires gets confused with the date of the coming into force of the directive itself.

The primacy of community law By virtue of this assumption, national courts are obliged to apply community standards even if these are contrary to the dispositions of the Member State.

b) Other results of specific dispositions in the text
The Member States are subject to a double obligation According to article 11 of the directive, Member States must have brought their internal law into line with the community standard before 31 December 1989 and have communicated to the Commission, also before this date, a certain amount of information relative to 'criteria concerning therapeutic classification of medicinal products... which are used by the competent authorities to verify the fair nature and transparency of prices invoiced for transfers within a group of companies, of the principal drugs or intermediate products used in the manufacture of medicines or finished pharmaceutical products' (article 8), and to 'legislative, regulatory or administrative dispositions relative to price fixing of medicines, to the profit of the manufacturers of pharmaceutical products and to the reimbursement of medicines by the national health insurance system' (article 11).

The Commission sees itself set a new task The Commission will have to submit to the Council, before 1 January 1992, 'a proposition including appropriate measures, with a view to putting an end to distortions or barriers which exist in the area of the free circulation of proprietary medicinal products with the hope of the further harmonizing this sector with the normal conditions of the internal market' (article 9).

This mission will necessitate the establishment of a preliminary report because the proposition for a new directive will have to be formed by 'the light of experience' only. The role that the Commission will be called to play, in the near future, appears once more to be essential, even if the standard procedure retained (proposition of a directive to the Council) gives it less freedom than a delegation of responsibilities.

The behaviour of the Member States and the industry is very tightly regulated The procedure for the price determination of medicines for human use will henceforth obey very precise rules. The same applies for the eventual inclusion of a pharmaceutical product or category of products in the national health insurance system. The detailed analysis of the procedures was shown in Tables 5.9 and 5.10.

2) Despite all these guarantees, the range of the directive will depend only on the effective use made of it by the industry
a) Two scenarios are possible
A status quo dictated by prudence It is obvious that the industry should take full advantage of a directive that gives it guarantees over the time permitted and the bases for decisions. They can, however, quite legitimately fear a guardian administration which has the privilege of having public power and because of this give up the benefits of a new tool, however promising it may be.

A more positive attitude It is, however, more probable that faced with the importance of the economic stakes, the pharmaceutical industry will overcome its apprehension and take advantage of a systematic strategy for exploiting the possibilities offered by the directive.

Thus we can ask the question, who will be in the best position to take advantage: small, medium or large laboratories, national groups or foreign subsidiaries? We can also think about the risks incurred: will they be of the same type and will they carry the same importance for everyone? One last question raises itself: how far will the industry demands go? Will they be content with explanation of their own dossiers only, or will they try to expose any eventual discrimination of products from competing laboratories? Will they clamour for public justification of decisions taken by the competent authorities, and in what measure will they oppose this practise because of the confidentiality attached to certain elements of a dossier?

With regard to this, the fourth preamble to the directive, aimed at obtaining 'a view as a whole of the national agreements on price fixing, including the way that these are applied in individual cases' and at providing 'public access to these agreements to any person concerned with the market for pharmaceutical products within the Member States', could form the beginnings of a reply. But the wording is too ambiguous; what is more it is not a disposition but only a consideration of the directive....

b) The effects of the directive will reveal themselves over two periods
In the short term Until now, decisions taken by the authorities regarding prices and reimbursement have often been too largely stamped by economic consideration: the first objective was to ensure better control over health spending; the second aimed at setting up local research and production centres, thus permitting the creation of jobs and the development of exports.

The administration and the authorities thus concluded reciprocal commitments of which the counterpart was the concession of more favourable conditions on prices. This practice obviously goes against the requirements of community law; the ambition of the Commission is to completely do away with this type of special advantage and the transparency directive was elaborated to guarantee, if not equality of opportunity, at least the equality of treatment between different groups in the pharmaceutical industry.

In the medium term Laboratories will be led to change their thinking and will develop a new industrial strategy; in particular the optimization of means of production will be looked at on a European scale, taking into account cost differentials for workforce, transport, energy.... The probable result will be a restructuring of production and research potentials, giving way to a policy of delocalization, inter-company agreements, even mergers.

162

Elsewhere, the relationship between the administration and the industry might invert itself; the latter, without hope of any specific advantage, will show itself more intransigent over the prices accorded to their new products, arguing in particular about the very large disparity of prices for medicines in Europe and menacing the authorities with non-commercialization in the home country. This emergence of 'orphan states' in Europe might serve as a spearhead for the consumers and make the position of the administration even more fragile.

5.4.4 Conclusion

On a scientific and technical level, the process of eliminating the obstacles to the free circulation of pharmaceutical products is well under way: the proposal concerning the future community system for marketing authorization should have been presented before the end of 1989, conforming to the envisaged timetable in the Commission's White Paper. The elimination of these obstacles on an economic level constitutes a new stage, perfectly illustrated by the transparency directive.

Other initiatives - directives on branding, restoration on the length of patents... will however be necessary to complete the work undertaken. The delicate problem of the opportunity to harmonize the different price and reimbursement systems in Europe will still exist. The Commission may not have said its last word on the subject, but progress can only be very slow when one takes into account the different political and economic option of the 12 Member States.

5.4.5 Notes

1 Judgements CENTRAPHARM-WINTHROP (1974), CENTRAPHARM (1975), ROUSSEL and others versus the Netherlands (1983), the EEC Commission versus FRG (1984), DUPHAR and others versus the Netherlands (1984), CLIN MIDY (1984), LUXEMBOURG versus BELGIUM (1986).
2 Draft decision of the Consumer Consultative Committee on the proposition of the directive concerning the transparency of measures governing price fixing of medicines for human use and their cover within national insurance systems. (Com. (86), 765 final - JO C 17 /1987)
3 Transfer prices: invoiced prices for the transfers (within a group of companies), of the principal drugs or intermediate products used in the fabrication of medicines or of finished pharmaceutical products.

Table 5.9
Measures Favourable to Foster Transparency

Type of case involved	Obligations incumbent upon the applicant	The obligations incumbent on the competent authorities and the consequences these imply		Other
		The time limits for reply in the case of a negative response	Information which must be provided	
1 Marketing authorization is only given after consultation on the price of the product by the competent authorities (article 2).	The holder of a marketing authorization asks for a price for a given medicine. He must transmit adequate information to support this request.	- The decision must be taken and communicated to the applicant within 90 days of the reception of the application.	- In the case of a refusal, the decision must contain a statement of reasons based on objective and verifiable criteria.	- The list of medicines for which the price has been fixed during the period of reference is published at least once a year, as are the prices which can be applied to such products.
The case of Belgium, Spain, France, Greece, Italy and Portugal		- If necessary a request for detailed additional information is immediately made. - The final decision must be made within 90 days of the second exchange of information. - In absence of a decision in those 90 days, the applicant may market the product at the proposed area.	- The applicant is informed of the existence and nature of the remedies open to him as well as the time-limits allowed for applying them.	- Publication is made by an appropriate body, in communication with the Commission.
2 The increase in price of a medicine is only authorized after preliminary agreement by the competent authorities (article 3)	- The applicant must deliver adequate information, including details of facts which having intervened since the medicine's last price fixing justify, according to him, the price rise requested.	- The decision must be taken and communicated to the applicant within 90 days of reception.	- If the rise is partly or wholly refused, the decision must include a statement of reasons based on objective and verifiable criteria.	- The list of medicines for which price rises have been accorded during the period of reference and the prices which can be applied to them in the future, are published at least once a year.
- The case of the Netherlands		- If necessary a request for detailed additional information must be made immediately. The final decision must be made within 90 days of the receipt of the new information. - If the number of requests is exceptionally high, the time-limit may be prolonged by 60 days. Notification is given to the applicant before the expiry of the original time allowed. - In the absence of a decision after the further delay, the applicant is authorized to apply the desired price rise in full.	- The applicant is informed of the existence and nature of the remedies available to him as well as the time allowed for their commencement.	- The publication is made by an appropriate body and is communicated to the Commission.

Type of case involved	Obligations incumbent upon the applicant	The obligations incumbent on the competent authorities and the consequence these imply		Other
		The time limits for reply in the case of a negative response	Information which must be provided	
3 There is a price freeze on all medicines or only on certain categories of them.				
a. The general case		- The Member State verifies, at least once a year, whether the macro-economic conditions justify the maintenance of the price freeze. If increases or decreases in price are carried out, they must be announced within 90 days.		
b. In the exceptional case where the holder of a marketing authorization for a medicine requests a derogation for a particular reason	- The request must include a statement of reasons.	- A decision must be taken and communicated to the applicant within 90 days. - When necessary detailed additional information is immediately asked for. The final decision must be made within 90 days, to begin from the date of receipt.		- If the derogation is allowed, it must be published immediately.
4 There exists a system of direct or indirect control of profits (article 5) The case of the United Kingdom		- The Member State must publish and communicate the following information to the Commission: a. The method or methods used to define profitability: return on sales and/or return on capital. b. The range of the rates of authorized profits. c. The criteria by which the reference levels of profit are individually granted to those responsible for marketing, as well as the criteria by which they will be allowed to retain profits above their given targets in the Member States concerned. d. The maximum percentage of profit that those responsible for the placing of medicinal products on the market are authorized to return over and above their target.		- In certain cases, the state sets to work a system of profit control. Articles 2, 3 and 4 of the directive thus apply if necessary.

Table 5.10

Measures Favourable to Transparency in the Field of National Health Insurance Systems

Type of case involved	Obligations incumbent upon the applicant	The obligations incumbent on the competent authorities and the consequence these imply		Other
		The time limits for reply in the case of a negative response	Information which must be provided	
1 A medicine is only covered by the national health insurance system if it figures in a positive list (article 6)				
a. The case of the inclusion of a product within list	- The holder of the marketing authorization must request the inclusion of his product within the list. He must submit adequate information to the competent authorities, if this is not the case, the time limit is deferred. - If the request for inclusion precedes the acceptance of price or if the two decisions result from the same administrative procedure, the time limit is prolonged by 90 extra days. In the case where the price must be fixed before inclusion within the positive list, the total time for the two procedures cannot exceed 180 days.	- The decision must be adopted and communicated to the applicant within 90 days of the receipt of the application - If necessary, a request for detailed complementary information is immediately transmitted to the applicant.	- A rejection of inscription must include a statement of reasons, based on objective and verifiable criteria, including if appropriate the views or recommendations of the experts, on which the decisions are based. - The applicant is informed of the existence and nature of the remedies open to him as well as the time-limit for their application.	- The reasons for inclusion on non-inclusion of medicines within the list must be published and communicated to the Commission before 31 December 1989. - The complete list of products covered by the national health insurance systems as well as the prices fixed for each of them, must be published and communicated to the Commission before 31 December 1990. The information must be updated at least once a year. - The diverse publications are made by the appropriate official publication.
b. The case of the exclusion of the product from the positive list			- Any decision of exclusion from the list must include a statement of the reasons based on objective and verifiable criteria, including if appropriate, the views of recommendations of the experts on which the decisions are based, and must be communicated to the person responsible for marketing. This person is informed of the remedies open to him as well as the time period allowed.	
c. The case of the exclusion of a whole category of medicines from the positive list			- It must contain a statement of the reasons based on objective and verifiable criteria.	- The publication is made by an appropriate body.

Type of case involved	Obligations incumbent upon the applicant	The obligations incumbent on the competent authorities and the consequence these imply		Other
		The time limits for reply in the case of a negative response	Information which must be provided	
2 A medicine or a whole category of medicines can be excluded from the range of the national health insurance system (existence of a negative list). (Article 7)				
a. The case of the exclusion of a whole category of medicines			- Any decision of this type must include a statement of reasons founded on objective and verifiable criteria, and must be published.	
b. The case of the exclusion of one medicine in particular.			- The decision includes a statement of reasons based on objective and verifiable criteria and if appropriate, the views or the recommendation on which they are founded. It is communicated to the person responsible who is also informed of the remedies open to him and the time-limits.	- The Member States publish and communicate to the Commission the chosen criteria for exclusion before 31 December 1989. - The publication is done by an appropriate body. - The competent authorities publish and communicate the list of particular medicines which have been excluded from the range of the health insurance system to the Commission before 31 December 1990. - The information must be updated at least every 6 months. - The publication is made by an appropriate body.

6 Health Care Management

Contents

6 Health Care Management

6.0 Introduction
W.J. de Gooijer

6.0.1 Introduction

The single internal market, viewed as a major growth-oriented project, will test the managerial skills of the economic and social actions, on the one hand, of recognizing and exploiting opportunities and, on the other hand, distinguishing between and resolving problems and unfounded fears. The fact that the Single European Act is silent on the subject of health care enhances the challenge facing health care managers (Doherty). Part of this challenge is the lack of consensus for political actions for making health care pave the way in the further evolution of a Citizens' Europe (Schutyser). There are however opportunities for development in a European way, if we are able to solve problems like the need for non-ambiguous European (health) care statistics and data registration, the growing shortage of health care personnel in many European countries, the improvement of salary- and labour conditions included, the frictions between the different social security systems that will arise from the evolution of a free European insurance market and the establishment of European medical centres of excellence beyond the country borders. To tackle these problems it is absolutely necessary that we have a database containing information on population needs and demands, service provisions to meet those requirements, the effectiveness of those provisions and the cost of providing them (Grimes). The information needs to provide comparisons of institutions, over population groups, over geographical divisions, and eventually, over countries.

Apart from this we have to realize that health care is a highly labour-intensive affair. Taking this into account it is a fact that worker participation is very differently institutionalized within the European Community. It is, therefore, not unrealistic to assume that as a consequence of 'Europe 1992' the development of worker participation will stabilize on the level of the country that has a lack in development compared to the other member countries (Van Zuthem).

6.1 Europe 1992 and the Consequences for Health Care
A first survey and discussion paper
W.J. van der Eijk et al

6.1.1 Summary

The integration of the European market is prompted by developments in the world economy. Multinational companies play the leading role in these developments. In the coming years, employers will make a bigger mark on many areas of society than ever before. There will be a resurgence of the 'spirit of free enterprise' in the next decade. This is also the case for the health care sector.

It is not so much the direct effects of measures from the European Commission in Brussels that will have an influence on health care. The secondary effects on the process lying behind the 'Europe 1992' phenomenon will, in their indirect way, have a far greater bearing on this. Both the 'White Paper' from Brussels and the Dekker Plan from the Dutch Government in The Hague can be seen as manifestations of this very same process.

Employers will probably influence health care in the areas of finance and insurance even more than before. We anticipate an acceleration in the decrease of levels of taxation and social premiums. In that case, pressure may increase on health care to organize the supply of facilities even more efficiently. Also, both employers and employees will be increasingly reluctant to fund a package of health care provisions as extensive as the present one. This will probably cause health care to become more directed towards 'cure', that is, more medically-orientated. We view this as cause for concern. If no change in policy is forthcoming within the next five to 15 years, a segmentation will occur within the existing health care sector. This will entail a hardening of the distinction between acute treatment and chronic care, which will spread throughout all the traditional areas of health care, altering current funding and management systems.

In this connection, three possibilities present themselves. The most probable scenario will involve the funding of acute somatic care from social premiums and insurance money and the funding of chronic care (together with welfare services) from tax revenue. The two sectors then created will possess separate management systems and negotiation circuits.

An increasing number of privatization and commercial initiatives will be taken in the areas of care of the elderly, welfare services and acute somatic care. In this last field specifically, privatization and commercialization will be particularly prevalent in the fields of hospital representation, guidance and counselling: many 'hospital consultancies' will appear and possibly compete with the Hospital Centre.

Health insurance and improvements in the efficiency of organization of health care services will progressively become more closely associated, falling under a single area of administration. Indemnity insurers will have to evolve into care insurers in order to survive. As a parallel, those who provide care will have to evolve into care insurers in order to hold their own ground. This presents an opportunity of high strategic importance for the Hospital Centre.

The primary issues in health care policy will be those of insurance and finance. The new game will be played, in a new arena, by 'agents' who have undergone metamorphoses or who have newly appeared. The weaker sections of society (the unemployed, patients and consumers) will, at least in the short term, still have no significant role to play. They will have to fight for their rights at a European level.

Employers, but also the Treasury and the Ministries of Social and Economic Affairs (with their attendant consultancies) will become of increasing importance to health care. The increased pressure on the collective tax burden will force health care to compete with other areas, among them social welfare and the Arts.

The increasing influence of employers and the constantly developing process of unification of the European Market will cause changes in the health care decision-making process. The trends are towards the dominance of finance and insurance organizations and towards a change from national to European and Euro-region level. New areas of negotiation and new spheres of influence will arise. This process has not yet been fully clarified.

Cartel formation will proliferate throughout the health care insurance world and more foreign companies will appear on the Dutch market. These will also begin to sign agreements with those who provide care in other countries. Companies will also start signing collective health care insurance agreements for their employees. Should the so-called Dekker Letter be implemented, health insurance funds may start operating as private health insurers. However, they will first have to amass sufficient reserves.

The evolution of pure medical indemnity insurance towards a more comprehensive care insurance will continue, because of the increasing importance of organizing care provision efficiently. Depending on the extent to which the health insurance market is opened up, comprehensive care insurance may even develop into an entirely new branch of insurance, separate from indemnity insurance. It may be productive to organize this on the same lines as the HMO in America. Alternatively, care services may be managed by the new health insurers themselves. In the long run, chronic care services and welfare services will increasingly be removed from the health insurance package.

A greater variety of medicines will be admitted onto the open market. Prices will be fixed according to a band system. The government will acquire a more important monitoring role in this, but will find it necessary to be flexible enough to able to step in quickly. The way medicines are distributed will alter. It is here that strategic possibilities for the Hospital Centre lie.

Foreign banks will start offering their services in the Netherlands. There will be mergers. Loans from foreign banks will become more attractive. It is anticipated that insurance companies will also offer loans to facilitate investment.

We do not yet know how the alterations in the VAT system will affect health care. From a macro-economic point of view, these adjustments will have a negative effect on the Dutch government's budget. Resources will have to be found elsewhere to compensate for this. This is why cuts may be expected; cuts which will also affect health care.

Foreign building companies will begin to compete on the Dutch market. Their projects will be temporary, staffed by foreign employees and will take place with social premiums in operation. Because of this, they will be able to undercut the competition.

It is not clear to what extent the planning regulations will continue to function and what exactly the consequences will be of border-crossing patient traffic, freedom of practice and residence for health care practitioners, a concentration of high-grade clinical functions and the signing of agreements between insurers and those who provide care in foreign countries. Follow-up research, in connection with the possible implementation of the third Dekker Letter and the Oort Plan, will be necessary.

6.1.2 Introduction

The level of publicity surrounding 'The Unification of the European Market in 1992' has recently increased. This has led to my initiative of a preliminary collection of data regarding the opening of European borders in 1992, and the consequences for Dutch health care. This proposition was first discussed within the National Hospital Association (NZR), where I worked at that time, in May 1988. It was decided to make a preliminary investigation into the possible consequences of the opening of the borders in 1992, in order to assess whether, on this basis, further research into specific areas of interest was merited.

In the following, I will present the results of the preliminary survey. This paper was originally prepared for the management and board of the NZR and National Hospital Institute (NZI). It was suggested that it might be useful to exchange contributions with foreign colleagues concerning the possible consequences for health care of the opening of European borders. This is in view of the fact that health care in all European Community Member States will inevitably be influenced by the positive and negative effects of the opening of the European internal borders. The reader should remain aware that this paper was compiled on the basis of the situation in the Netherlands, and is primarily intended as discussion material for the management and board of the NZR and the NZI; therefore I have included some more information about the situation in the Netherlands in 1988.

In 1986, the Dutch Ministry of Welfare, Public Health and Cultural Affairs decided to create the Steering Committee for Structure and Finance of Health Care. This committee was assigned the task of finding radical structural solutions for the financing difficulties of Dutch health care. The chairman of this steering committee was Dr. Wisse Dekker, former head of the Dutch electronics conglomerate Philips. Accordingly the committee was named the Dekker Group, after its chairman. In the context of the Dutch situation, it was striking that someone from the private sector became so actively involved with health care. When the findings of the Dekker Group were submitted to the Dutch Government, they replied with a series of three letters, later called the 'Dekker Letters'. The content of the Dekker Letters thus represents the reaction of the Dutch Government to the recommendations of the Dekker Group, the so-called Dekker Plan. A number of radical measures were proposed:

a) there will be a mandatorily deducted basic insurance package for all Dutch people plus a supplementary insurance. All insurers will be obliged to accept every applicant (a statutory duty of acceptance). Premium differentiation will be outlawed. The basis insurance package will not only cover costs directly incurred through illness, but also includes cover for the provision of related fields of care, such as that of the elderly and in the home. About eighty-five per cent of medical expenses will be covered in the basic insurance package, and the other fifteen per cent by the supplementary insurance. The premiums for these insurances will be paid by employees (partly on a percentage basis and partly on the basis of a statutory fee).

The Dutch health insurance market is currently divided. The sickness insurance organizations account for sixty per cent of the market (dealing with people with an income of less than Hfl. 50 000), with private insurers accounting for the other forty per cent (those with an income of more than Hfl. 50 000). The idea behind this is to abandon the distinction between health insurance funds and private insurers. This should lead to fiercer competition between the insurers, which is in turn expected to increase efficiency. The forty per cent of the market open to tender from private insurers will be reduced to around fifteen per cent.

b) Dutch health care should become more susceptible to the influence of market forces. Levels of health care are currently strictly regulated by government planning strategies. The intention behind this is to achieve greater efficiency by a tighter grasp of the purse strings plus deregulation of the planning system. Negotiations will also be set up in the Dutch regions between insurers and those who actually provide care, resulting in the conclusion of contracts concerning the extent, type and price of care offered.

c) The Dekker Plan will have consequences for the incomes of Dutch citizens. A second group, called the Oort Commission, has also been active in the Netherlands in formulating a new restructuring plan for the tax system. Since the 'Oort Plan' also affects incomes, the two plans will be introduced simultaneously. The Oort Plan proposes the incorporation of health insurance premiums into taxation. The majority of Dutch health care is currently funded from social insurance premiums contributed by both employers and employees.

European readers should realize that the health insurance package in the Netherlands is somewhat sizeable. In recent years the insurance package has been extended to include a great number of non-medical activities. This enlarged package incorporates various welfare services. Dutch in-patient care falls into four sectors: general and teaching hospitals, psychiatric institutions, care for the mentally handicapped and nursing homes (care for the aged falls under welfare). It covers a rather broad spectrum, and all four sectors are characterized by high standards. Dutch institutions are practically all privately run, as are the NZR and the NZI. Responsibility for care rests with the private sector. The Dutch government has a predominantly stimulating and subsidizing role, with a subsidiary monitoring function. The Netherlands is also known for its liberal attitude towards private health insurers (with forty per cent of the market).

In this paper, I will attempt to locate the 'Europe 1992' phenomenon in a wider framework. This is the process that underlies the publication of the White Paper from Brussels. I will further define the correspondences with the field of health care. With this process in mind, I will present three possible scenarios for the development of health care. Following this, we intend to formulate the possible conditions that may become important when considering the future orientation of the NZR and the NZI.

175

After defining a general framework, I will attempt to interpret the proposals from Brussels[1] which may be related to health care, giving regard to their effects, and to locate them within the above framework. In this respect, I will not only examine the content of measures proposed or accepted, but will also incorporate opinions of relevant external officials. Possible consequences for the Hospital Centre will not be ignored.

I stress the role of employers strongly in this paper. In the interest of clarity, it should be pointed out that this term also refers to multinational companies and to the influence of an atmosphere geared towards private enterprise, and to the resurgence of enthusiasm in the private sector.

Finally, I will enumerate the options available to the Hospital Centre and to the in-patient care sector, in order to deal with the developments attending Europe 1992 adequately.[2] I recommend the development of follow-up activities.

6.1.3 Global Developments

A search for the roots of the phenomenon 'Europe 1992', will soon arrive at the 'White Paper' written by Lord Cockfield.[3] This paper begins with 300 measures (later reduced to 280) suggested in order to achieve a single European economic market, with a free flow of people, goods, services and capital.[4] With these suggestions a schedule has been drawn up, with 1 January 1993 as the target starting date. Every two years the respective national government bodies must present an evaluation of progress, at national level, in implementing decisions from Brussels. In the Netherlands, however, Parliament has proposed that this should be done annually by the Government, and also that, henceforth, each reading of a new bill should have regard to its possible relationship to the process of unification of the European Market.

By the 27 April 1988, 69 of the suggestions made in the White Paper had been approved by the European Council of Ministers, and 126 remain under consideration. The European Commission has at present submitted 208 of the 286 suggestions to the European Council. It is questionable whether the Council will be able to deal with all of these in time.

This White Paper has not appeared out of thin air. It has come into being after a number of leading businessmen from large European multinationals (Dekker from Philips, Agnelli from Fiat, and so on) gathered together to form a think-tank concerned with Europe's future world status in economic competition, in particular with Japan[5] and the USA. New policy developments were necessary to avoid Europe falling behind, with various attendant social and economic consequences.

Thus the initiative originates from a circle of leading European captains of industry. The European Commission's appreciation of the concern of these businessmen prompted the publication of the White Paper. The starting principle in both circles was the status of Europe in competition with Japan and the USA. A secondary benefit of a strengthening of this status would be an improvement in the employment situation.

In order to be able fully to evaluate the Europe 1992 phenomenon and adequately to assess the state of play, it is, in our view, important to recognize that a certain category of leading European are initiators ('agents') taking as a guiding principle the strengthening of Europe's ability to compete against Japan and the USA (the 'objective').

At the heart of the Europe 1992 phenomenon we are thus concerned with the agent multinational and the objective, strengthening of the ability to compete. Correctly to identify agents and their objectives will tell us more about changes already in motion as well as those that still lie in the future.[6]

The fact that Europe 1992 is a momentous historical event with its roots in the corporate world is easily explained. On a global level an economic struggle is running rife,[7] in which increased mutual dependency, internationalization and increase in scale constitute a process that private enterprise, particularly the internationally-minded company, was the first to encounter. The European private sector quickly became aware of the possibility of, or rather the need for, an integrated European market.[8] In the light of these developments in the world economy, it becomes easier to appreciate that it is the private sector which is the substantial force behind the move towards abolishing internal borders. After the economic integration has taken place, a certain measure of political integration will become necessary. The role of the new supranational government will be to create a suitable environment and an infrastructure for the newly integrated economic market.

Major companies are the most important agents in this newborn power vacuum, with its dearth of pre-set rules for power-play and market forces at the European level. It is widely accepted that in situations where uncertainty and insecurity about the location of power run rife, those who assert themselves, use their initiative and set their objectives firmly in their sights, will be able to take command and determine the rules of the game. Ultimately, it should be taken into account that European decision-making rarely attains an optimal level, and is often somewhat unclear, both at supranational level and between supranational and national governments.[9]

Our fundamental assumption is that the leading entrepreneurs of European multinationals will inevitably be the ones to determine policy, or at least retain an important guiding function, with employers,[10] the European Commission and the various Ministries of Economic Affairs[11] following in their wake. It is their objectives that will define the face of Europe, therefore it is essential to keep a close eye on these objectives.

Consumers and patients have as yet no significant role to play at either a national or a European level. Just as, at the turn of the last century, employers and employees had to fight for their respective positions in the then power vacuum, the time has now come for a repeat performance at European level.

6.1.4   Possible Consequences for Health Care

The (large) companies will attempt to strengthen their ability to compete by:

a)   creating a larger market;
b)   decreasing production costs and wages;
c)   focusing on high-quality training, research and innovation;
d)   improving quality.

It is mainly the second objective[12] which will affect health care: the employers will press for a decrease in gross wages. Because of the need for a balanced relationship between gross and net wages, the structuring of gross wages will have to be re-evaluated. After all, a reasonable level of purchasing power, that is, a sufficient net income, is not only in the interests of employees, but also of equal importance to employers. Important components of the gross wage include taxation and social premiums. Given this background, it is to be expected that in future, taxation and social premiums will be lowered.[13] It is precisely here that the 'link' with health care is to be found. After all, social premiums represent an important part of health care funding. This, at least, is the case under the present system.

I expect the employers to make their mark upon the organization of health care,[14] increasingly pressing for the lowering of, amongst other things, social premiums (and a more efficient management of services). They will use the lower collective tax burden in most other EC countries to back up their argument. Harmonization of social security systems will become an important political issue in the future, already the case with the lowering of taxes.[15]

Given this background, Europe 1992, like the Dekker Plan, is merely an emphasis and manifestation of a political process already being encouraged or, if you will, dictated by developments in the world economy. Strengthening of the ability to compete is becoming a more and more legitimate political argument, now that people possess an increased consciousness of the need to survive economically. A number of considerations manifest themselves here:

a) Employees will become less willing to contribute to the current health and welfare package
b) It will be necessary for employers to contribute more to health care. In fact this amounts to an alteration in the direction of cash-flow: privatization. However, it is also in employers' interests that health care remains affordable to employees and that the relationship between gross and net wages remains in proportion
c) Both employers and employees, as well as those directly involved in the labour process, will begin to pay more attention to what they get for their money
d) This means pressure on health care to operate both more efficiently and effectively will increase. Companies, health insurers and special interest groups may want to conclude their own collective agreements and/or adopt control of cure services themselves
e) This means that employers will have a greater interest in maintaining a healthy work force than in caring for people no longer involved in the labour process. That is to say, employers will increasingly begin to question the need to subsidise the chronically ill, the aged and all those who no longer work. They will be less and less inclined to contribute in these areas.[16] However, it is in their interests to facilitate the return to work, fit and well, of their employees. This is why the distinction between acute somatic health care ('cure') and chronic care or aid ('care') will become more defined. This will lead to a cutting back of the health care package with a bias towards cure-directed services, as well as changes in what are usually understood as welfare and social services[17]
f) In order to maintain an acceptable standard of acute care, chronic care and social services, whilst social premiums and taxation are being cut back, citizens/voters and the authorities will be forced to chose their priorities with regard to patterns of expenditure. This means that the EC countries, each according to their own individual practices, will have to choose priorities with regard to expenditure yet to be allocated. In practice, more choices will have to be made than was previously necessary. For instance, should more money be devoted to art subsidies or to care of the mentally handicapped? Thus, health care will be exposed to even fiercer competition from other sectors in society.

The trends outlined above may well result in the emergence of a more clearly defined distinction between acute somatic care and chronic care. This will also manifest itself in the future structuring of funding and insurance. The question is what consequences this will have for the way the various areas of health care will be organized. In the following chapter a number of possible scenarios will be detailed.

6.1.5 Possible Future Developments

Because of economic developments on a global scale, employers, or rather the influence of a climate favourably disposed to the private sector, will increasingly make their mark on health care.[18] This is especially the case as regards the collective tax burden. The health care package will be cut back at the expense of chronic care, which will tend to be accommodated in the welfare and social services package. Within the political arena, heavy competition will arise with other areas of expenditure, like the Arts, housing, preservation of the environment and so on. The process of segmentation which entails the hardening of the distinction between acute and chronic care, will permeate all health care sectors, irrespective of traditional divisions. Put simply, this is the probable outcome if no modification is made to current policy.

However, other variants are possible. Employers are primarily interested in reducing social premiums and taxes (structure of gross wages). It is they who will be in a position to exert influence at the negotiating table in the area of social premiums. On the other hand it is Government and Parliament, with the wishes of the electorate in mind, who will be the more dominant negotiating party in the area of taxation. At first sight, it appears irrelevant which component of the gross wages is cut, as long as the sum total is indeed reduced. From a purely mathematical point of view, it is merely a cosmetic exercise to finance health care more heavily from taxes than social premiums, or vice versa (so long as the overall expenditure remains the same).

There are, however, two different considerations, on the basis of which three different scenarios may arise:

a) The direct interest that employers take in the health of their employees. There is no direct interest in providing care services for sick employees no longer able to take part in the labour process, except a moral one. Employers, but also employees will increasingly question the need to contribute to funds of no direct profit to them. With the advent of a business-orientated culture and the persistence of the cult of the individual, I expect a weakened feeling of solidarity.[19]

b) Strategic considerations: the method of funding determines the terrain on which actions take place. Employers (and increasingly employees as well) will continue to want to exert direct negotiation on the form of the collective tax burden. The implementation of the Oort Plan will be of great importance in this respect.

1) Scenario 1 - The Corporate Model: In spite of the segmentation of acute somatic care and chronic care, both will still be funded from social premiums and insurance funds. For both, but especially chronic care and welfare aid, employers will exert pressure for cuts to be made to the package, especially with regard to its welfare aspects. These latter services will largely be offered on a commercial basis. Health care will become more medically-orientated. Once they reach the negotiating table, those who represent health care will find themselves hindered by the need to defend an extensive package.[20]

The additional benefits of acute somatic care (automation, technologization, planning, protocol and so on) are much more significant than those derived from the caring and nursing sector, which is seen as having a much more traditional and practical character. Employers have less direct interest in this latter sector.[21]

In this event, care of the mentally retarded, as well as the majority of nursing and mental health care, will be placed under heavy financial pressure. In view of the size of the package they defend, and the growing influence of their partners in negotiation, representatives of health care will find themselves in a somewhat uncomfortable position. Pressure on chronic care may be alleviated by means of a special insurance package for this category of serious risks, such as the 'VOR'.[22] Among other groups, the Dutch health insurers' organization advocates the funding of this 'uninsurable' category of risk from insurance money rather than from tax revenue.[23] Insofar as this is concerned, private insurers may be considered coalition partners by the health care lobby.

2) Scenario 2 - The Government Model In this scenario, all health care will be funded from tax revenue. When tax revenue is assigned a specific target destination, it is possible to use the term 'national insurance'. In this case, health care will find itself facing the Government as its primary negotiation partner. The influence of the segmentation process will not be so strongly felt. The necessity of defending a large package will once again cause difficulties in negotiation. This may be aggravated because the package of services will be continually extended into the welfare sector. In addition, all health care will have to begin competing to a greater extent with social security, the Arts, agriculture, and so on.

In this event, it is highly likely that pressure on the collective tax burden will be difficult to avoid. It is to be expected that employers and employees will find themselves with interests in common, and will bargain with the government as if they were partners in coalition. The implementation of the Oort Plan may be considered a step towards embracing this Government model. However, there is still uncertainty as to what exactly should be done with the funds collected for health care under the Oort Plan. It is feared that there is no specific target destination for the revenue collected. In that case, health care will experience competition from welfare, the Arts, agriculture, and so on. A cumbersome negotiation process is likely as well as one over-strongly influenced by ballot-box decision-making.

3) Scenario 3 - The Mixed Model: Acute somatic care will be funded by social premiums and insurance, whereas chronic care will be funded from tax revenue. Thus two funding systems will come into being, with two separate arenas for negotiation. Consequently, the process of segmentation will have a great impact. Because the packages in question will have become relatively small, a more favourable negotiating position will ensue in the two separate arenas with their differing authorities. Employers will be the most important negotiation partners for acute somatic care and the Government for chronic care.[24] In this event, it would seem that both kinds of care, accommodated in their separate negotiation arenas, will be easier to defend. The successful functioning of acute somatic care is directly in the interest of employers. Chronic care will be in a more favourable position in negotiating with the government, which faces political choices and has a greater interest in concepts of solidarity. Since, in both cases, the packages in question are smaller, the negotiation position should improve (in comparison with other sectors).

In this scenario, significant segmentation will occur, but not interfere with the maintenance of 'cure'. It has been suggested that chronic care funding should be made independent of tax revenues. Conversely, others believe that 'care' will be more fully safeguarded against the whims of the electorate if covered by an insurance system.

6.1.6 The Possible Consequences for the Dutch Hospital Centre: A First Orientation

Because employers will probably gain a larger influence on health care, and because insurance and funding will become the dominant factors, it may be anticipated that the following functions of the Hospital Centre will become important considerations:

a) its function as an employer,
b) its funding, management and investment function and,
c) its role as arbitrator.

Also, the future method of financing adopted will have an influence in determining the way health care will be run. In scenario 3, the so-called Mixed Model, two different management systems come into being. The management of the Hospital Centre will have to anticipate this development adequately.

1) Function as employer Insurance and funding issues are closely bound up with collective bargaining policies and other optimalization issues. In its capacity of representing health care employers, the role of the NZR (National Hospital Association of the Netherlands) will be to discuss this so-called budget or volume policy with its financiers: the workforce and the government. It is anticipated that this function of the NZR will become more and more important. It should be added that this function may have to be redefined. At present, the NZR has a dual role. On the one hand, it functions as a negotiation partner for employees; on the other hand, the NZR protects the interests of health care in its entirety, including those of employees, patients and consumers. If the NZR were to adopt the function of a health care insurer, this would cause its (strategic) position and, therefore its role, to change again (seen paragraph 2 (below) and 6.1.7 (2)).

2) Funding, Management and Investment Function The NZR, in its capacity of employer, should be able to secure, by negotiation, a sufficiently substantial initial budget for the health care institutions; in its funding capacity, it supports these institutions with various management services, by obtaining resources for investment and by protecting other resources. It is expected that in the future, the Hospital Centre will be asked to support health care institutions more and more in managing their finances. Therefore this function will grow in importance.

In this connection, a pilot study concerning the feasibility of setting up an independent insurance and/or investment company may well be considered useful (perhaps in collaboration with existing insurance companies and banks).

In this way, the Dutch Hospital Centre might become an insurer and financier, and would thus be in a position to create investment by distributing loans.[25] A second benefit of this option would be the possibility of anticipating the growing tendency for the gap to narrow between the practice of medical indemnity insurance, run strictly on a commercial basis, and the increasingly efficient organization of care services, resulting in the creation of a comprehensive care-orientated insurance package ('care insurance'). See also paragraph 6.1.7 (2).

In the event of an alteration in the funding and insurance system, attention to the provision of guaranteed research funding will be necessary, especially for those hospitals conducting research (teaching hospitals and larger general hospitals). This funding will have to be kept separate from funds used for the day-to-day running of hospitals.

3) Arbitration I expect health care institutions to make greater demands on the arbitration function of the NZR. In a more business-orientated climate, with survival becoming an even more apparent reality, arbitration will be a more frequently necessary resort in the event of conflicts, and in cases where there is need for legal aid.

4) Miscellaneous Functions I anticipate that the future demand for support of institutions will fall particularly under the following headings:

a)   management support for institutions and
b)   meditation in the event of disputes and so on.[26]

Thus, the Hospital Centre will find itself sharing a market with various kinds of agencies and consultancies. Competition with commercial agencies will be more prevalent.

The present function of *quality control and improvement* will be developed in such a way as to be adapted to fit in with the scenarios and functions described above. That is to say: its shape will be determined by those who will be paying for health care. This function will decline in importance for the Hospital Centre. The shaping of this function will mostly be at a regional level, as part of the market mechanism.[27]

For the same reasons, the present function of *planning*[28] will be subsumed under other functions, and will become increasingly determined within each region. Planning, as it has traditionally been carried out in health care, will no longer be effective. The concept of marketing will have to be taken into account as planning develops.

It should be expected that the *research function* will also be carried out on a more commercial basis.[29]

The various factors detailed above will have consequences for the future structure of service provision for health care institutions.[30]

6.1.7   The Measures from Brussels

The economic integration of Europe has been awaited for many years. This delay has especially hit the European business world, particularly the multinationals. In 1984, they expressed their concern to the European Commission. Besides voicing their concern, they also submitted a paper indicating how one single integrated European Market could be achieved. Their concern was appreciated by the Commission, and the list submitted served as the basis for what later became the 'White Paper' by Lord Cockfield; this contains just under 300 proposals. I have researched which of these proposals may, directly or indirectly, have consequences for health care. So far I have selected 24 proposals. In addition, there have been talks with a number of external officials. On the basis of this selection and both internal and external discussions, I have come to formulate the following areas of attention.

It should be mentioned that the text has been structured in such a way as to offer as many issues within the areas of attention as possible.

1) Top-grade Clinical Facilities Especially as far as top-grade clinical facilities in the border regions are concerned, changes can be expected in patient traffic. Even though, on the basis of existing international agreements regarding social health insurance, it is already possible for patient traffic to cross borders, and no new guidelines in this field can be expected from Brussels, the creation of Euro-regions will have an influence on the orientation of their inhabitants. It is expected that existing possibilities will be exploited to greater advantage.

There are existing guidelines concerning traffic. Insufficient data was available for us to be clear about the scope of these guidelines, therefore the exact nature of their influence on international road and air ambulance traffic (neonatology and organ transplants come to mind) should be further investigated.

Social health insurers especially, would seem to be in favour of creating a number of 'Centres of Excellence' at a European level. That is to say, a concentration of high-grade medical facilities. They hope that in this way, the costs of, for example, heart operations and neurosurgery can be brought down. Should a stage actually be reached where health insurers systematically set up these centres at a European level, this would mean that the fundamental principle in the Treaty of Rome that health care should be carried out on a national basis, would have been abandoned. Health insurers have agreed to adhere to this principle in the Treaty of Rome in future. However, they appear to want to make an exception for their Centres of Excellence.

2) Border-crossing Patient Traffic As noted in paragraph 6.1.7 (1), changes in patient traffic may be expected in the border regions. The whole situation will hinge on the options insurers offer to their customers. Because these options are as yet unknown, I have only been able to assess those claims valid on the basis of the Dutch AWBZ (Exceptional Medical Expenses (Compensation) Act).

3) Freedom of Practice With the exception of paramedical professions, at present all qualifications within the health care sector are recognized in every EEC Member State. Restrictions on freedom of practice and freedom of residence will be eliminated by the measures from Brussels. These measures prohibit discrimination on the grounds of nationality. It is the combination of freedom of practice and freedom of residence that may have effects on the employment situation. Until now, no link has existed between the two. The guidelines control the mutual recognition of foreign qualifications. This means that if a qualification is issued in one European country, it should be valid in all other EC countries. However, it is the case that Member States sometimes specify conditions concerning the freedom of practice, which will then count for everyone in practice. One is reminded of the system behind planning and licensing. It is questionable, however, whether the planning and distribution of licences may be considered to constitute restriction of trade. The Court of Justice in Luxembourg provides a forum for complaints in this connection. The European Commission encourages citizens and the business community alike, to exercise their right of complaint if they are 'suspicious'. I am not convinced that significant changes in the nature of the job market are likely, should the present planning system be maintained. Radical changes will only occur if the proposals of the third Dekker Letter are implemented.

However, it is true that since foreign specialists will now be in a position to settle in the Netherlands with greater ease, specialists with a Dutch qualification will, in principle, lose their monopoly of the job market. Since this will probably only occur on a small scale, it is unlikely to lead to a lower level of tariffs. (Statistics have shown that, up until now, migration has only taken place on a very small scale: only a couple of hundred people per year are concerned among all professional groups.) It should be noted here that health insurers may sign contracts with employees abroad (for further reference, see paragraph 6.1.7 (4)

The combination of the effects of

a) concentration of top-clinical resources,
b) freedom of practice and freedom of residence,
c) border-crossing patient traffic, and
d) signing of agreements with those who provide care abroad,

will require careful monitoring and should be explored more fully by a follow-up study (see recommendations: 8, 13 and 19). Within our assignment, I have confined myself to a pilot study, since as yet little data is available.

4) The Insurance and Banking System[31]   The guidelines from Brussels will make it easier for foreign insurers and banks to offer their services in the Netherlands. However, insurers are bound by the guidelines to retain twenty-four per cent of their assets in reserve. If, after the implementation of the proposals in the third Dekker Letter, Dutch health insurance funds become private insurers, they will have to build up this level of reserve assets as well. The framework for this to be possible is being set up. Thus, it is obvious that the third Dekker Letter is crucial to this area.

I think it significant that Wisse Dekker, one of the members of the interested group of businessmen, was also the chairman of the commission that devised the proposals for restructuring the health care industry.

The Netherlands is an attractive market for foreign health insurers (forty per cent private). With the exception of Belgium and West Germany, the private sector in other Member States represents only two - seven per cent. Government health care systems exist in most Member States.

Incidentally, extensive government involvement can be used to discourage the admission of foreign health insurers. This is because, under the present situation in Dutch health care, it would be difficult for foreign health insurers to accuse the Dutch planning and accreditation regulation of constituting trade restrictions. There has been more and more talk about the privatization of health care in the other Member States. For example, if it were left entirely to Mrs. Thatcher and the UK Conservative government the bulk of the NHS would be sold off.

In Dutch health insurance fund circles, it is felt that the basic health insurance package should be regarded as a strategic instrument to exclude unwelcome foreign influence. The statutory duty to accept applicants, the prohibition of premium differentiation, and so on are mentioned as methods to achieve this. The Association of Dutch Health Insurance Funds,[32] together with its EC sister organization, intends to argue, via the AIM[33] in Brussels, for the threshold for foreign insurers to be raised. Also within AIM, the health insurance funds are holding internal discussions about the possibility of cutting their costs by funding a number of European 'Centres of Excellence', for high-grade medical functions, to be administered by a body of their own, similar to the HMO in America.

It has been noted that Dutch health insurers are none too happy about the intrusion of foreign health insurers into an already overloaded health insurance market. The possibility has been suggested that foreign insurance companies would be prepared to forego the subsidy from the central fund, should the statutory obligation to accept all applicants and the prohibition of premium differentiation then be waived.[34] This does not only concern insurance companies from other Member States: in particular those from Japan, Switzerland and the USA appear extremely interested in the European insurance market. They see the Netherlands as an ideal bridgehead for this purpose.[35]

The hypothesis of foreign health insurance companies being prepared to forego the subsidy from the central fund and thereby to avoid the statutory obligation to accept each applicant and the prohibition of premium differentiation is rejected by the KLOZ (the Dutch organization that defends the interests of private health insurers). They consider it legally impossible. EC insurance companies cannot be excluded from the Dutch market on the grounds of their nationality. They must, however, comply with Dutch law. Just as with planning regulations, freedom of practice, and so on, no case has ever been brought to the Court of Justice in Luxembourg on these grounds.

In the near future, Dutch and European insurance companies and banks are expected to form cartels (see paragraph 6.1.3 and 6.1.4). A number of large (health) insurance companies will remain, some of which will form partnerships or merge with other European conglomerates.

In the insurance world, some feel that damage risk should be assessed at a regional level. This implies that, for example, a Dutch company seeking to operate in France would either be required to open an office there and immediately acquire the necessary expertise, or take over a French insurance company. Insurers of this opinion are less afraid of takeover and cartel formation.

The private insurance companies held an entire day of talks on the effects of opening the European borders on Dutch health care insurances. During these talks, they surveyed the whole of the Dutch health care market and concluded that few changes were likely, simply because any foreign insurance company can already operate in the Netherlands. There are already many foreign companies in the market. They merely have to comply to the solvency conditions (which are supervised by the Insurance Regulations Office) and put down a deposit.[36] A certificate of professional competence is also required. These areas are regulated by the WTZ (the Dutch law on admittance of insurers to the field of health care insurance) and the WTV (law on admittance to indemnity insurance). The Association of Insurers,[37] however, is of the opinion that, although foreign insurers are already free to operate on the Dutch market, the opening of the borders will still encourage them to become even more active in the Netherlands. This might be the result of a cartel formation being anticipated. Insurers hope that, in this event, they would be able to protect themselves by improving their market position.

According to KLOZ, the Dutch health insurance market has been left fairly open to competition. West Germany and France are examples of EC countries that have made up so many regulations in this area as to render the market inaccessible to foreign insurers. Dutch insurance companies are currently attempting to make this restriction of trade an issue at the European Commission.

KLOZ takes the view that Dutch insurers are likely to succeed in the foreign market, rather more than foreign insurers will in the Dutch market. This is because there are

185

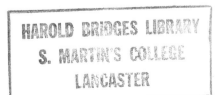

hardly any private health insurers in the EC, and therefore a corresponding dearth of expertise.

Thus there is, in actual fact, very little free market space available in the EC for the private health insurers. Even in the Netherlands, this space will not grow with the implementation of the Dekker Plan. Thus the market is strictly regulated, and this is because health care in Europe is considered part of the welfare system. The Association of Insurers has asked the European Commission to monitor the extent to which the welfare system is privatized.

According to KLOZ, the present guidelines from Brussels will hardly have any direct influence on the insurance systems. However, a number of secondary effects can be expected. Two factors play a part in this; surplus of facilities, and the greater shaping role of employers on health care.

The primary influence of employers will be towards a more efficient organization of care. Well-organized care is therefore in their interest. Employers feel that resources are often wasted. Since, according to them, a surplus of facilities exists, they will increasingly be in a position to select those providers of care that function most efficiently. This is in view of the fact that companies are expected to begin signing more collective agreements for their personnel with those who provide care. This not only applies to companies, but also to insurers and special interest groups in society (for example anthroposophers). The trend is towards organization on HMO lines. In fact, the most characteristic aspect of this development is the tendency for purely medical insurance (indemnity insurance) to move in the direction of more general care insurance. That is to say; a merging of insurance and the organization of efficient care provision. According to this view, a smaller number of care insurers will remain in existence (such as the 'OHRA' and 'Zilveren Kruis' companies). If those whose interest lies purely in the indemnity insurance sector (for example 'Nationale Nederlanden') do not adapt, then there is a real chance that they will not survive. Cuts are expected.

Alongside the remaining care insurers, large companies and insurance companies will also offer care under the auspices of their management. A firm like Philips is able to calculate reasonably precisely the indemnity cost they will incur for their personnel. For companies like this, the signing of collective agreements on behalf of personnel as well as the incorporation of care under their own management is expected to be beneficial.[38] That is to say, it serves their self-interest. Pressure will be placed on employees to abandon their mutual solidarity. In any event, the employers will acquire more influence on all areas with society. This will be the new spirit of the times.

When the above developments transpire, it will be necessary to take the creation of separate clinics designed for specific high-grade care functions into account. For example, the Netherlands is known for its dental and oral surgery, and clinics specializing in this are therefore quite likely to be founded. In the long run, this could radically change the organizational structure of hospitals. This is particularly true for top-clinical and high-grade functions.[39] KLOZ does not share the view that of all the top-clinical facilities in Europe, only the Centres of Excellence will remain. The size of the patient population is too great for this to happen.

In addition, KLOZ refers to the fact that an increasingly aged population is developing. In the future, the elderly will have been used to a higher standard of living, with greater purchasing power. These elderly people will have different needs from those of today, and probably consider the quality of health care a higher priority. There will be a larger market for health care and social services, with the emphasis shifting away from clinical care towards maintaining care within the home, for as long as possible. Private initiatives are to be expected, and insurers will monitor this trend in the market carefully.

Private insurers take the view that the sectors of care of the mentally handicapped, nursing homes and the mental health care, ought to be funded from social premiums or, to put it another way, out of national insurance rather than taxes. The size of this high-risk package must not become an electoral issue. In fact, the risks in this area are relatively stable and predictable, that is easy to calculate. In addition, insurance companies are expected to begin to make loans. This may be important should hospitals wish to make investments. Many of those interviewed expect that will be a harmonization of the social insurance systems in the long run. In contrast to the current situation in the Netherlands, a greater distinction is likely to develop between the funding, insurance and management aspects of acute somatic care. The mutual effects of these processes on one another need to be monitored.

Finally, it may become an attractive prospect for Dutch in-patient care to take out bank loans, particularly in the UK and Belgium, where interest rates are much lower. According to the Cecchini Report growth in the financial services industry is going to accelerate, because of the creation of a large single market with great potential for expansion. A lot of mergers in the banking industry are expected, creating a higher standard of efficiency. The smallest decrease in insurance costs is expected to be in the Netherlands (together with the UK and Luxembourg), which, according to the Cecchini Report, points to a high competitive status.

5) Tax Systems and VAT Levels[40] VAT payments will take on an increasing importance for health care funding. This is because, in a number of countries in the EC, VAT is charged on goods and services either directly or indirectly relevant to health care. Under harmonization of payments and duties, there may well be a VAT charge levied on health care. This would entail a considerable rise in health care expenditure. (Dutch health care institutions and practitioners are not currently liable for VAT payments. VAT on medicines is six per cent. I am not aware of the situation in other countries). There is a secondary factor in the background: the relationship between national and supranational governments. More control over policy will be transferred to Brussels, which will demand larger financial resources. This will cause changes in the taxation system, and VAT will be an important factor here.

In any event, a review of the VAT system will be disadvantageous for the Netherlands. According to the Dutch Treasury, budgetary problems will be created here, because of the high existing VAT tariffs in the Netherlands. A reduction in VAT is expected. The resulting shortfall in revenue will have to be made up from other areas. The result could be additional government cuts. This will probably not result in an increase in direct taxation, which might inhibit Dutch companies' ability to compete effectively (no support will be found for an increase in taxation, since both employers and employees would object to a bigger wedge being driven between net and gross earnings). Future plans for regulations in this area are as yet unknown.

A few surprises can be expected here, as will become apparent from the following example: during talks with the VNZ (Dutch Association of Health Insurance Funds), I am told about the VNZ computer department being found liable for VAT by the Dutch Treasury, simply because this department also caters for third parties.

6) Medicines There are two important guidelines here: first, guidelines concerning the rationalisation of prices, and second, guidelines concerning the definition of what a medicine is.

Measures regulate the admission of new products to the market. At present, it is more or less the case that each country registers the admission of a new medicine individually. This is done in the Netherlands by the 'Medicine Monitoring Board'. The idea behind the EC guidelines is to harmonize the procedures under which new medicines are admitted. Ideally, when a new form of medicine is admitted to one EC country, it should be admitted throughout the entire EC, and should not have to undergo a different procedure in each country.

At present, most medicines are covered by national insurance. Thus, genuine price calibration does not take place. An international pricing policy is sought, with restrictions to be put on what can be defined as a medicine. These guidelines have reference to the social insurance package. In this connection, it is important to remember the Duphar case, brought to the Court of Justice in Luxembourg. The verdict resulted in criteria being laid down for the negative lists for medicine that have been compiled by the health insurance funds.[41]

In principle, freer admittance of medicine to the market will become possible. The new medicine guidelines introduced on 1 January 1989 also allows governments to impose price blocks. Besides this, a price-fixing policy will be introduced. This means that if the price of a medicine is higher than the set price, then the consumer will have to pay the difference. Many people anticipate a fall in the price of medicine.

Another area to be focused on is the expected changes in the distribution system. In the present situation there is the question of parallel import. If it is found that medicines can be bought more cheaply from a factory in Spain, this will have an influence on the present lines of import. The question arises: what influence will this have on the wholesale trade? In this connection, the Medispatch case comes to mind, in which the company wanted to have hospital laboratory tests and experiments carried out more cheaply in Belgium. Other hospital charges would then rise. For this reason, the VNZ (Dutch Association of Health Insurance Funds) opposed the Medispatch plans at the time. The extent to which hospitals farm out their functions to third parties is likely to increase, in view of the financial pressure. However, it is difficult to predict accurately how often this will occur.

7) Technology Assessment In general, the policy will involve the concentration of knowledge, research and innovation, especially at the top end of the scale. Practical research in the medical and technological fields will be fused together to forestall the duplication of investment (and therefore, inflated and uncompetitive prices). A fast information exchange system will be required to coordinate these areas. This may be a useful opportunity for the Hospital Centre.

A decision about who will coordinate Developmental Medicine at a European level is important to the hospitals and the insurers, as well as to the Dutch Ministry of Welfare, Public Health and Cultural Affairs and that of Education.[42]

8) Ethical and Cultural Norms and Values Only one guideline exists with direct reference to this. It concerns personnel medicals. What effect this will have on, for example, the policy on AIDS, remains unknown. This requires further attention.

The so-called Bio-card is worthy of note here. This is a card with an electro-magnetic strip on which a full run-down of medical information can be stored, and called up on a computer. There have previously been discussions at EC level about the Bio-card, but no decision on policy could be reached. The Royal Dutch Medical Association (KNMG) strongly opposes the Bio-card, on the grounds that abuse is possible, for instance when passing through customs.[43]

In general, it is to be expected that political discussions about topics of an international character that concern health care, will result in the adoption of those norms and values that accord with the realization of the aims of the business community. This will be achieved under the guise of harmonization. Parallels can be drawn with Dutch judicial policy on drugs and traffic offences. The Dutch government has been forced to compromise in these areas in order to come to agreement with the German government.

9) European Decision-making Policies Concerning Health Care The 1992 phenomenon is part of a process of economic integration that transcends national frontiers. Freer commercial traffic will limit the decision-making capacity of national government.

The liberalization of the economic market will compel governments to bring their economic and monetary policies closer together at European level.

The question arises: how will these developments affect health care? At present these areas are largely administered by the Directorate-General of Social Affairs in Brussels, coming under 'research' rather than 'policy'. The importance of full communication between the Dutch Ministries of Social, Financial and Economic Affairs, rather than with the Ministry of Health, has already been stated. At present moves are already under way towards the fixing of premiums and tariffs being dealt with by such bodies as the National Economic Development Council (SER) and the Joint Industrial Labour Council (Stichting van de Arbeid).[44] This trend is supported by recommendation 1.a.

10) Miscellaneous Finally, it should be pointed out that there are no measures from Brussels with a direct bearing on the monitoring and stimulation of planning and/or standards. In this paper, I have been focusing on the possible secondary effects of these measures, for example the effects of patient traffic crossing borders, the effects of the concentration of top-grade clinical functions, freedom of practice, the increasing importance of marketing and the tendency for quality control to be connected, at a region level, to the working of market forces.

6.1.8 Excerpt of Relevant Recommendations with regard to the EEC-Hospital Committee

Here I will show how the Hospital Centre can anticipate future developments. On the one hand these recommendations come from the consequences of the measures of the White Paper from Brussels and on the other hand from developments behind the White Paper and of which the Dekker Plan is also a manifestation.

1a) Reorientation Present Lobby-practice It is recommended to promote the interests of the intra-mural health care (via the employers organizations) at the Ministries of Finance, Economic Affairs and Social Affairs. This promotion of interests will not only have to take place on a national level, but also on a European level. Promotion of interests should also take place on the level of the counterparts of the above-mentioned

Ministries of the European Institutes. Taking into account the more prominent role of the European Parliament and the European decision-making procedures, this organ also deserves the necessary attention. Intra-mural health care must not miss the opportunity to participate in the recent discussions about the 'social dimension of Europe'.

1b) Reflection on the Position of the EEC-Hospital Committee The role and position of the EEC-Hospital Committee has to be overhauled. It is recommended to utilize the EEC-Hospital Committee as a better policy instrument - with the status of private enterprise - to influence decision-making in Brussels.

1c) Analysis of the European Field of Force It is also recommended to attain a deeper understanding about the decision-making processes in Brussels and those between Brussels and The Hague. A practical survey is advised as to the (future) position of health care within these decision-making circuits. In this perspective the positions and objectives of the leading players have to be studied. It is necessary to invest now in a survey in order to present proposals later on.

1d) Conceptual Support of Lobby To acquire a deeper understanding of the relevant subject and because of the above-mentioned lobby work it is recommended to initiate additional policy-preparing activities within the NZR-office, possibly in close cooperation with (the participants of) the EEC-Hospital Committee. Taking into account that the employers look after the total sum of the social premiums and tax components which comprise the gross wages and do not differentiate from the different components of which the social premiums have been built up as such, it is advisable to get a better view of the costs of the intra-mural health care in relation to the amount and quality of the product, also in comparison with those of other EC-countries. The Dutch Christian Employers Organization (NCW) let the NZR know that they consider this a responsibility of the NZR. The outline plan is to look only after the costs, but also after the volume and quality of the delivered health care.

2) Segmentation It is recommended that attention is paid to the interaction of the process of harmonization of the European social security systems and the process of segmentation.

Examination of how to cope with the process of segmentation is advocated; which preferences exist with regard to the source and system of financing and insurance and the steering system belonging to it. It is recommended to initiate a survey on the financing and steering systems of health care in the other EC-countries in close cooperation with the EEC-Hospital Committee.

3) Cohesion with Dekker Plan It is recommended that consideration is given to the opinions of the NZR with regard to the implementation of the Dekker Plan in cohesion with the mentioned and endorsed statements in this document (obligation of acceptance, differentiation of premiums, international agreements and contracts with health care suppliers abroad and the process behind the White Paper).

It needs to be taken into consideration whether the Hospital Centre has something against the arrival of foreign health care insurance companies and if so, what? In that perspective the future position of the Assurance Chamber has to be kept in mind (to a greater extent than simply checking with the solvability, because of harmonization with the Assurance Chamber in other EC-countries).

4) Foreign Patients, Personnel and Border Crossing Contracts (suppliers abroad and hospital functions) Investigation is recommended of the consequences of opening up the European internal borders for border-crossing patient traffic and the freedom of professions in combination with the freedom of establishment of professionals, and to contract foreign providers of health care. In this perspective also, the consequences of concentration of top-clinical supply have to be taken into account as well as the establishment of foreign institutes for health care in the Netherlands and the deregulation of the planning system of health care facilities (WZV).

5) Level of Institutes Translation is recommended of the now-surveyed consequences of Europe 1992 on a macro-level, to the possible consequence for the institutions. The management of the institutions will have to be instructed with necessary information and skills to cope with these problems in advance. The translation of macro-level to the level of the institutions has still to be completed.

6) Public Relations It is recommended to increase public interest for the position of health care with support of an active PR and lobby policy. This is in view of the greater competition anticipated with other social and cultural provisions.

7) VAT It is recommended to advocate to the government and employers organizations that changes in the VAT system may not lead to VAT pay-off by the institutes for health care. Moreover, it has be presented that services rendered to outside organization will be subject to VAT. This will have to be implemented by the Ministry of Finance. Do health care institutions in other EC-countries have to pay VAT?

8) Research It is advisable to consider whether the Hospital Centre should set up a 'rapid-information-exchange-system' to prevent double research and investments. If possible this may be done in collaboration with the Royal Dutch Medical Association, the Ministry of Health or the EEC-Hospital Committee. The question is, who is going to coordinate the development of medicines on a European level?

9) Emergency Admissions It is recommended to develop proposals arranging emergency admissions of foreigners.

10) Ethics It is recommended to observe decision-making in Brussels and to pay close attention to ethical aspects (AIDS, euthanasia, Bio-card, biomedical experimentation, patient policy and so on). It is advocated in this respect to collaborate with the Ministry of Health, the Royal Dutch Medical Association and the National Patients and Consumers Platform.

11) Traffic It is advisable to examine the various traffic measures on possible consequences for border-crossing by air and by road ambulance (neonatology and organ transplants).

12) Radiation Effects It is recommended that the organization of an informal workshop and small circle with other organizations involved in health care should take place. Private enterprise in health care transformed into government beaurocracy should be avoided.

Following that, a major congress for all EC involved persons and institutes/institutions in health care has to be set up, to profile health care in Europe in more detail.

On the basis of this first survey, recommendations and discussions, a policy has developed in which a *'plan-de-campagne'* for the NZR will be presented.

6.1.9 Notes

1   This refers to the 280 or so proposals in the 'White Paper' drafted by Lord Cockfield.
2   This term represents various other descriptions: 'Europe without borders', 'The unification of the European market', and so on.
3   The former British commissioner to the European Commission for European Integration. The 'White Paper' was published in 1985.
4   In order to put these suggestions into practice fully, the so-called European Act was passed. It serves as a kind of lubricant for the decision-making process. With the exception of issues of tax and finance, this act may be implemented with an authorized number of votes and does not require unanimity.
5   Here Japan should be seen as only one among the up and coming nations of the Far East, which include South Korea, Taiwan and Singapore. These countries are characterized by low wages, high productivity, high quality products, and the accumulation of knowledge. High technology research and innovation are their definite strengths.
6   In the meantime, several new agents have begun to pull their weight in the economic arena, including the European institutions, the various national governments, and also, later, the unions, employer's federations, consumers and so on.
7   The concept of 'struggle', in the sense of the mobilization of all resources available in order to survive against one's competitors, will not be explored here. It need only be said that Japan had formerly confined itself to the duplication of Western goods, whereas it now purchases western research and innovates in the high tech field, thus repaying the western world with the creation of employment, an objective set at an ideological premium in Europe.
8   The acquisition of a sizeable market opening is not the only objective. Lower production costs, that is lower wages, higher standards of quality, the accumulation of knowledge and innovation, especially in the high tech fields, are also important factors. It is, in turn, possible to translate these objectives into the fields of industrial relations, education and research.
9   The term 'leakage of funds' is inclined to crop up here, referring to the tendency of money to flow from national to supranational level.
10 Small- to medium-sized companies should also be mobilized.
11 In the past six months a countermovement has emerged with the motto 'the social dimensions of Europe', led by the Commission's chairman Delors, the French president Mitterand and the (divided) European unions. The Commission has recently suggested a statement dealing with the social dimensions of the internal

market, to form the basis of a discussion amongst all the social partners of the Member States.

12 If these objectives are to be striven for, unification and harmonization must be considered important subsidiary aims. Equalization must take place to create the single market, but harmonization of social, legal and taxation systems, with their attendant social, ethical and cultural standards, is also necessary. With respect to political decision-making about international health care problems (AIDS, euthanasia, and so on), I would venture to say that those norms will be introduced that will facilitate the realization of the above objectives and subsidiary objectives. This, incidentally, is also true of, for instance, the work ethic.

13 In the Netherlands, these measures, or at least proposals to the same effect, are already being put into action.

14 The first significant manifestation of this trend was the appointment of one of the concerned European 'captains of industry' as chairman of the Dekker Commission. This group was assigned the task of formulating far-reaching proposals with regard to the infrastructure of Dutch health care. In addition, employers are generally expected to make themselves felt in many other sectors of society as well.

15 It has been suggested that harmonization in the areas of finance and taxation is not always necessarily in the interests of major corporations.

16 Recently, even amongst employees, statements have been heard implying that some workers might abandon solidarity if higher wages were offered.

17 This means that, although chronic care and aid will be considered a welfare service, some of its components will be privatized (for example social services and care for the aged, home care, and so on).

18 This is also true for other sectors in society.

19 The interests of employers and employees tend to become increasingly associated. Also it is likely that the unemployed and special interest groups of patients will increasingly express themselve through Government and Parliament. This is true for the consumers as well, but this group will also exert its influence via insurers, if there is any question of market forces coming into play.

20 In the field of negotiation, 'the smaller a package, the easier it is to negotiate ... the larger it is, the more difficult', is a valid motto.

21 Both in scenario 1 and in scenario 3, research funds should be kept separate from funds intended for the maintenance and management of health care institutions.

22 The so-called VOR (Insurance for Uninsurable Risks) is an initiative of the National Hospital Association of the Netherlands (NZR). The present Exceptional Medical Expenses (Compensation) Act (AWBZ), originally had the same aim: the insurance of large and high risks such as chronic illness. In the course of time, more and more only marginally connected services were added to this AWBZ-package, causing it to exceed its intended scope.

23 The Dutch organization that defends the interests of private health insurers is called KLOZ.

24 In view of the fact that policy is becoming increasingly dominated by insurance and financing, the most important governmental negotiation partners will be the Ministers of Finance and Social Affairs.

25 Strategically speaking, the killing of two birds with one stone in this way is greatly advantageous for the NZR's position. Furthermore, it will facilitate anticipation of

the grouping of pure indemnity insurance and organizational efficiency in care provision under a single command.

26 This does not necessarily imply that other NZR functions, such as innovation in both care and general fields, will disappear.

27 At present, state supervision plays an important part in the protection of standards of Dutch health care. According to the Dekker Plan, the Dutch government should eventually have only a marginal monitoring role. The maintenance of standards will lie much more in the hands of insurers and those who provide care than at present. In future regional contracts between those who provide care and insurers, not only costing and levels of care will be taken into account, but also quality.

28 Planning will be deregulated and moved to a regional level. In the regions, increased exposure to the market mechanism will necessitate greater market orientation.

29 In the Netherlands, it is anticipated that the demand will arise for the flow of money in the direction of umbrella organizations, at present guaranteed, to become less free.

30 Because of increased outside pressure, the NZR will be forced to justify its existence on the basis of its representative function. The NZR is, after all, an association of in-patient health care institutions.

31 These proposals revolve around three principal maxims:
    a) harmonization of the standards of management control, in order to protect the consumer,
    b) mutual recognition of the way in which each Member State implements these standards,
    c) supervision and control, from their own home country, of financial institutions functioning abroad.
    This implies that banks and insurance conpanies will be free to offer services on the basis of a single licence issued in their own country, provided they are able to observe the guidelines which relate to their assets. The insurance guidelines are mostly concerned with high risk (mass insurance). Health insurances are not mentioned specifically.

32 VNZ - Vereniging van Nederlandse Ziekenfondsen.

33 'Association Internationale de la Mutualité,' the Association of European Health Insurance Funds (and non-profit making insurers).

34 Premiums are deposited in a central fund. From this, the money is then allocated to the health insurance funds, in accordance with the previously agreed scale of payment.

35 The Netherlands is known for the tolerance of its investment and business climate towards insurers. Moreover, it is sometimes regarded as the distribution centre for Europe.

36 The Association of Insurers anticipate that the tasks and responsibilities of the Insurance Regulations Office will be extended in order to achieve a greater harmonization with similar institutions in the other Member States.

37 This group represents the interests of all Dutch insurers, not only health insurers.

38 The introduction of the Dekker Plan entails a statutory obligation for companies, in the situation described, to accept all applicants, including non-members of the personnel.

39 A topical example is the recent development in which the Rosendaal Municipal Council plans to build a high-technology eye hospital in an industrial zone.

40 The sixth VAT guideline from Brussels is going to be readjusted to treat the buying and selling of goods across the community's internal frontiers in the same way as that within a single Member State. The second part is the foundation of a clearing house to ensure that VAT revenues are received by the treasury of the Member State where the goods are finally consumed. Moreover, there will be two VAT bands: the normal tariff of between fourteen and twenty per cent plus a lower rate of between four and nine per cent for essential goods. Standardization of these tariffs is being aimed at within the EC.

41 The health insurance funds have compiled lists in which certain medicines are recommended on the basis of their quality and cost. The prescription of identical medicines of a higher price is discouraged.

42 The Dutch Ministry of Education funds the training and research functions of teaching hospitals.

43 The Royal Dutch Medical Association (KNMG) protects the interests of doctors and medical staff.

44 These are two Dutch consultancy bodies in the social and economic field.

6.2 A Healthy Europe Too?
K. Schutyser

At the end of the magical year 1992, a *free economic market* should be implemented, as agreed upon in 1958, when the European Economic Community (EEC) was established by six states. Since 1958, the same states set up the European Atomic Energy Community (Euratom) and, since 1952, the European Coals and Steel Community. Since 1967, these three Communities have merged under a single executive power and expended from six to 12 states.

This European Community remains a practical and limited stepping stone for integration in the domain of Coal and Steel, nuclear energy and economics in general. Since World War Two, the dream of a wider politically-integrated Europe has been fostered, but the formal rearrangement of the three Community Treaties in the Single European Act of 1986 could only reactivate the European idea economically. After more than 30 years the free Common Market for goods, persons, services and capital should be finalized by the end of 1992, when about 300 regulations will have been implemented.

Besides this reactivated economic aim this Single European Act of 1986 makes a functioning of the EC-institutions more flexible. However, the sphere of the mostly economic competence of the EC only knew limited expansion, especially where research and development, regional development and monetary and environmental policy are concerned. The wider 'Citizens' Europe' which, since 1984, has been growing in the sphere of culture, tourism, youth, education and even public health, could not be ratified in the formal texts.

Historically, public health and health care were, so to speak, not explicitly mentioned as objectives in the three Treaties, except for the health protection in the Euratom Treaty. By the Single European Act of 1986, amendments were made to the EEC-Treaty, so that now public health verbally appears as a modest objective in the texts. A modest objective indeed: the 1989 budget of the EC provides only one per thousand for health care projects.

Nevertheless, even before 1986 the various organs of the EC acted restrictively in three public health matters:

First, in executing the free-market-regulations, health care was dealt with.

a) The right of free establishment (including conditions for their education) was regulated for doctors, nurses, dentists, midwives, pharmacists. Other health care professions are registered under a general directive. In January 1988, the doctors of the EC even proclaimed via the 'Orders of Doctors' a European Ethical Code, so as to prevent any deontological impediments regarding the freedom of establishment.

b) The free market regulations concerned also medicines and medical appliances. Various directives were formulated for medicines and in June 1989 for human blood. Where medical appliances are concerned, European intervention is limited to the thermometer and safety measures for electronic equipment.

Second, health care was part of the social policy. Social policy was explicitly mentioned in the EEC (economic) Treaty. A number of European social measures refers to health care: a recommendation for a European list of occupational diseases; regulations regarding health care of workers travelling within the community, as well as all measures concerning their safety and health at work with special regulations for mine-workers and radiation protection.

Third, the EC authorities gradually paid attention to other domains of public health that were not directly connected with the specific tasks of the economic and social policy of the Treaty. The meetings of the ministers of Health of the EC have recently given a new impulse. The powers of the EC grew with regard to the following matters:

a) Drugs: cooperation against the use of drugs started from 1972.

b) Smoking: since 1977, the Europe's attention to the harmful effects of tobacco led recently to a directive stating that from 1993 onwards, each packet of cigarettes should mention that 'smoking damages your health'. In Brussels in May 1989, the British Minister of Health voted against this, because he did not consider the European Community to be authorized.

c) A Cancer Programme: 'Europe against Cancer' has been developed since 1987 and focuses on preventive actions such as the 'European Week Against Cancer' and a European Code against cancer.

d) Alcoholism: is another topic and so is

e) AIDS: since 1986, there has been an AIDS action programme that draws attention to the spreading of this disease which threatens the lives of 100 000 European citizens by 1990.

f) Organ Transplantation and

g) Other Diseases received attention as did:

h) Patients' Rights: the approval by the EC Hospital Committee of a European Charter for the Rights of Hospital Patients in 1979, led five years later to a resolution in Parliament. The European Commission was ordered to formulate a European Charter of the patient. This has not happened so far and neither for the rights of children in hospitals, which were also discussed in Parliament. (The

European Office of the World Health Organization in Copenhagen has recently been very active in this field and circulates a draft Declaration of Patients Rights). Although the European Parliament agreed that the general right to the best medical treatment is a fundamental right in the whole Community, the basic EC-right concerning fee movement of patients has not turned into a universal reality for all European citizens so far. It does exist but reimbursement of health care costs is only foreseen for employees and their families under certain conditions. On 29 September 1989 the Council of Ministers asked the Commission to study the introduction of a European card for emergency care, starting with the recognition of all national social security cards within the Community. A European health card or European medical passport has also been prepared since 1986 and actually there is circulating a proposal for a council Directive on the introduction of a standard emergency call number throughout Europe by 1992!

i)   For Handicapped People: lots of initiatives have been developed, also via the European Social Fund. Since 1988 a Helios-programme has led towards a coherent policy for handicapped people;

j)   In Research and Development: since 1977, a certain priority has been given to medical science and public health.

k)   Environment and Consumer Policies: have been activated by the EC-organs since 1972. Sometimes the domain of health was touched. In 1975, the Council acknowledged the right of protection of the consumer's health. Since 1984, there has been an alarm procedure between the Community and Member States for serious incidents during the use of consumption products.

The sum of these interventions cannot easily be qualified as a genuine European health policy. Whether or not 1992 will bring about a healthy Europe depends only partially on the 300 measures which are or should be taken in the light of the realization of a free Common Market. Some of these measures are of course associated with public health. Sanitary controls are a difficult obstacle as a number of custom restrictions have to be modified before the end of 1992. Also, if some Member States decide to use privatization or commercialization of health care as a tool to reduce costs in the budgets of social security, a lot of health care regulations which are currently nationally competent and outside the market, could become, in that situation, 1992 subjects. Meanwhile, even specialists of EC-law and those of health care law (the combination of these two specialities is until now very exceptional) are asking many questions about the detailed consequences of community law and its 1992 measures on national health care systems. This concerns free competition, free service, free establishment of health care professionals and free movement of patients.

However, the further possible evolution of European health care is not really bound to the strict 1992 objectives and date, but to the wider European evolution which will even reach beyond 1992. There are three linking points:

a)   In the EC-Treaty especially, public health has now been more explicitly mentioned since the Single European Act of 1986. This increases the changes for further progression in the years to come also, of the European technological research and development policy which has now been made possible, and whose executive programme 1987-1991 consists of many topics concerning public health care: quality of life, prevention, diagnostics, consequences of an ageing population and medical research on cancer and AIDS. In the biotechnological action programmes, health problems are treated as well, and in the telecommunication programmes, one specifically deals with Advanced Informatics in Medicine (AIM). Research specifically pays attention to developing countries and their public health as well.

b) Together with safety the health of the workers at the workplace is explicitly mentioned in the EEC-Treaty since the Single European Act and on these grounds a recent directive has already been formulated (June 1989). This leads us to the very delicate question of the social dimension or the social face of the 1992 European United Market or to the even more delicate matter of the evolution of a social Europe. At the beginning of 1989 the Economic and Social Council has taken cautious advice concerning a Community charter of basic social rights. Here, the strong contrasts between European representatives of employers and employees are hidden, especially with regards to European collective agreements and to the right of participation in enterprises. The Commission already came to draft a 'Social Charter', which became an explosive topic in the European Summit of December 1989 in Strasbourg. Indeed, according to the British government, some of the matters dealt with exceed the current powers of the EC. As health is treated within these basic social rights, the evolution of a social Europe will surely have to be observed by those responsible for health care.

c) By way of this Social Charter, which remarkably mixes up the social rights of workers and of citizens, one enters the already-mentioned, much broader 'Citizens' Europe' in which public health, however, does not get explicit priority by the Commission's action programmes 1988. Education, on the other hand, does. Public health even proves to be a delicate matter where the growth of EC competence is concerned. The lack of consensus between the European ministers of Public Health with regards to cigarettes in May 1989 illustrated once more that there is caution and even opposition between the Member States to the idea of turning health care into a principal objective of an explicit European integration. Together with justice, culture, education and welfare, public health is nevertheless an important part of the inevitable expansion of Europe for companies and their employees towards a Citizens' Europe. How quickly this will happen and how soon public health will play an active part in that evolution, can, in practicable terms, not be predicted at this time. It depends not only on the political will of the Member States, but also on the will of million of citizens, their associations, political parties and on the evolution of the role and the powers of the European Parliament. Meanwhile, it is not easy for the many health care workers and institutions and for their European associations to get actively involved in the varied and fragmentary EC-activities in the health field. In the Economic and Social Committee, there are no 'reserved seats' for them, and apart from some accidental technical advisory committees with a majority of experts, they have no institutionalized contacts with EC-institutions.

One of these European associations for health care is the Hospital Committee of the European Community. Since 1966, a number of hospital associations within the EEC have set out to confer with each other and have proved that basic questions about hospitals and the wider field of health care can mostly be answered from a European perspective. The Hospital Committee made important studies and recommendations on EC-hospital and health care professions terminology, rights of the hospital patients, hospital costs, planing and management, clinical budgeting, medical-ethical problems of health care, as well as the recent recommendations concerning child care in hospitals, AIDS/HIV (1989) and organ transplants (1989). An exchange programme for Young Hospital Administrators started in 1981 with EC subsidies, which in 1989 was extended in a non-subsidized way to older hospital employees. The 1989 Plenary Assembly in Lisbon decided that the EC-Hospital Committee should set out some very concrete European hospital actions in the years to come. They will be promoted under the name HOPE, HOspitals for EuroPE. These HOPE-actions will necessitate a more intensified contact and consultation with the existing colleague-associations in the field of European health care, so that hospitals are given the opportunity to advocate their specific roles, contributions and problems in the wider developments of European health care. **This does not mean that the 12 countries should obtain one uniform hospital legislation as soon as possible, nor that hospitals claim a central role in a uniformed European health care system.** Multiformity is undoubtedly an historic and positive reality in the health care and hospital sector in Europe.

In the European hospital world, there is currently no consensus on possible political actions for making health care pave the way in the further evolution of a Citizens' Europe. On this matter, the Hospital Committee will certainly continue its reflection. There is certainly no lack of opportunities for development in a European way. Here are a few examples:

a) an obvious need exists for non-ambiguous European health (care) statistics and better (and cheaper?) data registration;
b) the growing shortage of health care personnel in many European countries and the recently (even by strikes) claimed improvement of the salary- and labour conditions, leads to questions about a European approach, or possible exploratory collective conversations between the European social groups of the hospital sector;
c) the evolution of a free European insurance-market will cause friction with the social security systems which have been organized up until now in a rather national way. There will be more questions on real free choice and social coverage of all the patients towards the health professionals and institutions and this not only in the border regions;
d) the question of European medical Centres of Excellence beyond the country borders has to be answered as well as the question of possible minimum-quality-norms, technology assessment and implementation of medical research results;
e) and probably the European Ministers of Health will, as they do already on Aids and drugs, join to tackle the problem of the ageing population with or without additional financial means and manpower and/or to exchange their national techniques to control the financial-economic growth in the health care sector, to realize preventive policies and to look for answers to the many ethical and legal questions raised by the biomedical and social evolution.

The 13 000 European hospitals with a staff of about 4 million are conscious of the fact that they are like a chain of continuous and high quality service to the 325 million European citizens and their primary health care. They want to continue that role. They ask for political transparency concerning the evolution in European health care matters, for a democratic role for the European Parliament in that evolution and of course for participation of the hospitals themselves in that process. A healthy Europe is indeed a matter of a healthy democracy as well.

6.2.1 References

Asso, M. (1986), *Twenty years of activities (1966-1986) of the Hospital Committee of the European Economic Community*, Acco, Leuven.

Bosscher, A.E. (1989), La coordination des régimes de sécurité sociale dans la Communauté, Communication au Colloque, *La segurança Social e a Europa 1992*, Porto (Portugal), 12 Octobre.

Cecchini, P. (1988), *'The European Challenge - 1992: the benefits of an Single Market'*, Gower Publishing Company Ltd, Aldershot, 1988.

Commission of the European Communities, *XXIInd General Report on the Activities of the European Communities*, 1988, Office for Official Publication of the European Communities, Luxembourg, 1988.

Commission of the European Communities, *Europeans, you have rights*, Office for Official Publications of the European Communities, Luxembourg, 1988.

Commission of the European Communities, *Social Europe. The social dimension of the internal market*, Office for Official Publications of the European Communities, Luxembourg, 1988.

Council of Ministers of Public Health, *Conclusions on texts decided since 1986*, O.J. n° 89/C 185/g.e.v.

Crijns, L.H.J. (1988), Het sociaal beleid van de Europese Gemeenschap in de afgelopen dertig jaar (1958-1987), in *De Gids*, **2**, 119-132.

De Schoutheete de Tervarent, Ph., *L'Europe politique*, rapport présenté par le représentant de la Belgique auprès des Communautés Européennes à un Colloque 1992 de Cepess, Bruxelles, 1 février 1989.

European Communities, Economic and Social Committee, *Basic Community Social Rights, Opinion*, Brussels, February 1989.

European Parliament, The Health systems of European Community Countries, Research and documentation Papers, Environment, Public Health and Consumer Protection Series, N, **12** 1988/9.

Hospital Committee of the European Economic Community, *Hospitals in the E.E.C., Organisation and terminology*, Gyldendal, Copenhagen, 1988.

Institut Europeen d'education et de politique sociale, *Reports (not published yet) of the Colloquium on 'higher education and Europe after 1992'*, K.U. Leuven, 21 June, 1989, i.a.: on medical studies (H. Karle and T. Kennedy).

International Hospital Federation, *Hospital Management International '89*, Sabrecrown Publishing, London, 1989.

Massart, F. *et al.* (1988), *L'Europe de la santé, hasard et/ou nécessité?*, Academia, Louvain-la-Neuve.

Massion, J. (1988), L'hôpital et l'Europe de 1992, in *L'hôpital belge*, **194-195**, 74-81.

Nationale ziekenhuisraad, *Europe 1992 and the consequences for health care*, NZR, Utrecht, 1988.

Noel, E. (1988), *Les Institutions de la Communauté Européenne*, Office des publications officielles des Communautés européennes, Luxembourg.

Pollers, L. (1986), *Hospitals and health care in the European Community*, (1957-1985), Acco, Leuven.

Pors, A.G. (1989), l'Europe des hôpitaux: force et nécessités in Evènement Européen, November.

Schutyser, K. *Legal and ethical issues in health*, Contribution at the International Seminar 'Health for all' organized by the Confederacion Argentina de Clinicas, Sanatorios y Hospitales privados and the International Hospital Federation in Buenos Aires, on 16 and 17 March 1989 (will be published in 1989 in World Hospitals).

Tijdschrift voor Gezondheidsrecht (Dutch Health Law Review), 1989/5: *special edition on 'Europe 1992 and health care' treating national health care and Community law* (B.H. ter Kuile), *competition law and health care* (H.E.G.M. Hermans), *Chances and threats for health professionals in a free European market* (W.B. Van der Mijn), *1992 and social health-cost insurance* (G.A.H. Hamilton).

Storme, M., *Het Europa van de burgers*, report at the CEPESS-Colloquium '1992', February '89 in Brussels (Citizens' Europe).

Van Langendonck, J., *The role of the social security systems in the completion of the European internal market*, lecture given in Lisbon, October 1989.

Venturini, P. (1988), La dimension sociale du marche intérieur. Pierre angulaire de la construction européenne, in *Futuribles*, décembre, 3-22.

Wolfs, C. et Massion, J. (1989), Apport du Conseil de l'Europe à une politique globale de santé européenne, in *La Revue hospitalière de France*, **420**, 343-48.

6.3 Implications for Health Services Managers in Ireland
D.T. Doherty

At the end of World War Two Ireland, a small island community which had remained neutral during the war, was somewhat isolated from the rest of Europe in more than the physical sense. Our reaction to events was influenced by the attitudes of our English-speaking neighbours to the east and to the west of us. Our entry to the European Community was delayed until 1973 due to our economic dependence on Britain which necessitated our accession to the Community coinciding with that of Britain. By then the ideal of European union had begun to evolve and the Irish people anticipated that the pace of change would at least continue even if, in the words of Schonfield, it involved embarking 'on a journey to an unknown destination'.

The Irish people have, in plebiscites and in opinion polls, been supportive of our membership of the Community. We are now less dependent on the British economy as evidenced by, for example, the decision of the Irish government to join the EMS even though Britain has not. In a survey in 1988 eighty per cent supported the view that Ireland had benefited from membership of the Community.

The Irish people voted overwhelmingly in favour of the Single European Act and there exists a widespread expectation that Ireland will benefit from the creation of the single market. Many view the prospect of 'a frontier-free Europe' as extending far beyond freedom of movement of persons, goods and capital. They will expect the health services to match the success of the sectors which perform best in the single market. The fact that the Single European Act is weak on the subject of health care enhances the challenge facing health services managers.

The Irish health service entitlements and structures reflect the influence of our English-speaking neighbours to the east and to the west of us which I spoke of earlier. The services are funded, in the main, from general taxation and are organized in eight regions. The Regional Boards are responsible for the planning and delivery of all aspects of the health care and many social services. However, all of the major hospitals in Dublin and a small number in the provinces are self governing. One state-guaranteed Insurance Company monopolizes the private health insurance market. Thirty per cent of the population have opted for this form of insurance cover and may choose between private hospital care or the special facilities for private patients in publicly funded hospitals. One must assume that with the arrival of the single market, companies in other countries will be eligible to compete for a share of this market. Since the scope for increasing the size of this market is limited, non-Irish insurance companies may not consider it worth their while to enter the Irish market. The report of a government appointed commission on health care funding was expected to provide guidance on how our services ought to be reorganized and managed. Although the report would be concerned in the main with issues of a national character it was expected that the implications of the single market for our health services would receive attention also.

It is difficult to forecast if and how health service needs will change as a result of the introduction of the single market. A critical, largely to-be-resolved issue, is the importance to be attached to the social implication of the new Europe. It has been estimated that the level of poverty in the Community increased by twenty per cent between 1978 and 1988. There are well known links between poverty, high unemployment and ill health. If our economy were, for whatever reason, to perform less well than the economy of the Community as a whole, health service needs might well increase as a result. There is much concern in Ireland about the cost to our economy of harmonizing the rates of indirect taxes. As a major user of goods and services my organization stands to gain from a reduction in indirect taxation levels. But, because the organization receives the bulk of its finances from Government, any significant reduction in Government revenue is likely to result in a reduction in the allocation of monies to fund health services. The structural funds exist, of course, to support the infrastructural development needs of the weaker areas of the community. I was interested to see in the new rules of the Regional Fund published in February 1990 that for the first time, hospitals are mentioned as being eligible for support from the fund. Ireland, being one of the priority regions of the community, may stand to benefit from this change.

Health service structures, funding and eligibility issues are likely to remain the responsibility of national governments. However, citizens of the new Europe are just as likely to seek redress against inequalities in health care as they will in other areas. There are major variations at present between Member States in the resources devoted to health care and in health status indicators. The fact that life expectancy for men is highest in one of the Member States which spends least, *per capita*, on health care, only serves to illustrate how complex the entire health care issue is. Health care managers seeking guidance on the priority areas of the European dimension of their work are likely to identify inter-state collaboration and information technology as key areas. There are already many interesting projects underway which may serve to guide future plans:

a) Comac HSR has developed a proposal for assessing, evaluating and comparing services for adults with mental illness in different countries. Projects of this nature could usefully be undertaken in respect of many health services and if successful would be of considerable benefit to planners, managers and perhaps even to institutions charged with adjudicating on complaints of inequality from citizens.

b) The joint Council of Europe/WHO/European Communities Model Programme 'Promoting Health Education Amongst Young People' is an interesting example of collaboration directed at a topical issue causing grave concern - in this instance drug abuse.

c)   Europe's AIM (Advanced Technologies for Medicine and Health Care) Programme is currently supporting 37 research projects in the fields of medicine and health care.

d)   Cancer, being the major cause of death it is, has become the subject of a specific eduction/awareness programme 'Europe against Cancer' and has brought increased prominence to health issues at European Community level.

The level of information technology in hospitals is low everywhere in Europe compared with North America and Japan. That needs to be improved and to move on to develop data interchange standards. Managers need to recognize the key role information technology will play in the Europe of the future and actively consider how we can secure and apply the resources which exist to facilitate developments in that area. I see this as an area in which Irish health services managers are well positioned to contribute significantly. The computer industry is strong in Ireland and many of the major US computer hardware and systems companies have located research and development, as well as manufacturing facilities there. There are interesting developments taking place in our hospitals using state of the art technology and our health care delivery structures are sufficiently different from those in most other countries in Europe to make them interesting in the context of developing information interchange standards.

The presence of so many of the leading computer companies in Ireland presents us with an opportunity to join with them and health service partners in other Member States to engage in health research and new technology applications considered both relevant and eligible for financial support by the EC. I believe it behoves health services managers in Ireland, as elsewhere in the community, to contribute in every way we can to developing awareness of the European dimension of health care. By collaborating in devising comparative and evaluative methodologies, information technology applications and by promoting data interchange standards we are likely to have EC support in more than the financial sense and to be contributing to an increase in awareness of the European dimension of health care I have mentioned.

The provisions of the Single European Act relating to the freer movement of workers throughout the Community is of considerable significance in some Member States. The major concern in this area is the possibility of an increase in the spread of communicable diseases. I consider it highly unlikely that there will be any significant inward migration of workers to Ireland and I do not, therefore, anticipate any noticeable impact on disease patterns or health service needs on that account.

In relation to changes which will occur in regard to job opportunities for health care professionals, I foresee a number of problems and opportunities. The rate of taxation in Ireland is very high and the tax base is very narrow. Unless this situation is remedied in the lead-in period to 1992, it is likely that many of our better qualified young people, increasing numbers of whom speak one or more continental languages, will emigrate. If this happens the health services are likely to be one of the major sufferers. Already many of our acute hospitals are heavily reliant on junior hospital doctors from Third World countries despite the fact that our universities train more doctors than our services require. Many of our graduates pursue career development opportunities in the UK and North America and some return to take up consultant posts in their mid-thirties. Our hospitals have not so far attracted doctors from European countries in which doctors are unemployed. This may well be because our hospitals tend to rely on long established links with medical schools in India and Pakistan rather than to possibilities in Europe. It will be interesting to see if these patterns will change in the years ahead. The health care professions, especially nursing, have a strong appeal for Irish school-leavers; our training standards are high and our graduates are highly regarded at home and abroad. I am aware that the health services in other European countries are experiencing difficulties in securing nurses in sufficient numbers. It occurs to me that an opportunity exists for hospitals in Ireland to contract with hospitals elsewhere in Europe to train nurses on their behalf.

The opening up of the sectors of public procurement, until recently exempted from the community rules, and plans for the free movement of pharmaceuticals are of considerable interest to health services managers in Ireland. If we can tailor our contracts to attract more potential suppliers we may, in addition to attracting keener prices, assist Irish suppliers to compete in the larger community market place. Pharmaceuticals are expensive in Ireland. Many doctors have been reluctant to prescribe the generic equivalent of brand-named products claiming that ongoing quality control checks on the generic products, especially those of non-EC origin, are not adequate. Plans to introduce a single appraisal of all licence applications followed by a single decision to be valid throughout the community and changes in pricing systems may, therefore, produce cost reductions and more acceptable quality standards relating to generic products.

In Ireland funding for health services has declined, in real terms, each year since 1980. Efforts are on-going to shift resources from hospitals to community care. There is an on-going debate about the adequacy of our delivery structures; about the method of funding hospital and other service delivery agencies; about whether we have the volumes to justify organ transplant programmes of acceptable quality and whether, in any event, it may be more cost effective to buy such services abroad. It is a time of considerable change and uncertainty even without the changes which 1992 will bring.

A time of change is also a time of opportunity and challenge. The following extract from 'Social Europe - The Social Dimension of the Internal Market' describes well the challenge and opportunities facing health services managers being asked to play minor supporting roles in a major drama for which the plot has been written, but for much of which there is yet only an outline script.

'The success of the setting up of a single internal market as a growth-oriented project, will depend primarily on those economic and social factors who will be able to manage the necessary strategies and exploit all the potential effects of the dynamic process which will be set in motion'.

This presupposes that opportunities will be recognized, that the social implications will be correctly assessed and that a clear distinction will be made between real problems and unfounded fears.

6.4 A Database of Health Activity in Europe
C.B. Grimes

6.4.1 Introduction

A database of health activity contains information on population needs and demands, service provision to meet those requirements, the effectiveness of those provisions and the cost of providing them. The information needs to provide comparisons - over institution, over population groups, over geographical divisions and, eventually, over countries.

6.4.2 Information

Good information is the basis of effective plans and the means of monitoring those plans. Information on health services is required by:

a) The general public
b) Health care professionals
c) Health care managers
d) Academics
e) The Media
f) Politicians.

Information should be:

a) free from professional or political bias
b) up-to-date and readily accessible
c) comparable as regards time and in relation to other service providers.

Types of health care information:

Inputs	Outputs
Finances available	Costs
Manpower data	Productivity
Facilities	Efficiency
Capital resources	Effectiveness
Demography	Trends
Raw activity data.	Processed activity data:
	Numbers treated over a period
	Length of hospital stay
	Turnover interval.

Such information is required in all countries, but the different structures of services, terminologies and currency differences render comparisons difficult. Yet a lot can be learned from comparisons, and there is much that is common between services provided in one country and those in another.

Recent trends, particularly the escalation in the costs of health services, have put methods of providing those services under the microscope in most western countries. Moves towards greater separation between the agencies involved in planning and financing services and those providing services and the introduction of greater competition have called for more detailed information. This is particularly so in relation to clinical services and the imposition of cost limits, which has led to wide interest in Diagnostic Related Groupings, first introduced in the United States of America to help meet those requirements. Simultaneously the rapid strides made in information technology have made available the mechanism to provide the required information.

6.4.3 Information Inputs

These cover:

1) Finance

a) Expenditure:

Staff Costs	Medical, nursing, paramedical, support services
Materials	Drugs, dressings, medical equipment, food, maintenance of buildings and plant, office services and so on
Capital	New and upgraded buildings and engineering services and large scale equipment (for example X-ray machines)
Income	Fees, sales of services and so on.

2) Activity

a) Inpatients
- Patients treated
- Average occupancy
- Day cases
- Lengths of stay
- Bed usage
- Turnover intervals
- Physician episodes.

b) Outpatients)
Accidents &)
Emergencies)
- New cases
- Referrals

c) Day Patients

d) Community Services
- General Practitioner attendances and treatments
- Community Nurse attendances and treatments
- School visits
- Preschool visits
- Home confinements
- Elderly
- Preventive medicine.

e) Ambulances
- Patients carried and mile covered.

f) Waiting Lists
- Numbers, specialities and waiting times.

3) Manpower

a) Manpower

- Professions and Numbers
- Skills mix
- Turnover
- Training needs and provision
- Forecasts.

6.4.4 Information Outputs

a) Costs

- Per patient day/per outpatient/per patient visited in community
- Per case/consultant episode
- Per treatment over diagnostic-related groups
- Per institution   - buildings, engineering
                    - support services (for example, catering)
- Per GP prescription
- Savings by greater efficiency.

b) Manpower

- Trends
- Costs per head over types.

c) Activity

- Comparison over time in:
 - numbers treated by speciality/disease
 - numbers waiting
 - bed use
 - length of stay
 - morbidity

d) Demography

- Populations served and characteristics (ages, sex, social and industrial categories)
- Population movement and effect
- Population forecasts.

6.4.5 The CIPFA Database (United Kingdom)

The Chartered Institute of Public Finance and Accountancy (CIPFA) is one of the six major accountancy bodies in the United Kingdom and covers all aspects of the public service. Its Health Service arm, the Healthcare Financial Management Association (HFMA) has a membership open to all qualified accountants working in the health field.

Over the past three years, CIPFA and HFMA have been building a database of health information and have published three volumes of data, the latest being 'Health Service Trends - Second Edition', launched in June 1989. A further publication was published November 1989, containing information on the financial out-turn of Health Authorities for 1988/89 and plans for 1989/90.

The database covers the following:

a) Information collected from:
 - 14 Regional Health Authorities
 - 200 District and Special Health Authorities (DHAs and SHAs)
 - Central government

- Independent agencies
- Organization for Economic Cooperation and Development (OECD).
b) Data concerning:
- Finance
- Activity
- Manpower
- Demography
- Independent Sector in UK
- National data from EEC countries, the US and other comparable countries.
c) Comparative data:
- between Health Authorities
- within the independent sector
- between a base year (usually 1982/83) and the latest year available.

The database is intended to provide a subscription service to:

a) Health Authorities
b) Local Authorities
c) Independent agencies including Management Consultants
d) Universities and Schools of Management
e) Trade Unions (for example, British Medical Association).

CIPFA acts in close contact with the National Association of Health Authorities, the BMA, the Audit Commission and Health Authorities individually. An advisory group representing officers of Health Authorities has been set up by HFMA.

6.4.6 Opportunities and Problems

Opportunities are beginning to present themselves for exchanges of information on a national scale. The Health Care Financial Management Associations in the UK and USA have been cooperating on exchange visits including seminars on data comparison. Some early work has taken place with the EEC Hospital Committee. A number of developments have taken place in Europe and in other western countries using Diagnostic Related Groups.
   The French data base 'Eco-Sante' appears to have similarities to the UK programmes. Further opportunities may arise from:

a) Extension of DRG work
b) Use of European Currency Units as a conversation process for exchange differences, noting the stability of the European Monetary System. (This could replace the use of dollars which is the common currency employed by OECD, but which lacks stability in relation to exchange rates.)
c) The effects of 1992.

Problems relate largely to definitions and differences in types of service provided in different countries, language and currency difficulties.

6.4.7 Essentials of a Database

To be effective a database must be:

a) Timely
b) Built up from local data which is recognized by those whom it affects - preferably by using locally published data
c) Processed quickly within an established system
d) Published quickly
e) Capable of using incomplete information in a controlled manner. Times does not always permit one hundred per cent data to be collected.

6.4.8 The Future

Health Service providers in all EEC countries can benefit from wider knowledge of the ways in which Member States provide their services. In particular, there are lessons for:

a) Economy and efficiency in the provision of services
b) Maximum benefit from input resources:
    - Staff productivity
    - Best buys
    - Optimum use of buildings and equipment
c) Alternative treatments
d) Planning of services
e) Meeting challenges of the future.

Early steps can be taken in setting out:

a) Common terminology
b) Common lay-out of information
c) Better communication.

6.4.9 Proposals

CIPFA is prepared to work with European organizations to take this subject further. Its interest is exemplified by the publication 'Health Service Trends - Second Edition. In particular, early steps to identify the common ground with the French system and any other European systems available could be profitable.
1992 seems to give the opportunity for significant progress.

6.5 New Developments in Workers Participation in Europe 1992
H.J. van Zuthem

Workers participation is accepted in all countries in the western world. Participation within this respect means participating in decision-making processes within organizations. The most common form is the works council. The influence of the works council is not the same in every country; the differences are impressive. This has important implications for Europe after 1992. I shall elaborate on this point later on.

The role of the unions is accepted in the western world, but the differences in this field are impressive too. We should not forget that workers participation as part of the decision-making processes within organization is not the only form of participation. In this respect the history of power distribution in labour relations, for instance, assigns an important role to workers unions. Up till now, the unions, as workers representatives, also participate in decision-making processes; on national level, on the level of (the) branches and also within organizations like companies, hospitals, and so on.

Workers participation is a normal aspect of modern labour relations, but it does not have the same meaning in every country. Workers participation is still a matter of development: sometimes evolution, sometimes revolution. In any case, it is a matter causing tensions and conflicts in many situations. What are the reasons for these tensions and conflicts?

In my opinion they are as follows:

1) In some countries (for example in West Germany and in the Netherlands), a process of decentralization of bargaining is going on. The reasons for that are well known. More and more we see a tendency to create a relationship between wages and other conditions and the profitability of the enterprise. Another reason is the complexity of technological innovation. These problems are not the same in every company and this means that the unions have to carry on negotiations in every company separately. The same holds true for the implementation of flexible working hours, shifts, and so on.

On the other hand, the works councils have their own rights with regards to working conditions, working hours, and so on. There is a real danger that unions and works councils will become competing institutions.

There is a story of a union official who is very much concerned with workers participation and especially with the influence of the works councils. This official is a religious man and every morning he asks for more influence for the works council. But every evening he thanks the Lord that it did not happen.

2) There is another reason for the tensions and conflicts in the field of workers participation. Managers of organizations emphasize the effectiveness of their organization as first priority. Workers participation, however, takes time; sometimes a lot of time. For instance, member of works councils have to be informed and skilled. Nowadays there is a strong need for more efficiency, cost reduction(s), quality, and such like. Reallocation of production means is very often the result and this affects the interests of the workers.

After 1992 the possibilities or reallocation across the borders are increasing. We may expect a strong reaction from trade unions in protecting the interests of the workers. The internationalization of production can be disturbed by workers participation and also by the influence of works councils. This is another reason for conflict in the field of workers participation.

3) There is a third reason for tensions and conflicts.

Workers participation via unions and works councils is an expression of collective opinions and feelings, based on consensus about interests and goals. Nowadays there is a shift in our culture to a more personal and individualistic view regarding interests and goals. Modern personnel management (human resources management) stimulates this view by creating working conditions adapted to individualistic circumstances. Defenders of workers participation will criticize these developments by trying to make all kinds of individual arrangements in collective agreements. When this occurs in agreements with works councils, the possibility of conflict between unions and works councils will increase.

Viewing these three basic conflicts in workers participation we have to look for a solution in the concept of participation itself.

On the one hand, participation has to do with democracy; with the fundamental right of people to have a say in the conditions of their working life. This form of participation has basically to do with policy-making; in other words with goals, kinds of products, income policy and so on.

On the other hand, participation also means involvement in the implementation of policy, the daily work of everyone in the organization. Joint consultation on the shop floor is such a form of workers participation. The reason for this form of participation is not the fundamental right of democracy, but the need for efficiency.

We therefore have to make a clear distinction between participation based on the right of democracy, and participation as a need for efficiency. The history of workers participation shows that when this distinction is not made, a lot of confusion about participation can occur.

For workers policy-making is a difficult issue and it is much easier to discuss daily problems. Managers are responsible for daily productivity and they are afraid of a decrease in efficiency. Is there a solution to this problem?

In my opinion we have to work with the dual concept in the organization, based upon the two aspects of the decision-making process; policy making, and policy implementation.

What we need are two separate structures. The structure for policy-making is based on the norm of democracy and the structure for policy implementation is based on the norm of efficiency. In both structures we have to do with distribution of power and responsibilities. In the democracy-based structure, policy-making is a responsibility of every member of the organization, whereas in the efficiency-based structure, implementation is the ultimate responsibility of management. Power distribution is not an issue of democracy but simply a matter of delegation.

I am aware of the fact that my dual structure is no reality at this moment. Yet at least in some countries there is a development in the direction of a dual structure. Again I mention West Germany and the Netherlands. In these countries works councils discuss policy problems increasingly. They also have some influence on the composition of the supervisory board; more so in the large companies in West Germany than in the Netherlands.

It is very clear to me that in Europe after 1992 the importance of policy-making will extend. Not only business firms but also health organizations will explore the benefits of international cooperation. Cooperation across the borders will affect the interests of the workers. Re-allocation of employment is possible.

Before I elaborate on workers participation after 1992 I would like to mention the other side of the dual, namely the dual culture.

The structure of policy implementation is completed by norms like efficiency, inequality, expertise and appointments. I realize that not all workers are interested in policy-making, but works councils and workers unions will be so increasingly. Although, again, a dual structure and culture is not complete reality at this moment, it is around the corner.

What are the consequences for the behaviour of managers? In the first place, managers should help the workers to discuss problems of policy-making. Information, discussion and also decision-making are the elements of the process of policy-making. The rights of the workers are not the same in various European countries. However, it is necessary in my opinion that managers involve the workers in this process of decision making. If not, the resistance to change will increase.

Second, managers have to make clear vis-à-vis workers, works councils and unions that the implementation of policy is the primary responsibility of management. Implementation of policy is not a matter of democracy. Joint consultation about implementation makes sense, but the reason for it is efficiency, not democracy.

Finally, I would like to say something about the consequences of Europe 1992 for the institutions of workers participation. I would like to emphasize two aspects:

1) The European federation of trade unions decided in 1989 that there had to be co-determination or workers participation in economic and social organizations. This federation has chosen a system in which workers can have co-responsibility for the management of the organization. Arrangements in this field have to be the result of negotiation with the trade unions. If I am right, the European federation of trade unions wants the influence of the workers on policy-making via the right of consent. Elements of policy-making which the federation mentioned last year were: investment policy, allocation policy, cooperation with other organizations, strategic planning, social policy and appointment of board members.

The reason for the point of view of the European federation of trade unions seems quite clear. The unions are afraid of a re-allocation of business firms to countries with a soft regime in the field of workers participation.

2) Some time ago the European Committee presented a proposal with regards to a European business firm. In this proposal three regimes of co-determination (participation) are suggested:

a) at least one third of the members of the supervisory board are elected by the workers;
b) a works council with significant rights;
c) co-determination via trade unions.

As I mentioned, this is a proposal with regard to business firms. It is possible that other types of organizations will also receive a European legal status (rechtsvorm), for example a European hospital. I am not quite sure about the professional benefits of such a European institution, but it can perhaps prevent re-allocation of labour and employment due to improper reasons.

My conclusion is that after 1992 the discussion about workers participation will receive a new impetus. Not a radical movement in the direction of self-management or syndicalism, yet an important development with two elements; more uniform regulations and more influence of workers in works councils and supervisory boards.

7   Health Care Professionals

Contents

213

7 Health Care Professionals

7.0 Introduction
W.J. de Gooijer

As far as the contribution of different professionals to the development of health care within the European community is concerned, there is a need for quality regulations regarding health care practice at three levels - self regulation, national law and community law. These levels are narrowly related, both procedural and material matters. At present the regulation of professional quality in general tends to guarantee a certain minimum. In the perspective of 1992 it is important to take into account the necessity of improving professional quality throughout the EC. For this purpose a certification-system seems a suitable instrument (Oosterman-Meulenbeld).

As far as the doctors are concerned regarding this item we may say that Europe 1992 has already started. The directives on mutual recognition of medical diplomas were completed in 1975 and came into force in 1977. Up to the present time (relatively) little use has been made of the opportunities offered there. In addition, the social security systems have been expressly excluded from the establishment of the internal market. Europe 1992 is limited to private activities. As health care in the EC Member States comes partly, or entirely, under the social security system, it may be said that the systems within which doctors will have to work in the period after 1992 will still be determined principally by national Governments.

However, this influence may weaken in the long term. Europe 1992 will also turn out to be a major 'cultural' process, in which opportunities which already exist elsewhere and are not, or are insufficiently available in one's own country, will not fail to have an influence on the doctors' position in the market. The importance of European doctors' organizations will start to increase from an organizational point of view. Moreover, Brussels will be taking an increasingly critical look at the extent to which the Member States might use their systems of financing in order to defend themselves against external influences, which include the establishment by doctors from the Member States. In due course Europe's involvement in health care will increase in an indirect manner and therefore also have an influence on the position of doctors (Laffrée).

Finally, Europe 1992 will mean a change in the hospital's strategic environment. To cope with the changes and opportunities that will arise from this transformation, hospitals need to adapt their organizational structure. Decentralization will enable hospital management to optimize the control of cure and care. In this process of reorganization nurses seem well-suited to adopt managerial responsibilities. In a decentralized organization job-satisfaction among nurses will be increased and the high turnover among nurses can be decreased (Musch).

7.1 Chances and Risks for Health Care Professionals in the European Internal Market
S. Tiemann

The European Internal Market means free movement of persons, goods, capital and services. This will be a chance also for health care professionals. They will be able to practise in every Member State of the Community. This is especially important for health care professionals regarding the permanently increasing numbers of doctors, dentists and pharmacists in all Member States.

Maintaining the high quality of professionals' formation and specialization will be one of the most urgent questions for health care in Europe. The difficulty is, that formation still differs in the several Member States. Besides, some professions have no protection of title and other professions do not exist in all European states. Another problem is national restriction of access to the social security systems.

Health care professionals are the patients' confidants. This will be even more important in the European Internal Market with open frontiers and industrial orientation. Therefore professionals rules which guarantee the professional independence (fixed charges, restrictions of advertising, professional self-government) are necessary and have to be maintained in the European Internal Market. Such rules - properly formulated - are the best consumer protection. A European health care system with commercialized professions would be a disaster for public health.

Cooperation within Europe will be much closer. We will have a European information system on questions of health care and there will be a lot of common European searching(programmes). These are chances for medical progress and effective medical care. On the other hand, the patient and his privacy have to remain the focus of health care, therefore we need special European rules for the protection of data in health care.

Finally the **systems of social security will not be harmonised but - for reasons of free personal movement in Europe - approximated.** Every European citizen should be able to chose freely the health care professionals and their services he desires anywhere in Europe. As a result, even working conditions for professionals within these systems will change. It is up to the European health care professional now to demonstrate the adequate principle for health care in the Europe of the future.

7.2 Health Care Professionals and their Right to Practise in another Member State of the European Community
A. Oosterman-Meulenbeld

7.2.1 Introduction

The right to practise in another Member State has been elaborated by different directives based on the articles 49, 57 and 66 of the EEC Treaty. They set out the conditions that govern the right of health care professionals to work, to establish themselves and to supply services throughout the Member States of the European Community. So far directives have been issued on doctors, specialists and general practitioners, nurses responsible for general care, midwives, pharmaceutical chemists and dentists.[1] In January 1989 a directive on the mutual recognition of diplomas of higher education came into force which also applies to diplomas of paramedical professions like physiotherapy.[2]

7.2.2 Some General Remarks

The directives mentioned above not only govern the right to practise in another Member State but also create the possibility of rendering services without the actual establishment in another Member State. Nevertheless there can be some restrictions according to national or professional rules that are not in defiance of the EEC Treaty. A well known example is the condition that a specialist or a general practitioner must establish himself within a certain area of the hospital or general practice. The reason for this condition is that the presence of medical help is guaranteed within a short lapse of time.[3] The legality of such conditions has been confirmed by the Court of Justice of the EEC since the Court stated that the special character of certain services can demand special professional rules and control.[4] Another condition that is acceptable from the point of view of community law is the compulsory participation of doctors providing urgent medical help, such as is the case in Luxembourg.[5] The present legal obligation for general practitioners in the Netherlands to be in possession of a licence to practise, granted by the local authorities, is not in defiance of the EEC Treaty, provided that *de facto* the chances of obtaining such a licence are equal for general practitioners from other Member States.

There are other conditions that can be in defiance of the EEC Treaty like the provision in the French *code de la santé publique* that permanent employment as a health care professional in public hospitals is reserved for French nationals. The Court of Justice stated that the exception of article 48(4) of the EEC Treaty, namely that a Member State can refuse to hire non-nationals in the public service, is valid only for functions that are directly related to the public authority or the protection of the interests of the State. The reach of this provision cannot be made conditional on the character of the legal relationship between employer and employee.[6]

Once the health care professional is allowed to practise in another Member State, he or she is admitted to the national health insurance system of the receiving Member State under the same conditions as apply to the nationals. This means, for example, that in the Netherlands a doctor has the right to enter into an agreement with a sickness insurance fund since a contract is obligatory to get payment from the sick fund. In the present reorganization of the Dutch health care system this legal obligation will probably disappear in order to allow a more open competition between health care professionals and health insurers.

Because the knowledge of the foreign language is in the interests of both health care professionals and patients, the receiving Member State must, in instances that may occur, give the health care professional the opportunity to learn the foreign language.[7]

7.2.3 Doctors, Specialists and General Practitioners

An agreement between the Member States on the mutual recognition of the university courses from doctors and specialists was not too difficult to achieve because the professional organizations of doctors in the Member States had already made the necessary arrangements to meet the requirements of the directive. The directive does not contain provisions on the actual competences of the different specialists.[8]

If a doctor attends an officially recognized specialization course in another Member State with the preliminary permission of the competent authorities of the original Member State, the latter state automatically recognizes the specialization obtained in the other Member State.[9] Doctors (and dentists) can use this facility if in their own country there is a shortage of opportunities for specialization.

Eleven specializations are commonly recognized by all Member States and thirty-six only by two or more of them. Indeed it is the case that every Member State is tied to the directives. This is even so when a Member State has asked to strike out a certain specialization and the Council of Ministers has not yet accepted this proposal.[10]

7.2.4 Nurses and Paramedical Professions

Unlike the medical profession, there were more difficulties with the directives on the nursing profession. First there are big differences in vocational training in nursing in and between the Member States, and second, nurses are not so well organized in professional associations as doctors are. Because of the differences in vocational training in general nursing, the directives contain minimum requirements on the duration of the vocational training and the theoretical and practical skills that must be acquired during it. The differences in paediatric and psychiatric nursing are even greater than in general nursing, so it is only recently that the advisory committee has been able to put forward a proposal for these specializations.[11] However it is uncertain whether these proposals will lead to directives because of the recent general directive on the mutual recognition of diplomas of higher education mentioned above. It is the first directive on the free movement of health care professionals that confines itself to the principle of mutual recognition without a preliminary coordination of national schooling and training courses. The directive applies to diplomas that are obtained after a post-secondary study of at least three years. If the schooling courses and practice in the original Member State are quite different from those in the receiving Member State, the latter can require a special term of probation *or* the passing of a proficiency examination. This examination can also refer to acquaintance with the deontological rules which apply to prospective health care practice. A proof of good conduct can also be required. The directive had to be implemented in national law by the Member States before January 1991. Because the directive applies to all diplomas of higher education, there is no reason why those specialized nursing diplomas which are not yet covered by a directive should be excluded from it.

7.2.5 Midwives

The preparation of the directives on midwives took a long time because the differences both in schooling and in practice are quite important between the Member States. Therefore the directives specify the different ways of schooling (with or without a nursing diploma) and describe the field of competence of midwives.[8]

7.2.6 Pharmaceutical Chemists

The directives on pharmaceutical chemists state that the right of establishment does not include the right to become the holder of a pharmacy. This provision was necessary because some Member States try to restrict the number of pharmacies on their territory.

7.2.7 Dentists

The directives on dentists were rather difficult to elaborate because in some Member States dental activities belong not only to the competences of dentists but also, albeit mostly unused, to that of doctors. Besides, the competences vary considerably from one Member State to another. Because some Member States feared that dentists would transgress their competence, the directives embody the provision that the activities of the dentist can be restricted in accordance with the national legislation of the receiving Member State.[8] Although some experts hold the opinion that no significant migration of dentists may be expected after 1992 because of the national differences in language, culture, social system, fiscal facilities and so on, Dutch dentists have already taken particular advantage of the directive by establishing themselves in other Member States.[12]

7.2.8 Summarizing Conclusion

From this brief survey it appears that the EEC objectives on the freedom to work, to establishment and to supply services have been attained satisfactorily regarding health care professionals. Although the free admittance to professions in health care requires specific attention for manpower planning at a national level, only a few difficulties have arisen so far in this respect. The possibility of mutual assistance through rendering services without actually moving to another Member State could be exploited further. It offers major possibilities for combining forces when it comes to highly specialized techniques in health care and could even result in mutual agreements on the repartition of super-specializations between Member States.

7.2.9 Notes

1 Doctors and specialists 75/362 and 75/363, O.J. 1975 L 167. General Practitioners 86/457, O.J. 1986 L 267. Nurses 77/452 and 77/453, O.J. 1977 L 176. Midwives 80/154 and 80/155, O.J. 1980 L 33. Pharmaceutical chemists 85/432 and 85/433, O.J. 1985 L 253. Dentists 78/686 and 86/687, O.J. L 233.
2 Dir. 89/48 O.J. L 19.
3 For example, Dutch General Practitioners must, according to the rules of the professional association, be at the patient's home within a quarter of an hour.

4   The Van Binsbergen case 33/74 E.C.R. 1974, 1299.
5   Written question 2865 in O.J. C 208 1989.
6   Commission vs France case 307/84 E.C.R. 1986 p. 1734-1740.
7   E.g. see directive 75/362 art. 20 for doctors in O.J. L 167, 1975 and directive 77/452 art. 15 for nurses in O.J. L 176, 1977.
8   J. de Vries, 1983, 'De erkenning van artsen, verpleegkundigen, tandartsen en verloskundigen in de Europese Gemeenschappen'. *Tijdschrift voor Gezondheidsrecht*, mei/juni, 109-118.
9   Commission of the EEC doc. III/D/1904/79.
10   Commission vs Belgium Case 306/84 E.C.R. 1987, 683-687. Although Belgium had already requested that the Belgian specialization in tropical medicine should be struck out of the directive, it was condemned by the Court because the duration of the specialization in tropical medicine had to be four years according to directive 75/363 and in Belgium the duration was only one year.
11   Commission of the European Communities document III/D/1832/4/85 and report on psychiatric nursing in the European Community doc. III/D/700/7/82.
12   Europa van Morgen, 12 April 1989, 210. While in 1988 only seven dentists of other EEC countries came to Holland, mostly to increase their specialization, and 239 Dutch dentists received a declaration to practise in other Member States (mostly Germany and Italy).

7.3   The Expanding Role of the Nurse as Manager in Europe
C.K. Musch

7.3.1   Introduction

Hospital managers in Europe are being confronted with a system of developments that shows similarities in most countries of EEC. The welfare state is no longer able to pay for the high standard of health care that has become customary. It is becoming increasingly difficult to deliver good care to those who need it for a price society can afford. Governments within EEC roughly formulate the same goals to control the health care system (Hospital Committee, 1983; Beske *et al.*, 1987, Godt, 1987). During the last decade most EEC countries started to re-structure the health care system. Policies are directed at cost-control. In most cases the method to achieve this is to influence the *prices* of health services as well as the *utilization* of health services. This can be a double-edged sword. A *per diem* price per bed will fix the budget; by reducing the number of beds a considerable reduction of the budget should be obtained. In today's jargon it is evident that these two aspects need interfacing.

Hospital management at the moment is often confronted by conflicting policies because this interface of planning and financing is far from optimized. In some cases planner and financier are totally different institutions.

a)   A major development in the financing of the system is the trend towards holding hospital management accountable for achieving results. Budgeting systems including that accountability are being introduced. Hospital management is having imposed upon it the obligation to show results. These results are often formulated in quantitative, even financial terms.

b) The utilization (and thus the supply) of health care services is regulated by the planning of hospital beds. Within EEC there is almost no other instrument for planning hospital care. Sometimes permission to purchase and use sophisticated health technology is legislated for as a means to prevent the uncoordinated use of very expensive machinery.

c) Planning on a more regionalized basis is being introduced in virtually all countries of the EEC. In most cases this will mean that hospital management will have to operate in a new political environment.

d) Quality of care is fast becoming an issue of public concern. Because there is less and less money available it is becoming increasingly important to spend the remaining money in a better way. Hospital management must find ways to deal with this in such a way as to convince potential patients. There is growing evidence that nurses participate heavily in quality assurance programs (Systchenko & Fabry, 1988).

e) Health technology is showing rapid development. Apart from restrictions imposed by either government or financiers, hospital management is seldom fully equipped to be able to judge the necessity of proposed purchases or the amounts of money involved.

f) The trend towards consumerism in society is also taking place within the health care system. Patients are organizing themselves into special-interest groups to obtain specific forms of care. These groups have often gained enough influence to be put on the political (and therefore the financial and medical) agendas.

g) A point of special interest is demographic factors. More and more people are needing help because of their age, and fewer and fewer people are being born to take care of them.

h) Of those being born, fewer and fewer are willing to join the nursing profession. Although this problem differs between the countries of the EEC there seems to be concern in all countries. A recent article in Germany expressed this feeling of concern rather dramatically by advocating that measures be taken to fight the calamity threatening the nursing profession (Lauffer, 1989). Not only is recruitment a problem. An area of major concern is the high personnel turnover (for example Shoemaker & El-Ahraf, 1983; Smith & Falter, 1988; Lauffer, 1989). In a series of articles the assistant editor of the British Medical Journal concluded that nurses were voting with their feet: 'Two Decembers ago one London hospital ward was unable to find its Christmas decorations. Not one nurse was still working there from the year before', (Delamothe, 1988).

The consequences of these developments seem clear. Hospital management is entering unknown territory. The demands on the organization are far more complicated and hybrid than they used to be. It is true there are still the usual problems, but these are getting tougher. Then there are the new problems and challenges. More and more hospitals will have to compete, not because the laws of supply and demand are being introduced all over Europe, but because money will go where there is quality. Patients will go where there is quality. Personnel will go where there is an organizational climate that will keep them from having to vote with their feet. Governments and financiers will put budgetary restraints on those hospitals not working within the agreed financial framework. This will mean less possibilities for maintaining a steady pace in developing care.

STRATEGIES FOR REDUCING EXTERNAL CONSTRAINTS

Controlling domain	Status
Create, join, participate in industry associations	P

Choosing a particular domain	status
Expand geographically	P
Internally develop/implement new services	P
Adopt new services through acquisition	P
Eliminate weaker services	P

Establishing external linkages	status
Establish joint ventures with other organizations	MIA
Alter input/output ratio (raise prices)	P

OPERATIONAL OPTIONS TO REDUCE COST

Modifying organizational structure	status
Create major functional units	I
Decentralize decision-making	P
Reallocate personnel to maximize productivity	I
Sub-contract out	I
Reduce administrative personnel	I
Develop aggressive marketing units	P

Modifying organizational process	status
Make major innovative changes	P
Reward employees based on predefined performance	P
Increase employee participation in decision-making	MI
Implement cost-conscious purchasing	I

* Status key: I = implemented; MI = may implement without approval; MIA = implement with approval; P = prohibited.

Figure 7.1 (after Sobczak, Fottler & Chastagner)

Sobczak *et al.* analyzed the methods for containment in France (Sobczak *et al.*, 1988). Their findings are rather illustrative for the managerial leeway that exists in a hospital in a centralized system. The tools available to this hospital are not very comprehensive. It is almost impossible to implement strategies aimed at finding an answer to external developments, because such strategies are explicitly prohibited. On the operational side the picture is somewhat less hopeless, but here also there are a number of limitations. Any entrepreneur would be astonished at these restrictions on operating a business.

Hospital management in these cases is bound hand and foot by rules and regulations. A WHO workshop recommended decentralization to prevent the danger of stifling creativity and making hospital administration cumbersome and costly (Beske *et al.*, 1987, 11). In the next section we will look at decentralization within the organizational structure.

7.3.2 Decentralization

The external developments (which should not be seen as threats but as opportunities) make it necessary to develop a cohesive internal structure. In organizing this structure the internal developments should be taken into account. An important part in this organizational restructuring is played by the nursing departments, by far the largest group of employees in the hospital.

To be able to respond better, which means to react faster, to changing needs in health care a decentralized organizational structure is necessary. By decentralizing, the quality of management decisions is improved. It has been found that this has a positive effect on the economic performances of companies (Vancil, 1979). In the WHO workshop mentioned above it was recommended that doctors and nurses should experiment with systems of clinical budgeting to promote cost-consciousness (and therefore cost-effectiveness, CKM) (Beske, 1987). Decentralization makes it possible to create a better balance between control (as a factor of both cost and quality), cure and care at a lower organizational level.

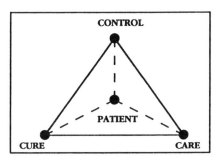

Figure 7.2

Experiments with decentralization are taking place in most countries within the EEC, (for example Gypen, 1988; Musch, 1988; Samuels, 1989). Sometimes the experiments are not aimed at decentralization *per se* but are very definite in trying to introduce models of participative decision-making (for example Schmidt-Rettig, 1989; Genin *et al.*, 1988) which serve the same goals: cost-containment, the control of quality and the reduction of high turnover among personnel, especially among nurses.

Not only will decentralization enable the hospital to react faster, better and in a more innovative and appealing way. A very important goal of decentralization of authority within the hospital is personnel-retention, especially among nurses. Research has shown that one of the key instruments in increasing personnel-retention is to increase job satisfaction. In a study among the 148 hospitals in California on the effects of decentralization it was found that the hypothesis stating that decentralization enhances both job enrichment and job enlargement can be accepted. They also found an increase in personnel retention with a congruent decrease in conflict. The majority of the decentralized hospitals in question (sixty-one point one per cent) gave worker satisfaction as the main reason for decentralizing (Shoemaker & El-Ahraf, 1983).

When responsibility and authority are decentralized a new chain of command is needed. Traditionally the Management Boards of many hospitals in the EEC counties are composed of three members: an administrative, medical and nursing director. There are some other arrangements, for instance in Belgium, Luxembourg, France, Denmark and Holland (Hospital Committee, 1983, 55). By forming well-defined medical units around the medical specialities (for example Medicine, Surgery) a new axis will become the backbone of the hospital.

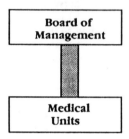

Figure 7.3

The medical unit can, in practice, be termed a division, a directorate or a production unit. These medical units will have to be managed by a team that mirrors the top-level Management Board: an administrator, a nurse and a doctor. Decisions concerning the management will have to be made by deliberation between these three members. In that way, guarantees are put into the system to ensure that all aspects of a problem will be taken into consideration. The managing team should be able to allocate personnel and resources, according to the production or quality, as agreed upon by senior management. In the UK a revitalization of National Health Service is under way, known as the Resource Management Initiative. It is being implemented at different sites on a test basis. Within these sites different solutions are used to tackle the problem of leadership (Chandler, 1989).

Within one of the teaching hospitals of the London area, Clinical Directorates have been installed. Some of these Directorates are managed by a senior nurse who is also the business manager. In situations like these a split accountability is to be found. There is a professional accountability to the director of nursing services and managerial accountability to the Management-Board.

In the University Hospital at Utrecht decentralization has been taken even further. The teams managing the medical units (called divisions) consist of a nurse, a doctor and an administrator. The team has joint responsibility towards senior management. There is no longer a director of nursing services, because that department, together with personnel and budget has been decentralized as well (Hoek, 1989).

To make decentralization work, a supporting infrastructure should be put at the disposal of the managing teams. This infrastructure has two aspects:

a) Service units, supporting medical and nursing processes, for example laboratory, X-ray, physiotherapy, social work. Because of their unique orientation towards the medical units the service units should be given the same organizational status.
b) Facility departments, facilitating organizational processes, for example housekeeping, logistics and purchasing.

The typical staff activities will be grouped in staff departments: finance, legal and personnel.

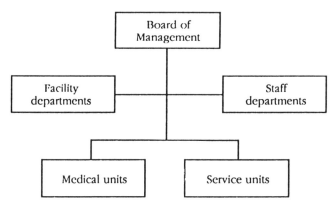

Figure 7.4

Cohesion within this organizational framework is maintained:

a) by participative processes for formulating policy (Dowd, 1988)
b) by introducing contract management between the medical and service units and senior management as well as within the units themselves (Musch, 1988; Hoek, 1989)
c) by creating a task-oriented structure for advising senior management. The decentralized management has an important role to play, because staff will be cut back drastically in a decentralized organisation (Hoek, 1989)
d) by creating an information network that delivers relevant information (Musch, 1989).

Within the units further decentralization should take place. These units usually consist of sections like wards, outpatient clinics, ICU's and sections for diagnosis or treatment (for example the haematology laboratory or the section for nuclear medicine). The units are the organizational level where real interfacing takes place between the cost, care and cure. As such, the sections form the real cost centres. For each of these sections, management has to be provided for. In the University Hospital at Utrecht teams were appointed to manage these sections. The teams consist of a nurse and a head physician. If necessary they can call on the staff of the unit they belong to. Experience shows that nurses are more enthusiastic about and therefore more cooperative towards the new responsibilities (Musch, 1989).

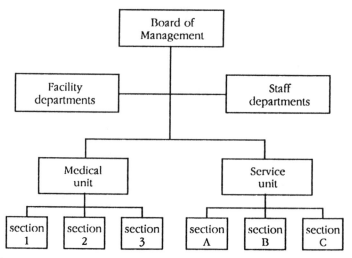

Figure 7.5

7.3.3 *Nurse Management Development, (NMD)*

Theories are being developed to deal with the dual responsibility which such a system implies (Anderson, 1989; Blair, 1989). The synthesis of these two aspects has even given rise to the Theory of Bureaucratic Caring: 'blending traditional management views and the nursing perspective' (Ray, 1989). At this point in time it is evident that nurses do not yet possess all the necessary skills from both domains, and this poses some threats to the nursing profession.

In the view of Knollmueller (Knollmueller, 1979), nurses who are not adequately trained in administrative and managerial skills tend to distance themselves from patients and personnel because their attention is geared towards the new responsibilities. In short, there is a danger of the nurse becoming a bookkeeper rather than a member of the managerial staff. Like every trained professional accepting the role of leadership, nurses will have to learn new skills, while at the same time some old skills must be unlearned (Gleeson *et al.*, 1983). Figure 7.6 shows this in diagram.

This calls for a specific Management Development Programme for Nurse Managers. In this programme the usual managerial skills, like cost-benefit analysis or human resource management, should be dealt with. But it will also be necessary to develop nurses' conceptual abilities. Special emphasis should be put on training nurses in working in a collaborative environment with physicians. This will require the nurse to be able to stimulate, and to motivate the medical co-workers. Sometimes the collaboration will take the form of negotiations and nurses will have to be trained in that particular tool of management. In this multi-disciplinary approach attention should also be given to aspects of health policy and health technology assessment (Grant, 1989).

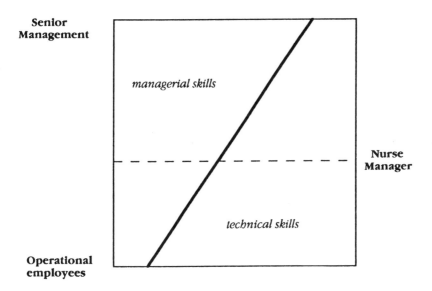

Senior Management

managerial skills

Nurse Manager

technical skills

Operational employees

Figure 7.6

Among the modern tools being developed for hospital management, DRG's (Diagnosis Related Groups) are emerging as an important classifying instrument. In Belgium the DRG, by Royal Decree, is supplemented by a Nursing Minimal Data Set (NMDS) (Sermeus, 1989). In the performance-oriented financing systems, being introduced in Europe, it will become important for nurses to gather information necessary for their part in the care-giving, because nursing care is one of the parameters for measuring performance. By contributing to the overall performance of the hospital, nurses will be entitled to play a part in management.

The introduction and development of the Nursing Minimal Data Set as part of a DRG system will therefore have to play in the NMD programme.

7.3.4 Critical Success factors

The better documented experiences relating to the involvement of nurses in decentralization of hospital management suggest that it is possible to formulate some critical factors determining the success of nurses in their managerial role.

1) Proximity Of all the professionals surrounding the patient, nurses are the ones constantly working in the presence of the patient. Nurses are never far away from the subject of their attention and are therefore able to react promptly to the needs of patients, employees and colleagues. In managing units and sections the need for this proximity is self-evident. Managing people implies a relationship. Presence and proximity are necessary conditions for establishing such a relationship.

2) Integration Medical professionals, working within a professional bureaucracy, direct their first loyalty to their profession and to their peers. Coupled with their 'sacred clinical autonomy' (Godt, 1987) this makes them stand aside from the organization they work for. Among the medical profession this lack of internal organization is being noted: *'Un premier constat montre que des trois partenaires - administratif, soignant, medecin - seul le dernier n'est pas organisé, hiérarchisé'*, (Diet, 1988). The organization is viewed as a facilitating agency ('Them') enabling the physicians ('Us') to do their jobs. Nurses on the other hand are trained for and selected by their social capabilities. Empathy (Ray, 1989) concern and commitment are factors governing their organizational behaviour (Bergot *et al.*, 1984). Because of these integrative capabilities nurses are well suited to lead and motivate people. Human resources form the most important investment of any hospital. Employees should be led by people giving them a sense of belonging.

3) Continuity The day to day presence of nurses on the floor of their sections gives their discipline great continuity for the patients. The nursing discipline is a highly visible continuous service to the patients. But not only in the day-to-day business is there continuity; it exists also in the hierarchy that constitutes the nursing discipline. This hierarchy consists of well-defined areas of authority and responsibility (Markham, 1988). Within this hierarchy problems are carried forward to the level where they can best be dealt with. Nurses are trained in dealing with this hierarchy; they go about it in an orderly way and they accept the rules of this system. The system would disintegrate if nurses were to bypass the hierarchical levels whenever it suited them.

4) Emancipation Nurses are in the middle of a process of emancipation. This is not only oriented towards their profession (for example Haldi, 1986; N.N., 1986; Clauwaert & van Eeckhout, 1984; Schmidt-Rettig, 1989).

This emancipation also has political aspects. Nurses have found a way to be put on the political agenda in Holland by using a method which until recently was considered unethical: they decided to strike. The professional status of nurses seems to be enhanced by some of the same factors that used to exist within the medical profession. Their professionalization will lead to 'formally recognized knowledge, made certifiable and interchangeable through diplomas' (De Swaan, 1988, 233).

On the other hand there seems little danger that the nursing discipline will fall victim to what is called by De Swaan: 'the reluctant imperialism of the medical profession.' (De Swaan, 1988, 238). This points to the tremendous influence gained by the medical profession in the distribution of the means of the welfare state. Important elements of the social security system need the cooperation of doctors. The emancipation of nurses is directed towards other goals. If there is such a thing as a "law of arrears that boost", it is certainly applicable to the emancipation process of nurses. Characteristically nurses are meeting the new challenges with confidence and elan. These challenges offer possibilities for innovating the profession. Unlike those who fight the developments in health care tooth and nail, nurses will gain influence and professional status by participating in changes taking place in hospital management.

7.3.5 Concluding Thoughts

Hospitals will have to be better equipped to deal with the challenges they are faced with. One of the ways to enable hospitals to deal more effectively with developments in their strategic environment is to decentralize authority and responsibility. Nurses can play a major role in this organizational process because they are by vocation, by position and by training well suited to accept new responsibilities. What is needed is a specific Nurse Management Development (NMD) programme to train them in the needed skills. Nurses can enter the decade after 1992 with confidence and élan.

7.3.6 References

Anderson, R. (1984), A Theory Development Role for Nurse Administrators, *Journal of Nursing Administration*, **19**, (5), May, 23 - 9.

Bergot, Ch. *et al.* (1984), Fonction de gestion du service infirmier, *Gestions Hospitalières*, **233**, Fevrier, 119 - 120.

Beske, F., Delesie, L., Rutten, F., & Zollner, H. (1987), *Hospital financing systems, Report on two WHO workshops*, Institute for Health Systems Research, Kiel.

Blair, E.M. (1989), Nursing and administration: A syntheses model, *Nursing Administration Quarterly*, Winter, 1 - 11.

Chandler, C. (1989) Separating some of the Issues, *Management Process*, **1**, (2), April, 16 - 17.

Clauwaert, G. & Van Eeckhout, S. (1984), Het verpleegkundig beleid in beweging; Reflekties omtrent tendenzen binnen het verpleegkundig management in Vlaanderen, *Het Belgisch Ziekenhuis*, **172**, 33 - 40.

Delamothe, T. (1988), Nursing Grievances, *British Medical Journal*, **296**, 2 January, 25.

Diet, J. (1988), Le chef de service, chef d'entreprise, *Gestions Hospitalières*, **279**, Octobre, 581 - 83.

Dowd, R.P. (1988), Participative decision making in strategic management of resources, *Nursing Administration Quarterly*, Fall, 11 - 18.

Genin, M.G., Mourdon, C. & Nicollet, M. (1988), Service Infirmier: notre expérience, *Gestions Hospitalières*, **278**, Août/Septembre, 501 - 4.

Gypen, T. (1988), De matrix-structuur als organisatie-model ter implementatie van het K.B. 407, *Het Belgisch Ziekenhuis*, **194/195**, 28 - 9.

Gleeson, S., Nestor, O.W. & Riddell, A.J. (1983), Helping nurses through the management threshold, *Nursing Administration Quarterly*, Winter, 11 - 16.

Godt, P.J. (1987), Confrontation, Consent and Corporatism: State Strategies and the Medical Profession in France, Great Britain and West-Germany, *Journal of Health Politics, Policy and Law*, **12**, (3), Fall, 459 - 80.

Grant, Colin (1989), Management Development for Health Care, *European Healthcare Management Association*, Dublin.

Haldi, N. (1986), Die europäischen Krankenschwestern mussen umdenken, *Krankenpflege*, **4**, 79 - 80.

Hoek, H. (1989), Unitmanagement, *C3 Cahier, Jaargang 1*, **4**, October.

Hospital Committee of the EEC, Hospital Planning and Management, Proceedings 1983/1984.

Knollmueller, R. (1979), What Happened to the PHN Supervisor? *Nursing Outlook*, **27**, October.

Lauffer, E. (1989), Kampf dem Pflegenotstand, *Krankenhaus Umschau*, **4**, 250 - 56.

Markham, G. (1988), None but the Brave, *Nursing Times*, **84**, (27), 33 - 4.

Musch, C.K. (1988), Veranderingsmanagement, *C3 Cahier, Jaargang 1*, **1**, November.

Musch, C.K. (1989) De verpleegkundige als ondernemer, Proceedings Verpleegkundig Informaticacongres, Academische Uitgeverij Amersfoort, Amersfoort.

N.N. (1986), Die Krankenpflege von heute und morgen, *Krankenpflege*, **2**, 77 - 81.

Ray, M.A. (1989), The theory of bureaucratic caring for the nursing practice in the organizational culture, *Nursing Administration Quarterly*, Winter, 31 - 42.

Samuels, D. (1988), From sister to manager, *Nursing Times*, **85**, (16), 45 - 6.

Sermeus, W. (1989), Hospital Care Financing and Nursing in Belgium, Proceedings of EFMI-Working Conference '89 on DRG's. UZ, Ghent.

Shoemaker, H. & El-Ahraf, A. (1983), Decentralization of nursing service management and its impact on job satisfaction, *Nursing Administration Quarterly*, Winter, 69 - 76.

Schmidt-Rettig, B. (1989), Perspektiven auf dem Gebiet der *Krankenhausökonomie und des Krankenhausmanagements*, *Das Krankenhaus*, 3, 111 - 14.

Smith, E.D. & Corso Falter, E. (1988), The nurse shortage: Coping through cooperation, *Nursing Administration Quarterly*, Fall, 40 - 4.

Sobczak, P.M., Fottler, M.D. & Chastagner, D. (1988), Managing retrenchment in French public hospitals: philosophical and regulatory constraints, *International Journal of Health Planning and Management*, 3, 19 - 34.

Swaan, A. de (1988), *In Care of the State*, Cambridge Polity Press, Cambridge.

Systchenko, B. & Fabry, J. (1988), Evaluation des soins hospitaliers, *Gestions Hospitalières*, **280**, Novembre, 715 - 18.

Vancil, R.F. (1979), *Decentralization: Managerial Ambiguity by Design*, McGraw-Hill, Homewood, Ill., 8.

8 Public and Private Health Insurance

Contents

8 Public and Private Health Insurance

8.0 Introduction

W.P.M.M. van de Ven

Several questions were put to the speakers in the session 'Public and Private Health Insurance', such as: Will the individual EC-members keep their autonomy with respect to 'social health insurance' after 1992? What is the definition of 'social health insurance'? Will the use of health care facilities in another EC-country have to be reimbursed by the public health insurance authority? Will the internal EC market stimulate a convergence of social health insurance premiums and benefits? Will there in due course become a compulsory European Health Insurance? Will the internal market lead to a competitive health insurance market? If so, what kind of pro-competitive regulation is needed in order to meet society's aims with respect to health care?

A remarkable finding is that none of the speakers was able to give a formal definition of 'social health insurance'. Van de Kasteele and Elsinga mentioned as important aspects of it:

a) the character of the insurance, which comes into being on basis of a law, and not on basis of an insurance contract;

b) the compulsory nature of the scheme by government-stipulated groups of persons;

c) a contribution related to wage or income;

233

d) the benefits fixed by the government.

Mrs. Sahmer, however, put forward that it is incorrect to consider the compulsory nature of health insurance schemes as a necessary condition for 'social' health insurance. She stated that under certain regulations, as in the Federal Republic of Germany, voluntary private health insurance can also be 'social' health insurance.

According to Maynard 'social' health insurance implies solidarity, universality and minimal price barriers to health care consumption for the majority of health care services.

8.0.1 Public versus Private

The public or private character of health insurance appears to have far-reaching consequences in Europe after 1992. With respect to 'social' health insurance the international coordination is regulated by the European Community Regulation 1408/71. It is expected that for the time being, 'social' health insurance will be mainly a national affair. Private health insurance companies, however, are obliged to observe the so-called first and second European directives on non-life insurance business. These directives relate to competition elements and regulate insurance technical matters like solvability requirements. The second directive provides the possibility of supervision by the supervising authority in the EC-country of domicile also for services rendered in other EC Member States.

The different ways in which Community Law treats public and private health insurance might lead to a divergence between both, especially with regard to elements of solidarity.

8.0.2 Time-bomb under Solidarity?

As Mrs. Sahmer stated, the inherent harmonization is designed to make it possible for European insurers to launch cross-border operations from their own headquarters into any other EC Member State with the long term objective being that this can be done in accordance with the legal provisions pertaining to the insurance transactions in the country of domicile. Existing differences in national practices, for example, the supervision of insurance companies, the approval of insurance terms and premiums, the formation and coverage of reserves for benefit payment, the investment in fixed assets, certain principles of operation like the separation of insurance lines and the actuarial computation, are to be largely harmonized.

If this will result in a strong competitive European market for health insurance, it is to be expected that this will lead to options such as risk-rated premiums, no-claims bonuses, exclusion of pre-existing conditions, risk selection, no continuity of coverage, and so on. Existing elements of solidarity will then get into danger. This will not only hold for Germany, but also for other European countries with substantial voluntary (supplemental) health insurance, like for example the Netherlands (where about forty per cent of the population has a private health insurance on a voluntary basis), France, Belgium or Ireland. Therefore, one should seriously ask the question to what degree the harmonization of the regulation of non-life insurance puts a time-bomb under the solidarity in private health insurance. If this is true, it is advisable to put all essential health care benefits into the public health insurance system in order to be sure that nobody will be prevented from access to care for financial reasons. An alternative would be, as Mrs. Sahmer and Van de Kasteele and Elsinga suggested, to include private health insurance in the discussion on social security within the European Community.

8.0.3 Medical Tourism?

With respect to public health insurance the focus in the coming years will be more on the increase in coordination than on integration of the different insurance schemes. This coordination is regulated by EC-regulation 1408/71. Article 22 of this regulation enables publicly insured persons to receive medical care in another Member State. In that case they are covered for the services and benefits as applicable in the country in which they stay. As Mr. Van den Heuvel said, this does not mean a free circulation of patients, because payment is still subject to the necessary authorization by the patient's national insurance organization. Whether or not this authorization is given depends crucially on whether or not the patient is in acute medical need. Nevertheless one should seriously ask the question to what degree this regulation can lead to a 'medical tourism' within Europe. Isn't it attractive for a patient who is in 'acute medical need' and who lives in an EC-country with a restricted public health insurance benefits package or with long waiting lists, to receive the necessary medical treatment in another EC Member State with a broad benefits package or without (long) waiting lists? Doesn't such a regulation offer the opportunity to specialized Centres of Excellence to attract patients from all over Europe? Finally, doesn't it offer to entrepreneurial hospitals and physicians who are confronted with over-supply in their own country, the opportunity to treat patients from other EC Member States at the expense of the public health insurance system of the homeland of the patients? The future will show us to what degree such medical tourism will take place and what its consequences will be.

Furthermore it is important to realize, as Maynard correctly pointed out, that without portability of health care benefits, labour movement will be circumscribed and the advantages of division of labour in a large EC market may be vitiated. Maynard therefore concluded, that if free mobility of labour is to be achieved, the portability of health insurance benefits across the frontiers of the EC Member States will have to be increased.

8.0.4 Convergence?

Will the EC market lead to a convergence of health insurance premiums and benefits? With respect to premiums one could wonder to what extent companies might gain an advantage by shifting their production lines to a Member State with less developed social protection. This is generally not regarded as an actual danger. As Mr. Van den Heuvel said, the decision of investors is influenced by many factors and it is very likely that vital factors like employee qualification, productivity and cultural environment for the executives will turn out to be at least as important as taxes and premiums for social health insurance.

With respect to health insurance benefits Van de Kasteele and Elsinga expect that in time there will undoubtedly come a convergence of insured benefits and services. They expect that the benefits in the northern countries won't grow too much in the future and that the benefits in the southern countries will come up to the level we now have in northern Europe. According to Maynard a 'core' set of benefits might be defined initially if only to concentrate minds.

8.0.5 European Health Insurance?

All speakers agreed that a compulsory European Health Insurance cannot be expected at short notice. Mr. Van den Heuvel pointed out the multiplicity of health care systems and the disparity of socio-economic possibilities and of cultural environment. Van de Kasteele and Elsinga mentioned arguments in terms of national orientation in the health care delivery field and the national emphasis on cost containment. In the long run, however, harmonization may be accomplished as a result of the evolution of the unified market. Maynard said that if a compulsory European Health Insurance ever arises, an insurance system based on the Canadian model seems to be a logical approach to achieve the collective objective inherent in the health care system of the EC Member States.

Looking at the US experience Kirkman-Liff stated that there is **no** intrinsic necessity for uniformity within a continent-wide system: uniformity is not essential from a macroeconomic perspective. However, a lack of uniformity means a lower level of social equity and solidarity within members of the same continent-wide community.

The choice is with the European citizens.

8.1 Health Care in Europe: Coordination or integration?
P.J. van de Kasteele and E. Elsinga

Before going more into detail about those aspects which the organizers of the Congress 'Health Care in Europe after 1992' asked us to survey, namely the influence of Europe 1992 on the health insurance systems in the countries of the Common Market, we would like to give a short description of the structure of the Dutch system of health care insurance and which elements are important in that system. In this way we hope to give you an impression of the background from which we are looking into the future.

8.1.1 Present Dutch Health Care System

The Dutch health care insurance system comprises four elements:

1) The Exceptional Medical Expenses (Compensation) Act   Insurance under the Exceptional Medical Expenses (Compensation) Act (AWBZ) is statutory: everyone meeting the criteria set in the Act is compulsorily insured, whether or not they wish to make use of the treatments and services offered, and must pay the relevant contributions. The Act covers the whole population resident in the Netherlands against 'exceptional medical expenses', mostly long-term care and catastrophic illnesses. This includes nursing homes, psychiatric hospitals and so on. The contribution to the insurance scheme is related to the income of the insured. For employees the contribution is paid by the employer; no contribution is payable in respect of under-15s and over-65s, at least up until now. This will change the next year. The insurance scheme is implemented by the health insurance funds, private insurers and the agencies that operate the statutory insurance schemes for civil servants.

2) Health Insurance Act (Sickfund Act)   The insurance scheme of the Health Insurance Act, the sickfund insurance, is a statutory insurance for employees with a wage below a certain limit, at this moment approximately ƒ 50 000 (Dutch florins) per annum. All employees who meet this criterium are compulsorily insured and must pay the statutory contributions. Retired employees remain in this insurance scheme. The insurance scheme covers a broad spectrum of 'normal' medical services, hospital admission, general and specialist medical treatment, dental care, pharmaceuticals, and so on. The contribution consists for the greater part of a percentage of the wage-income of which a part is paid by the employer. The other part of the contribution consists of a flat rate contribution per person. Around sixty per cent of the Dutch population is insured under this Act.

3) Private Insurance   Employees with a wage-income of over ƒ 50 000 (Dutch florins) per annum, self-employed people and civil servants employed by the central government, can insure themselves privately. This is a normal civil insurance contract. Nobody is obliged to take out this insurance coverage, and the private insurance companies are not forced to accept anybody; they can make their own acceptance policies. A private insurance contract generally covers the same medical services as the sickfund insurance scheme. Only for dental care is there usually a smaller coverage.

For the insurance one has to pay a flat-rate contribution per person. Children mostly pay at half-rate. About thirty-five per cent of the Dutch population has a private insurance contract.

4) Statutory Health Insurance Schemes for Public Servants   Civil servants, employed by city and provincial authorities are insured against medical expenses as part of their employment contracts. This insurance scheme generally also covers the same services as the sickfund scheme. The contribution also consists for the greater part of an income-related contribution of which the employer pays a share and of a flat-rate contribution which the employee has to pay for himself. The insurance scheme is implemented by eleven agencies. Around five per cent of the Dutch population is insured by this scheme.

8.1.2 'Change Assured'

Since the purpose of this session is not to focus on separate countries, but to look at developments in health care insurance and financing from the perspective of European integration, we will now give only a short description of the proposed changes in the structure and finance of Dutch health care, which we, the Dutch government, are trying to implement stepwise.

In August 1986, the Dutch government (the Cabinet) appointed an external committee that was instructed to find ways to improve the structure and financing of the health care system. This Committee on the Structure and Financing of Health

Care (the Dekker Committee) had six months in which to formulate its recommendations. In March 1987, the Dekker Committee published a report entitled 'Willingness to Change' which contained their proposals for fundamental changes in the present health care system that would result in a new system of financing and ensuring a basic insurance for the whole people and an enhancement of market-oriented activities.

After a prolonged and difficult decision-making process, the Cabinet presented its final reaction to the Dekker Plan in the policy paper called 'Change Assured' in March 1988; Parliamentary debates followed in June 1988. The first steps towards the new health care system were taken on 1 January, 1989. Full implementation will take at least four years and should be finalized by 1992 at the earliest, but will probably take a few years more.

The principal aim of the Cabinet's proposal, as set out in the policy paper 'Change Assured', is the creation of a health care system which combines the essentially social character of a health care system with effective mechanisms that guarantee cost-effectiveness and efficiency (a form of regulated competition). The main elements of the Cabinet's proposals are 1) a restructuring of the insurance system and 2) a greater role for market elements in the health care system. Both elements will briefly be described.

1) According to the Cabinet's proposals, some important changes in the insurance system will become operative in the next few years, resulting ultimately in a system of a basic and a supplementary insurance. The compulsory basic insurance package will cover most provisions in the field of health care (hospitalization, the GP, specialist, and so on) as well as social care services (homes for the elderly, family care, certain forms of home care, and so on).

The optional supplementary insurance package, which will account for nearly fifteen per cent of the total cost of health care and social care services, will include medicines, physiotherapy and dental care for persons over the age of 18.

The basic insurance plan will be financed partly by an income-dependent premium and partly by a flat-rate (nominal) premium. The income-dependent premium will be collected by the tax services and paid into a Central Fund. Out of this Fund it will be distributed among the insurance companies on a predetermined basis related to the proportion insured of the population by this insurer. The nominal premium will be paid directly by the insured to the insurance company.

After the restructuring process there will no longer be any distinction between health insurance funds (sickfunds) and private insurance companies, as there is in the present system. There will be only one type of insurance company, and the insured will be free to choose his insurer. In principle insurers will be obliged to accept all applicants and charge all persons insured by that company the same fixed premium.

2) The Cabinet's aim is to reduce direct influence of the Government and thereby the volume of legislation in the health care sector. The Cabinet hope to realize this through enhancement of the role of market elements and of self-regulation, thereby promoting flexibility, efficiency, the consumer's freedom of choice, individual responsibility and differentiation between different forms of care. The insurers and the providers of health care in particular, will have to become increasingly aware of their joint responsibility with regard to the volume, price and quality of the care provided.

Some illustrations of market elements in the new system are the freedom of insurance companies to contract with health providers (competition between providers) and competition between insurance companies with regard to the level of the nominal premium charged to the insured. Evidently, the market-oriented approach cannot provide solutions to all the problems facing the health care sector. Government regulations will still be needed in important areas, such as the quality of health care and the provisions of the basic insurance plan.

This short description of the proposals for change in the Dutch health care system makes it clear that an analysis from the perspective of 'Europe 1992' is of great relevance, both with respect to the new insurance scheme and the element of market orientation, including competition.

8.1.3 European Coordination: the Present Situation

When we look at the existing coordination framework in Europe we see two different systems for the private and the social health insurance schemes.

1) The private (health) insurance companies are obliged to observe the so-called first and second European directives on non-life insurance business. This means the First Council directive of 24 July 1973, on the coordination of laws, regulations and administrative provisions relating to the taking-up and pursuit of the business of direct insurance other than life assurance (73/239/EEC) and the second council directive of 22 June 1988 on the coordination of laws, regulations and administrative provisions relating to direct insurance other than life assurance and laying down provisions to facilitate the effective exercise of freedom to provide services and amending directive 73/239/EEC.

We do not want to go into detail on the contents of these council directives. Generally speaking on the one hand they regulate insurance-technical matters, like solvability requirements, liquidity requirements and similar matters. On the other hand they relate to competition elements, the possibility of operating an insurance company in the different countries of the European Community and so on.

2) Social insurance schemes are excepted from these directives. Neither internationally, nor nationally does a formal definition of a social insurance scheme exist, therefore we are not able to offer more than the description of some characteristics of social security schemes. Important elements are:

a) the character of the insurance, which comes into being on basis of a law, and not on basis of an insurance contract;
b) the compulsory nature of the scheme by government-stipulated groups of persons;
c) a contribution related to wage or income;
d) the benefits fixed by the government.

The international coordination of social insurance in the countries of the European Common Market, the social sickness insurance included, is regulated by the European

Community Regulation 1408/71. The people insured under a statutory insurance scheme of a country in the European Community are under the operation of this regulation also insured in the other countries of the European Community. They are covered for the services and benefits as applicable in the country in which they stay.

Privately insured people are not included in this coordination. They have to take out their own international insurance coverage.

8.1.4 Europe 1992

On trying to estimate the influence of Europe 1992 on the existing system of health care insurance, our first impression is that not so much will change immediately.

Social health care insurance is excepted from the European directives for the non-life insurance branch. The possibilities of free services in Europe after 1992 have no influence on the implementation of the social health insurance schemes of the different countries. One is not forced to accept foreign companies in the system, at least as far the social health insurance is concerned. As the international coordination for social health insurances already exists, no direct change will be necessary, or is to be expected.

For the private health insurance sector Europe 1992 means in principle a more competitive environment. We have yet to discover whether this will crystallize. The private health insurance sector in most European countries is relatively small, and at least in the Netherlands, more regulated than other insurance branches. In Holland this meant losses for this sector in the past few years. Although after 1992 it will be more easy for foreign insurance companies to operate in other countries, it is possible that less than rosy profit prospects means that they will be cautious in really moving into the market.

Because private health insurance is but a small factor in the total health insurance in Europe the development in this sector after 1992 will have but a marginal effect.

Whether *long term change* is to be expected in the system of social health care insurance as a result of Europe 1992, is another question. Our answer is a qualified yes.

When we look at what has happened in Europe since the Treaty of Rome in 1955, first with the agricultural policy and after that on other parts of economic policy, we see a slow but sure trend towards integration. However, nothing changes very quickly.

The countries of the European Community have very different systems to cover the cost of health care. We have only to think of the National Health system in Great Britain, the compulsory insurance scheme in Italy and the system of Mutualities in Belgium, to realize our different approaches. It is not to be expected that these countries will choose quickly in favour of one uniform system after 1992, and drop their own existing schemes which have been in place often for a long time. As we pointed out before, social insurance schemes are masked from competition. Because international coordination between these schemes is already in place, there will be only gentle pressure to realize international integration in the short term.

The difference in the social health care insurance schemes also means that the costs of health care services are shared in a different way in each country. There is a mix of contributions, tax payment and co-payment, that differs by country. The difference in benefits of the national schemes also means that this mix differs.

The greater possibilities for international competition after 1992, will probably mean a trend towards more equal labour costs in each country. This will apply to the sum total of the labour costs, however, and not to every part included in the labour costs; this means that there is no automatic mechanism that influences directly the social health insurance premium.

Moreover, there are differences in the organization of the social security schemes in the different countries. In Holland we have a clear distinction between insurance against the cost of health care and insurance which covers income benefits in case of sickness or disability. In some other countries these elements are included in one insurance scheme.

From these differences I conclude that a convergence of social health insurance contributions is not only not very soon (if ever) to be expected, but is also not a meaningful concept. The national schemes differ too much.

What we have said up till now does of course not mean that nothing will happen. In time there will undoubtedly come a convergence of insured benefits and services. On the basis of the so-called 'Norm-treaties' under the auspices of the International Labour Organization and the Council of Europe, there are already minimum standards which must be observed by the individual countries in their social security laws. It does not mean that these laws should contain exactly the same benefits. That may still differ from country to country. The difference in economic development between the southern and northern countries of Europe makes it plausible to expect that first of all we will see a convergence of services and benefits covered by the social health care insurance legislation. The benefits in the northern countries will not grow too much in the future and the benefits in the southern countries will come up to the level we have now in western Europe. That, and a more even distribution of health care facilities will be necessary before we can ever think of a compulsory European Health Insurance scheme.

The last-mentioned factor, the supply of health care facilities, is an element that should be explicitly mentioned. Health care delivery is, generally speaking, a local phenomenon. Although some medical specialists or hospitals have an international reputation, so that patients come from afar to receive treatment, that is more the exception than the rule.

Most patients are treated near their homes. There seems to be not much scope for international, competitive services; no international 'mail order' treatment. Besides, in many countries the feeling is that the making of a profit in health care delivery is unethical, which certainly acts as a brake on free competition in this sector.

The structure of the 'market for health care services' is a problem too. This 'market' is characterized by an inelastic demand, and a situation in which one can speak of the existence of forced consumption. The knowledge of the patient of the need for, or the quality of, the services supplied is mostly non-existent. This means that health care delivery does not easily fit into a market concept with real free competition. As a result, where real free competition does exist in health care, for example in the supply of pharmaceutical products, not everyone is happy with the result of that market process. What we try to introduce in Holland with the Dekker Proposals is more regulated competition and not really free competition.

The last element we want to mention is the development of health care costs, and the containment of its growth.

The costs of health care delivery have increased very fast in the last decennia, faster than the growth of the national income. This has happened in nearly every European country. The causes of this increase are, to enumerate just a few: the increase in services covered by the social insurance system; medical-technological progress; and the circumstance that health care delivery is a very labour-intensive process (which will hopefully stay that way). In nearly every European country cost-containment measures have been taken in the past ten years, with the aim of at least slowing down the growth of health care costs.

We cannot say that these measures have met with great success everywhere. Because of the importance of the effect of the increase in health care costs on the increase in labour costs and in that way on the development of the national economy, this element could also mean that governments will not be eager to delegate their authority in this field to Brussels.

Summarizing our line of reasoning so far, we would conclude that seen from the present situation, at first sight a real integration (that is unification) of European health insurance systems seems to be still far away, if ever to be reached. We can mention arguments in terms of:

a)   present differences in financing and organizing health care in the European countries;
b)   national orientation in the health care delivery field;
c)   national emphasis on cost-containment.

8.1.5 Some Principles on Coordination/Integration

After having sketched the present situation and the possible developments in the (near) future, let us now finally try to formulate some general principles on European integration with respect to health care finance and organization.

1)   Too often European integration is perceived as a threat instead of a challenge. International exchange of goods, products and services can be as beneficiary to health care as it is to other parts of our economy. We should not by definition be afraid of possible change as a result of Europe 1992.

2)   Within the present national and European regulation the difference between a social and private health system is very important.

This is reflected in the different European directives and regulations for these sectors. Generally speaking, the private health insurance directives focus more on the private insurance companies, with the objective of equal possibilities to do business. The European regulations for the coordination of the social insurance schemes focus on the socially insured persons with, as the objective, international coverage.

3)   In the Netherlands we try to realize a social health insurance system that is carried out by privately-organized health care insurers. This system is a more or less unique combination of social and private elements in health care organization and finance which should hopefully lead to a combination of the positive elements in both systems. Seen from the perspective of the present (European) regulation it leads however to many juridical questions such as: which directive/regulation should be

applied; what are the opportunities for foreign insurers and suppliers of care? and so on.

4) European integration is not a goal in itself, nor is national autonomy on the organization of health care. What we should try to do on the European level, is to define the general goals and conditions for a European health care policy, including a vision on the organization and financing of health care. This could include elements such as:

a) basic coverage for everyone;
b) regulation on payments (premium/taxes) according to income;
c) basic quality regulation.

Should there be a consensus on these principles of health care finance and organization in the first place each country could organize its own system in this way. After that there would probably be less obstacles for international exchange of goods and services than there is at the moment. Only in the end is it to be expected that we will achieve a really integrated European health insurance scheme.

The Dutch 'Dekker Proposals' are to a certain extent a step in this direction: the government clearly defines its goals and conditions and then it is up to the insurers, insureds and providers of care to take up their own responsibilities within this publicly-defined framework. European integration could be beneficiary in this respect: why not allow a German insurance company or a Belgian hospital to enter the Dutch health care market? As long as they - just as their Dutch 'colleagues' - follow the national/international rules, they have the same rights.

One can seriously doubt whether such international exchange will reach a large scale; probably not, but that is not the relevant point. More relevant is that European integration provides the opportunities for the possibility of international exchanges at the borders where countries meet. That might stimulate competition and cost-awareness in health care throughout the whole country even without any real, all-embracing international exchange.

On surveying the whole field we conclude that in our view the focus in the coming years will be more on the increase in coordination than on the integration of the different insurance schemes to one European Health Insurance system. That will still be very far away.

8.2 The Impact of the Single European Market on Private Health Insurance in Germany
S. Sahmer

The German private health insurance industry being the largest within the European Community - both in number of insured persons and in premium income - I have been asked to give you an outline of the expectations and apprehensions that are associated with the European integration in my country.

Contrary to the situation in the public sector - where harmonization of the different European systems of social security is not on the agenda for the time being - the incorporation of private health insurance has advanced rather far already. Since the sixties, there have been several directives of the European Commission in Brussels concerning the insurance industry, the latest being the second non-life directive on freedom of services from June 1988. As economic enterprises, private health insurance companies are fully subject to the free movement of services that is currently being implemented at EC level.

The inherent harmonization is designed to make it possible for European insurers to launch cross-border operations from their own headquarters into any other EC Member State with the long term objective being that this can be done in accordance with the legal provisions pertaining to the insurance transactions in the country of domicile. Existing differences in national practices - concerning, for example, the supervision of insurance companies, the prior approval of insurance conditions and premiums, the method of premium-calculation - are to be largely harmonized since they constitute obstacles to the free movement in the opinion of the EC-Commission.

This starting point, however, does not seem adequate to the particular function that private health insurance fulfils within the national systems of social security. Let me take the example of my own country:

Unlike the other member countries of the European Communities where insurance against sickness is provided either by obligatory membership of the entire population in a state health insurance or by a state-run national health service, the Federal Republic of Germany has a health insurance system based on the principle of pluralism. State and private insurance providers operate side by side, sometimes competing with, sometimes supplementing, one another, each with their own precisely defined tasks and responsibilities. The point of this dual system is that the state on the one hand meets its social responsibility by making available the necessary insurance service to those in need of protection at affordable premiums while, on the other hand, ample room is left for the individual to make his own provisions for the future and freely select his very own combination of insurance cover. It is this principle of subsidy that the entire German health insurance system is based on today.

In principle, the law requires that all persons undertaking paid employment must be insured against sickness. However, that compulsory insurance ceases to apply, in the case of both white- and blue-collar workers, where an employee's income reaches a certain level which is adjusted annually in accordance with movements in average earnings. As a result of this cut-off limit for compulsory insurance, employees may choose between statutory and private health insurance and may change from one sector to the other:

a) employees whose occupational income exceeds the cut-off limit for compulsory insurance from the start may belong to the statutory insurance scheme as voluntary insureds during a short transitional period; beyond that, however, they are not subject to compulsory insurance;

b) as a further consequence of the cut-off limit for compulsory insurance, employees whose earnings are initially below the limit, but then exceed the limit as a result of an increase in wages or salaries, are no longer subject to compulsory insurance. They may then either remain members of the statutory health insurance scheme as voluntary insureds, or choose to take out private health insurance;

c) conversely, employees who have already left the statutory health insurance scheme, but who are brought back within the scope of compulsory insurance by an increase in the cut-off limit, may be exempt from compulsory membership of the statutory health insurance scheme.

In addition to white- and blue-collar employees, there are other occupational categories which are not subject to the statutory health insurance scheme and where no compulsory insurance applies. Consequently, the self-employed and members of the professions operating independently are left to make their own arrangements for health insurance provision. Likewise, civil servants who are in receipt of sufficient medical expenses cover as a result of benefits provided by their employers are not subject to compulsory membership of the statutory insurance scheme. Civil servants and the self-employed may not belong to the statutory insurance scheme on a voluntary basis, even where their remuneration or income falls below the cut-off limit for compulsory membership. In the case of pensioners, compulsory membership of the pensioners' statutory health insurance scheme which, in principle, comes into force on retirement, no longer applies where pensioners have not been members of the statutory health insurance scheme for the greater part of their working lives. The provision of cover for all those people is the exclusive responsibility of private health insurance.

There are further population groups, for example students, trainees and part-time workers, who are subject to compulsory membership of the statutory health insurance by law, but who may be exempt in the majority of cases.

This dual system of state and private health insurance introduces market economy elements, especially competitive incentives, into health insurance and demands special efforts in terms of both efficiency and price-worthiness. The option of alternative or supplementary private health insurance coverage makes it possible for the state to limit itself to providing insurance coverage to those in need of protection according to the principle of subsidy and, as a result of that, to counteract the central problem of all health insurance systems in the western industrialized countries - the expenditures for the health system that have for years been rising much faster than the general levels of prices and wages. The lack of such a corrective mechanism has led to a situation in other EC-countries where members of the state health insurance were not only faced with excessive premiums but also considerable deductibles. Foregoing the benefits due to them from the state health insurance they sometimes even sought private insurance coverage.

This field of activity opened up to private health insurance implies, on the other hand, certain obligations. For instance, private health insurance has to guarantee the same standard of security as in the public system. The private health insurer together with the German Insurance Supervisory Authority have reacted to this demand by a particular actuarial technique and a material state control that led to the principle of specialization (which means that health insurance business may not be operated together with other branches of insurances), to the approval of conditions and premiums prior to their application in the market, to the calculation of specific technical provisions and to lifelong policies by waiving the right of cancellation in the insurance conditions. In addition, private health insurers take care to provide cover for so-called 'bad risks' as well, that is for people with pre-existing conditions, which is possible whenever a whole group of the population is assigned to private health insurance, and which we have done several times in the course of the implementation of the health care reform.

All this shows a considerable amount of regulation in the field of private health insurance which, in our opinion, is opposed to the European Community's concept of developing a Single European Market. Market principles are only effective within limits in the private health insurance sector, the reasons being as follows:

a) Private health insurance is part of the social security system.
b) The field of action for private health insurance is determined by the degree of freedom for private provision granted by the legislator.
c) As a result, private health insurance is differently organized in each of the member countries of the European Community. It extends from exclusive coverage for certain professional groups and groups of people in the form of comprehensive medical expenses insurance through supplementary insurance for those areas not covered by social insurance to an alternative form of insurance existing in parallel to the state system and based on personal initiative.
d) The products offered by private health insurance are tailored to fit into each national social security system.
e) The standards to be satisfied by the private health insurance companies in the individual countries (such as lifelong contracts which cannot be terminated by the insurer, premiums not dependent on age, specialization) are derived from their purpose within the social insurance system. They are specified by the social insurance system and thus cannot be influenced by the insurers. For example, the legislator can only designate entire groups of people for private health insurance if it is certain that they will obtain the same security standard as under the state system.

The European Commission's attempt to harmonize these different conditions as a prerequisite for the free exchange of services is neither meaningful nor possible. Basically, this presupposes a harmonization of all the social insurance systems. However, both the European Commission and the national governments have clearly rejected any such intention and instead pleaded for coordination of the various systems with due consideration for the natural structures and property states. In addition, the only health insurance cover required in any country is that meeting the national requirements. A Dutch 'standard package policy', for example, would be meaningless for a French person seeking cover for the deductibles prevailing in the French system. The proposed harmonization in the terms of definition and calculation of technical provisions does not solve the problem either. How can a British health insurer, for example, form old-age provisions for contracts concluded in Germany through the rendering of free services, when British law does not allow for any such provisions?

Moreover, from a purely practical point of view the free exchange of services will prove relatively insignificant in health insurance. The frequency of claims and the nature of the insured event make it necessary to have a permanent contact address within the country, which is not covered by the free services directive any more but demands an establishment in the country of activity. The health insurance business also demands a specific 'infrastructure' in each country, such as integration into the socio-political debate, integration into the hospital and medical care system and fulfilment of certain socio-political functions by also insuring bad risks, for example. This 'infrastructure' cannot be provided by insurers who are only active in the service sector. At the same time, it's mere utilization by the service insurers place the domestic health insurers at a competitive disadvantage.

For all these reasons, we consider a European harmonization in the field of private health insurance as inappropriate as it is in the public sector. Private health insurance can only be coordinated alongside the respective national systems of social security. As long as this target has not been reached, the operation of private health insurance business has to follow the rules in the country of activity in order to maintain the local standard of consumer protection and to guarantee policyholders the particular type of private health insurance cover that matches the respective national system of social security.

8.3 The Future of Health Insurance and Health Care in the European Community
Alan Maynard

8.3.1 Introduction

The impact of the Single European Act on the market for health care is difficult to predict. A market is a network of buyers and sellers, and thus the harmonization process may affect financial agents (insurers and budget holders), provider agents (for example hospital managers, pharmaceutical suppliers and doctors) and the contractual relationships between these agents. The difficulty of addressing these issues in a short paper was augmented by a checklist of questions (see Appendix 1) which contributors were asked to address.

Before addressing these issues and questions, it is essential to make explicit value judgements about the expected future course of political and economic integration in the EC. Here it is assumed that such integration is politically and economically inevitable and that the scope of any discussion should focus on how it will affect the market for health care.

8.3.2 What is Social Health Insurance?

In each Member State of the EC there is an implied (and sometimes explicit) contract between the State and its citizens about the provision of health care. Whilst the scope and nature of this contract is often poorly specified, it implies solidarity, universality and minimal price barriers to health care consumption for the majority of health care services. Health care is to be allocated on the basis of the patients' capacity to benefit from care as mediated by doctors.

In the public health care sector, the finances are not related to actuarial risks over the life cycle. Indeed, the use of the term 'insurance' is inappropriate. As Meriam *et al.* (1950) remarked about the UK social security system, the 'adoption of the term "insurance" by the proponents of social security was a stroke of promotional genius' which clothed it 'with an aura of financial soundness'. It is likely that policymakers in other health care systems (for example France) will emulate UK mechanisms to equalize resource allocations (RAWP) and seek to evolve statements about national priorities in the health care sector.

The premia paid to the sickness funds of many EC States, like the national insurance contributions of the NHS, are payroll taxes whose incidence probably lies on employees (that is, they are part of wages). Whilst they are a convenient fiction to confuse gullible electorates, such 'insurances' are taxes and, as such, can be the subject of harmonization efforts like those for VAT, excise taxes and direct taxes.

8.3.3 Will Individual EC States retain Autonomy with regard to Social Health Insurance?

8.3.4 Will the Internal EC Market Stimulate a Convergence of Social Insurance Premiums?

If a common market for goods and services is to be created, as set out in the Treaty of Rome, taxes will have to be harmonized. This will require uniformity in the type of taxes which will be levied and a convergence in the rates of taxation over time. The latter trend will be induced by firms preferring to locate where rates are low and, in so doing, putting downward pressure on high tax rate areas and upward pressure on low tax rate areas. Such trends imply particular conditions about competition and production functions (economies of scale) in health care producer markets.

8.3.5 Will there be Compulsory EC Health Insurance?

If free mobility of labour is to be achieved, the portability of health care benefits across the frontiers of the Member States of the EC will have to be increased, that is 'contributions' paid in one state will create eligibility for benefits in another state. Without portability labour movement will be circumscribed and the advantages of division of labour in a large EC market may be vitiated.

What benefits will be made portable? There are many possible answers to this question which can be seen in other federal states. In the USA, federal programmes such as Medicaid (for some of the poor) and Medicare (for the old) vary considerably, with Member States of the union having discretion about the extent of benefits which are made available. In Canada there is a national health insurance system whereby all residents regardless of age, health status or income are entitled by federal law to be members of their provincial health plan. The precise rules of each plan vary. In Ontario, residents participate directly or via their employers. Benefits are determined by the Ontario plans fee schedule and they are comprehensive, if poorly integrated (Inglehart, 1986).

The scope of benefits in any EC health care system would be influenced by income and the efficiency with which resources are used. The Germans and the French spend twice as much *per capita* on health care as the British, but with little measured difference in outcome, the marginal product of health care expenditure is uncertain. The harmonization of health care would be facilitated by agreed core information systems about costs, processes and outcomes so that 'good practice' could be identified and practices monitored across countries. Such systems would enable decision-makers to be better informed about the efficiency of competing treatments.

Thus the definition of any common EC benefit package is unclear and dependent on the political goals and vigour of decision-makers. A 'core' set of benefits might be defined initially if only to concentrate minds. The size of this core will affect the extent to which there will have to be resource transfers from the richer to the poorer Member States.

To achieve the collective objective inherent in the health care system of EC Member States, an EC health insurance system on the Canadian model is a radical but logical approach. This would permit Member States to vary contribution and benefit packages but over time, it would enable states to equalize. Such a mechanism has the merit that it is an effective way of controlling costs.

8.3.6 Regulating Competition in the EC Health Care Market

If health care systems are harmonized in the EC, how can the behaviour of budget holders and providers be regulated to ensure efficiency? Efficiency can be pursued by state regulation, competition of 'leaving it to the Gods', that is, appealing to the professional mores of doctors to ensure that care is provided efficiently and equitably.

Enthoven has written extensively about how to ensure the success of 'managed competition' (1988, 1989(a), 1989(b). He wishes to create an environment in which the disincentives arising from third party payments are removed so that consumers, budget-holders and providers have strong incentives to behave efficiently.

To achieve this goal, Enthoven wishes to create a market where consumers can choose between competing health plans (budget-holders, buyers or financing agents) and those competing budget-holders can contract with competing providers, public and private, of all types (diagnostic and therapeutic) of health care, that is competition (or a striving for shares of the activity) is to be created on the demand and supply sides of the health care market.

Enthoven has advocated such arrangements for the USA for over a decade and his proposals have influenced policy-makers throughout the EC, especially in Britain and the Netherlands. However, the creation and maintenance of competition in health care markets is very difficult: providers naturally conspire to create and sustain monopoly powers which enable them to 'organize' patients and budget holders into choices consistent with their (the provider's) self interest.

To avoid this outcome, vigorous and extensive regulation of the health care market will be essential. At present the resource allocation process is obscure and the success of managed competition requires that it becomes transparent, and accountable to democratic control. Such characteristics imply that European society wants trade-offs about life and death and other goods and services to be explicit rather than settled out of the public domain by professionals.

For a market to operate explicitly and more efficiently there needs to be:

a) consumer choice, or if that is not possible, clearly identified purchasers (budget holders) who act as the patients' guardians in the health care market by identifying the health needs of the local population and the cost-effectiveness of competing ways of meeting these needs;

b) clear identification of the budget holder, with sharp incentives for her to use resources efficiently and with clear delegation of authority to prioritize amongst competing services and service suppliers. This process will involve deliberate and explicit decisions not to fund beneficial therapies which cannot be financed within the budget constraint;

c)   a pricing system to signal to purchasers which providers are providing what caring services at what cost;

d)   a system of provision contracts for care which specify price, volume and quality of care in terms of process and outcome (for example, for particular types of surgery specific minimum volume levels should be set to ensure the lowest possible mortality outcomes) and leave purchasers to buy from competing public and private organizations;

e)   a system of labour and capital contracts which facilitate flexible employment (for example, doctors who are inefficient or whose services are not required can be dismissed) and capital practices (for example closing 'surplus' hospitals and beds);

f)   division of labour amongst providers with some centres achieving significant economies of scale (for example centralization of pathology and other testing with quick returns of results by facsimile and other new information technologies). This will lead to cross-national boundary flows of patients and the need for 'money to follow the patients'.

Once created, the financial agents (insurers) will have an incentive to merge and collude, and providers will respond to similar incentives: the market will be characterized by oligopoly and oligopsony. There is little data about the optimum size of financier or provider, and thus it is not possible to know whether or not competition can be created with or without trade-offs with regard to economies of scale.

Additionally, market arrangements with competing financiers (or budget holders) may create sharp adverse selection problems. To avoid this, it will be necessary to set rules for the allocation of high-cost patients across insurers. Enthoven (1988) believes this will be possible in addition to maintaining managed competition, but others are more uncertain (Fuchs, 1988).

The English novelist, G.K. Chesterton, argued that Christianity had not failed, it had just not been tried! Enthoven parallels this argument in believing that competition in health care has not failed, it has just not been tried. Certainly like Christianity, competition is difficult to adopt and sustain! For it to thrive, a strong 'church' will have to be created to initiate and sustain competitive practices and accept the consequence of the 'rough justice' of the market place, that is, hospital closures and redundancy for doctors and other health care personnel.

8.3.7   Regulated Competition in the EC: the Dutch or British Model?

Both models, British and Dutch, are innovatory, radical and untried. In the case of Britain, the Government is reluctant to evaluate its proposals and has adopted an ambitious programme which will lead to implementation from April 1991. It is impossible to choose between the Dutch model (which seeks to create competition only on the supply and demand sides of the market) and the British model (which seeks to create competition only on the supply side of the health care market) at this stage. However, with careful evaluation much may be learned which will be of value to other EC States. Clearly for the first time purchasers will be able to identify what they purchased last year and assess their current needs at different prices from different providers this year. This requires much new information and its collection will facilitate provider audit as well as purchasers' choices.

8.3.8 The Consequences of EC Integration for the NHS

The harmonization of input markets has been slow to affect the NHS. The 'free movement' of doctors and nurses to the UK has been inhibited by relatively low pay, by language barriers and perhaps by positive but hidden discrimination based on implicit judgements about the skill qualifications of health care professionals from southern parts of the EC.

The 'free movement' of pharmaceuticals has yet to be achieved. Price discrimination is extensive and the prescribing patterns of doctors vary enormously across the EC. The use of an 'EC-FDA' to regulate safety and efficacy and an 'EC Health Insurance Programme' to control prices and costs would confront a familiar problem of trade-offs. Should the EC reduce pharmaceutical costs to facilitate the provision of cheap health care or raise these costs in order to protect the industry and reduce an estimated adverse EC balance of payments in pharmaceuticals in 1992 of $3 billion? Perhaps the EC will adopt the British system of subsidising the industry via the Pharmaceutical Price Regulation Scheme (PPRS), thereby inflating the costs of pharmaceuticals in the health care system?

The impact of the EC on NHS information systems has been limited. Resources could have been allocated to create an EC core information set. However, it seemed initially that people are to be left to 'reinvent' wheels and lose the opportunities for industry of economies of scale arising from common EC-wide criteria about costs, processes and outcome data. More recently the managers of the AIM programme are recognizing the needs for common core information sets and developing means to achieve them.

8.3.9 Conclusions

The health care systems of the EC have very different structures of finance and provision. However, the problems they create - disincentives arising from third party payers, little evaluation of the cost-effectiveness of competing treatments, cost inflation and the oligopolist monopolist-power of providers and the oligopsonist powers of buyers - are very similar. The search for 'solutions' to these problems in the Member States of the EC tends to be dominated by ideology and with all too little reference to evidence about the workings of competing buyer and provider incentive structures (see Maynard and Williams, 1984).

There is a propensity for fashion to dictate the direction of health care reform. The current fashion of managed competition is unproven but logical in its theory. How this will be translated into an EC health care system only time will tell, and great care is necessary if competition is not to undermine the doctor-patient relationship and the 'sense of duty' which dominates many exchanges in the health care market place.

8.3.10 References

Enthoven, A.C. (1988), Managed competition: an agenda for action, *Health Affairs*, Summer, 25 - 47.

Enthoven, A.C. and Kronich, R. (1989 (a)), A consumer-choice health plan for the 1990s, *New England Journal of Medicine*, **320**, (1), (part 1) 29 - 37.

Enthoven, A.C. and Kronich, R. (1989 (b)), A consumer-choice health plan for the 1990s, *New England Journal of Medicine*, **320**, (2), 94 - 101.

Fuchs, V. (1988), The 'competition revolution' in health care, *Health Affairs*, Summer, 5 - 24.

Inglehart, J.K. (1986), Canada's health care system (second of three parts), *New England Journal of Medicine*, **315**, (12), 778 - 84.

Maynard, A. and Williams, A. (1984), Privatisation and the National Health Service, in J. Le Grand and R. Robinson (eds.), *Privatisation and the Welfare State*, George Allen and Unwin, London.

Meriam, L. *et al.*, (1950), The Cost and Financing of Social Security, Brookings, Washington.

8.3.11 Appendix 1

Questions about Health Insurance:

1 What is the *definition* of social health insurance?
2 Will individual EC States retain autonomy with regard to social health insurance?
3 Will the internal EC-market stimulate a convergence of social health insurance premiums?
4 Will there, in due course, be a compulsory EC Health Insurance? For what benefits? Will rich states subsidise poor EC-countries?
5 If the internal market will lead to cooperation between providers, will this produce competition in health insurance? What pro-competition regulation will be needed?
6 If, in the long run, there is compulsory EC health insurance, will it follow the UK model or Dutch regulated competition model? What are the advantages and disadvantages of each?
7 What will be the consequences of integration of the EC Market for health insurance for the UK/NHS?

8.4 1993 and Health Insurance in the European Community
R. van den Heuvel

The prospect of 1993 seems full of promises. No area can escape the rising tide. Health, one of man's most precious assets, will not escape either.

Today, the building of an economic Europe is catalysing energies and producing an upheaval in all our thinking. Will this psychological excitement have an even greater macroeconomic effect than the simple mechanical consequences of market enlargement?

This is open to debate.

What do we mean by health insurance, protection against the risk of disease and health promotion?

To query the future of health care is to become involved in the future of cultural models. It is common knowledge that the European Community can claim to be the cradle of social insurance. In this field, we indeed take a leading place for the accessibility of care and all that springs from it. The result followed a process of evolution which had its painful moments. It was i.a. the social movement which was the motor of progress, even if quite different logic applied in each country.

8.4.1 A Protection with Many Forms

Every system is built to cope with its specific environment. Operational methods are very different between countries; the differences are even more marked because of state influence on social protection, and consequently also on private protection. Before looking at the future of these systems, we should first try to understand the way they work now. Let us start by looking at schemes of public protection, to which private schemes have come to be added.

1) Two Types of Schemes for Social Protection   The very first type of compulsory institutional social protection appeared more than a century ago in West Germany. Progressively, it was extended to practically all member countries of the Community, more particularly after World Word Two, as a consequence of the Beveridge Report.

To begin with only employees benefited in these schemes from protection based on solidarity. Eventually, this was extended to other sections of the population. This trend took place along two routes.

The first route depended on the extension of compulsory social assurance. This was the case for the systems now familiar in the central countries of the Community, that is to say the Netherlands, Germany, Luxembourg, France, and Belgium.

In Germany and in the Netherlands currently[1], protection is not compulsory for all. In West Germany, white collar workers earning more than a certain amount can exert a free choice between insuring in the public system or individually. By contrast in the Netherlands, those who exceed the qualified earnings level for compulsory insurance are excluded from social cover.

In the three other countries; France, Luxembourg and Belgium, social insurance protects the whole population, but with criteria differing by category.

This model of protection is mainly characterized in its financing mainly by social contributions; segmentation of cover, based on socio-professional categories; employees/self-employed; with management incorporating a variety of players including the mutualities. In Belgium and the Netherlands, sickness funds are the carriers of the system; in Germany too, the sickness funds are responsible for both the administrative and financial management of the system; in France the 'general' regime is managed by a public social security network, but the other schemes are partly managed by mutualities, private insurers and a professional union. Finally, in Luxembourg management of compulsory insurance is carried out by a public administration.

The second route depends on the widest generalization of protection and is familiar in countries in Europe's outer ring: UK, Denmark, Ireland, Portugal, Spain, Italy and

Greece. We can see three variations of this method, each of which corresponds to the particular circumstances of social protection in these countries.

In 1948, the UK, after the example of New Zealand and the Beveridge Report, created the National Health Service (NHS). This public administration is today the central authority for the supply and funding of medical care. The system is mainly financed by taxation and delivers uniform services.

Between 1971 and 1973 reforms in Ireland and Denmark set up an insurance type of protection financed by taxes and administered by public authorities. These reforms maintained a segmentation of benefits by category: in Denmark there are two categories of beneficiaries for which the claimant is free to choose, and in Ireland beneficiaries are divided into three categories depending on their incomes.

From 1978 reforms took place in Italy (1978), Portugal (1979), Greece (1983) and Spain (1986), which are not yet totally completed. These countries opted for systems of universal protection managed by the state. They are still mainly financed by social contributions, and the coverage is split by category.

In fact, there are as many systems as there are Member States. Now wonder that the - non mandatory - article 117 of the Treaty of Rome aiming at the 'harmonization of Social Systems' never came into effect and that this objective has even been abandoned *sine die*.

The Single Act, however, added an article 130A to the original text whereby the economic and *social cohesion* of the Community is targeted. This new article aims more particularly at narrowing the gaps between the different regions and at the situation of the lesser favoured regions. Later on we will return to this question.

Looking at the different systems of public protection makes very clear the diversity of systems. Situations are even more complicated when you look at private protection.

2) Private Protection whether Complementary or Alternative As social protection covers the largest part of health expenses (seventy to eighty-five per cent) it necessarily defines the possible extent of private protection. Private protection can be of two types, complementary or alternative, and also on a for-profit or an non-for-profit base, that is, on solidarity.

Complementary protection covers in part or as a whole the difference between the total cost of health care and coverage as services provided by the generalized or compulsory schemes (reimbursement by social protection). Complementary schemes do cover co-payments or services or citizens excluded by the compulsory schemes. This is especially the case in countries which introduced compulsory social insurance schemes, that is Belgium, France, Luxembourg, Germany and the Netherlands. To these countries, we should also add Denmark and Ireland which have protection by category within the route of generalized cover.

Alternative protection guarantees protection in parallel with national insurance or health services in the UK, Portugal, Italy, Spain and Greece. In these countries some people welcome the opportunity to have free choice of cover, or they try to avoid the inadequacies, such as waiting lists. This type of private protection is also available in Germany and until now in the Netherlands, to those who do not comply with the income conditions of the compulsory social insurance.

This short overview shows a multiplicity of types of coverage within the EEC. This multiplicity of systems is today one of the main obstacles to any policy of Community harmonization, but even more important in this regard is the disparity of socio-economic possibilities and of cultural environment.

8.4.2 Different Levels of Cover

Let us illustrate this situation, and look at the differences of cost and coverage in the following two tables. Table 8.1 shows the total level of spending on health as a percentage of Gross National Product and Table 8.2 shows the average cost of health in absolute dollar terms, by citizen, in each of the Member States. As the costs of health covered by all protection schemes represent around three quarters of the total cost of health, and as they follow in general the same development, these charts also indicate the trend of differences between the schemes around the Member States of the EEC.

Table 8.1
Evolution of the Total Spending on Health as a Percentage of the GNP 1960 - 1986

	1960	1970	1980	1986
Belgium	3,4	4,0	6,5	7,1
Denmark	3,6	6,0	6,8	6,1
Spain	2,3	4,1	5,8	6,0
France	4,2	5,6	7,4	8,5
Greece	3,0	3,9	4,2	3,9
Ireland	3,9	5,5	8,5	7,9
Italy	3,3	4,7	6,8	6,7
Netherlands	3,9	6,0	8,1	8,3
Portugal	0,9	1,8	5,9	-
United Kingdom	3,9	4,5	5,8	6,1
West-Germany	4,7	5,5	7,9	8,1

Source: OECD data

These figures prove that high national income and high expenditure for health are generally correlated as it was confirmed by the OECD and other studies.

This is also the confirmation of the 'Law of Engel': with growing income the part of it spent on primary needs does decline and the part used for health, culture and leisure rises. This explains in detail the leading position of the USA and Sweden on world health levels.

Inside the EEC the differences are even more significant: health expenditures in France and Germany, for instance, are four times more important than in Greece, three times more than in Portugal and twice as much as in Spain. Looking at these facts, we can see how complex it would be to structure any form of overall Community protection, at least in the short term. The recent reforms carried out in certain Member States tend to confirm this view. All are strictly based on local national circumstances without any Community perspective.

Table 8.2
Absolute Cost of Health by Citizen ($ PPR)

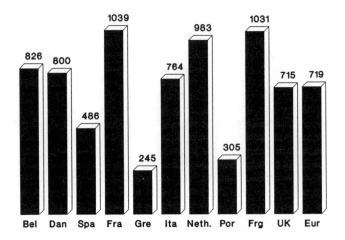

Bel	Dan	Spa	Fra	Gre	Ita	Neth.	Por	Frg	UK	Eur
826	800	486	1039	245	764	983	305	1031	715	719

8.4.3   Current Reforms: Strictly National

Today every country is trying to remedy the deficiencies of its own system, and improve the efficacy and efficiency of existing schemes. The main object of today's reforms is cost containment, and reduction in the growth of demand on the public budget.

In the Netherlands change has been blowing through health insurance since 1986. They began with a structural merger, regrouping all those compulsorily insured in one category: employees, self-employed and the elderly whose income was lower than threshold. Then Dr. Dekker's commission proposed in 1987 a radical reform of the existing protection system. The Dekker Plan was initially intended to produce a base of compulsory insurance which would effectively increase the share to be paid by the patient. Second, this reform aimed to introduce 'competition' as an incentive in the management of compulsory protection. Thus commercial insurers and sickness funds become competitors. Overall, the Dekker Plan followed a tendency which seemed, during the years of economic depression, to have been developed in several countries of the European community. It was called 'privatization' or 'desolidarization'.[2]

In Belgium the last draft laws owed little to the reforms proposed in the Netherlands. The aim was to renew the functional structure of the social protection system. Proposed legislation has set two objectives: to refine the organizational scope of the mutualities who manage both compulsory and complementary insurance service, and on the other hand to adapt the structure of the medical deontological bodies, especially in the fields of medical necessity control.

More transparency, democracy and responsibility are the themes of these reform projects. On a national and provincial scale, 'Round Tables' have been organized to start the process. They have allowed a wide exchange of view between the different

256

players in the health care field and could lead to a thorough reform by introducing the realities of financial responsibility of the insurance carriers.

In Germany, where cost containment was high on the agenda also, the Blum Reform took the name of their health minister. This has seen the introduction, since 1 January 1989 of 'basic amounts for some pharmaceuticals' and hospital fees. The savings will go to finance a policy of more home care.

In France the Minister of Health has been confronted with a partial collapse of the established system of tariff agreements. Today it is more and more difficult to use this technique to regulate urban medicine. The efficiency of agreements has been undermined by the growth of uncontrolled fees. The chosen objective has therefore been to restore a more effective fee-setting system.

In the United Kingdom, we see today a highly politicized climate generated by a new reform plan. The Government aims to improve the efficiency of the National Health Service by introducing incentives for better management. Implementation, principally in 1991, has attracted strong criticism from medical and nursing professions. They argue that the reform will involve discrimination between the sick. It is claimed that some patients will be able to afford private treatments while others will have to travel, sometimes long distances, to get their care. According to the medical profession, there could be other perverse effects to add to the widely-known waiting lists problem. An example might be the refusal of general practitioners to treat patients who require expensive equipment. It is still too early to evaluate the actual impact, however, since the new plan is not yet totally operational and it is not yet known how far the criticism is legitimate.

Finally we should consider the long-term impact of the radical changes in various National Health Services in the Mediterranean countries, which will permanently affect the sector. The upheavals in organizational arrangements are so great that aligning them later is sure to be a difficult and lengthy process.

This summary of the kinds of reform planned for health care schemes within the Community highlights the strictly national character of the measures being taken. These measures have nothing to do with a harmonization of the legislation of the Member States. As of now, there is no evidence of any strategy for future convergence. We are forced to conclude that in a foreseeable time there is no question of a single European system of health insurance or services.

8.4.4   The Single Act

To what extent is the Single Act going to close the gaps between social protection schemes? What risks do they cover? What are the future prospects for the private sector in the field of protection from illness? With the opening of the Single Market, these are the questions we are faced with.

1) Status Quo for Social Security   Up to the adoption of the Single Act which reformed the treaty originally creating the EEC, social protection policies remained the competence of each Member State. It will be practically the same after 1992 except for some legislation about working conditions, and protection of the workers.

But according to the new article 130A, is harmonization of the levels of social protection possible? Politically it will be extremely difficult to compromise between the Member States. Should we harmonize upwards or downwards? Either option will generate solid opposition and real problems of financing. In any case, what model should we choose? What criteria should we fix for the level of benefits? What time-scale should we plan for implementation in different states?

In any case unions, mutualities and political parties in the more developed countries will not tolerate seeing the degree of protection in their countries reduced in any convergency operation.

Without any doubt harmonization of the level of protection can be accomplished in the long term, without unifying the systems. It depends largely on the success - economically - of the Single Market. We should ask ourselves about the risks of relocation investments and of social dumping after 1992. To what extent might certain industries gain an advantage by transferring their production lines to a Member State with less developed social protection? Shouldn't we then expect effective deregulation of industrial relations agreements, with, as a target, a reduction in payroll overheads? How far is there an actual danger that any competition between different tax and social regimes would give an advantage to companies with the lowest levels of tax and protection?

- Investors may well not take into account such factors when planning their production facilities. It is much more likely that the vital factors like employee qualifications, productivity, and cultural environment will turn out to be at least as important as differences in hourly wages and costs.

However, several attempts were made to start with the convergence of the *level* of social protection: a 'guaranteed minimum', a 'common foundation', a social 'charter'. Finally the Commission adopted at the end of September 1990 a draft of Social Charter in the form of a 'Solemn Declaration' mainly about industrial relations and labour conditions. As far as social protection is concerned the text is rather vague: 'According to the proper conditions of each country every citizen is entitled to an "adequate" social protection' and further, the Commission thinks it necessary to guarantee a minimum income and a social assistance for those who are excluded from the labour market and for those such as the elderly, who do not possess the necessary means of subsistence.

After 1992, Member States' legal social security will therefore still be governed by the principle of national sovereignty and will continue to be coordinated by instruments coming from the Community. These have been designed to reinforce the principle of free circulation of persons within the Community. In the field of health, wage earners as well as self-employed people, and the members of their families, will therefore be able to preserve their national rights during a temporary stay in another member country (E 111). People near borders will benefit from a limited zone of care beyond national borders. Finally, certain patients are able to receive care abroad and still be reimbursed by their national social schemes (E 112). This is still subject to the necessary authorization by the patient's national insurance schemes, and some services like thermalism, can be excluded.

The effect of the grand Single Market could well intensify the mobility of patients. This is why the Commission is reviewing today whether it should adjust present coordination instruments to the realities of tomorrow.

2) What about a Free Market in Health? The Single Act doesn't change national rules, nor does it switch state competence to Community competence in the matter of social security. What difference, then, is this reform of the Treaty of Rome likely to make?

For an answer, we have to look at the 340 propositions and decisions set out in the 'White Paper'. Some of these could indeed have an impact on protection against the risk of sickness and health in general, for instance medical goods such as pharmaceuticals, high tech medication, equipment or devices, or free circulation of health care coverage in non-life insurance which includes sickness insurance. What will be the possible impact of these decisions on systems of health insurance or health services?

Let us look at the possible consequences:

2a) Medical professionals Free circulation of personnel will have only a limited impact. There are three reasons for this:

- First, simply look at the migration of doctors within the community. As a study by Professor Leon Hurwitz has shown, over a period of ten years following the application of directives authorizing free circulation of doctors, the overall migration within the community amounted to only 10 818 people (Spain and Portugal excluded).[3] As a percentage of the total number of doctors, that is only 0.21 per cent. Although in more recent years migration has accelerated, it remains marginal, just 3.4 per thousand doctors in 1986.[4] For some countries, however, there would be more important movements of dentists and nurses.
- Second, there are the cultural obstacles. These are particularly acute for medical professionals. Evidently medical and paramedical practice does not simply depend on technical know-how and a grasp of technology. What it needs is a quality relationship in which close knowledge of language and social and educational factors are key components.
- The third reason is simply economical; the attraction of better pay. This incentive to mobility can only come from Member States where the level of GNP permits it. In practice fees and salaries for health care are generally regulated by agreements. Moreover, there is a general oversupply of doctors in most European countries but a growing shortage of nurses.

2b) Medical Goods and Devices Alongside free circulation of medical professionals we should examine free circulation of medical goods. These include medicines, medical technology and devices and protheses or even software products for institutional care.

The pressure for harmonization of regulations in Member States faces a conflict between two major imperatives; guaranteeing social protection and upholding medical goods manufacturers' competitive position on the international scene.

Up till now, each Member State had always had the problem of meeting these national objectives, especially in the pharmaceutical sector. National authorities have insisted on pulling the strings both in fixing medicine prices and in calculating reasonable reimbursement conditions and prices by social security. They seek to keep a balance between economical and social interests.

Total freedom of medicine prices could produce in many countries a cost increase for the social system. So it will to the consumer. In fact, the use of generics can counter this effect. In West Germany since 10 September 1990 categories of pharmaceutical specialities are reimbursed by sickness funds at the prices set for generics. These categories are diabetes, 'circulatory deficiency', rheumatism, depression and cardiovascular problems. Five other categories will follow. In less than a month after this system became operational the industry cut down it's prices for comparable products by thirty to fifty per cent.

However, it is a false hope that market forces will automatically produce price reductions. Many of the producers are in fact oligopolist groups and the consumer cannot exert a real choice so that the demand-supply mechanism does not work.

Increasing European integration will probably increase the share of the medical sector in the economy. Authorities in the Member States will have to be vigilant. It is by no means impossible to imagine a flood of available capital rushing without necessity into private hospitals and health care facilities. Planning and regional priorities, already in place to control health costs, will have to be accommodated to avoid the diseconomies arising from any such movement and to safeguard the national cost-containment policies.

3) Private 'For-Profit' Health Insurance In view of the steadily faster development of new medical technology it is our opinion that the EEC needs a common research on efficacy and efficiency of these techniques and this perhaps in an adapted form of the Bureau of Technological Assessment (BTA) in the USA.

The third major effect of building a European Single Market could be in the private health insurance sector.

From the beginning of this decade, the market for private health insurance has been expanding in most Community countries. Annual growth of gross insurance premiums in the sickness sector well illustrates this trend.

Table 8.3
Annual Growth of Gross Insurance Premiums in the Private Sickness
Sector in Seven EEC Countries from 1975 to 1986
(in millions of national currency units)

Year	FRG DM	Belgium BF	Spain Ptas	France FF	Italy Lir.	Netherl. Fl.	United Kingdom
1975	6.521	852	15.447	2.416	18.000	2.600	82
1980	9.730	1.900	58.012	7.165	116.699	3.329	288
1982	11.900	3.003	79.607	9.475	168.746	3.729	390
1984	13.100	3.753	94.689	15.000	237.724	4.156	582
1986	13.630	4.816	115.148	19.253	328.279	4.429	798

Source: CEA

This development is partly explained by the growth in the health proportion of household expenditure (see Table 8.4).

Financing and spending on health care has therefore generated more demand for private cover. The development of 'for-profit' privatization is another part of the explanation. This trend of thought has increased criticism of state control and of generalized schemes of protection based on solidarity. These engendered a climate that favours deregulation and reduction of subsidies to the social sector. Besides the private sector is looking for new fields of activity. The existing markets are more or less saturated. Implementation of the directive on non-life insurance services (including health insurance) could encourage this trend especially in the countries where the legal systems are either inefficient because of insufficient coverage of increasing co-payments or by under-supply.

Table 8.4
Growth in the Health Proportion of Household Expenditure between 1960 and 1986

	1960	1970	1980	1986
Belgium	38	13	18	23
Denmark	11	14	15	16
Spain	49	46	26	29
France	42	22	19	21
Greece	44	46	-	-
Ireland	24	22	-	12
Italy	17	14	18	22
Netherlands	-	16	21	21
Portugal	-	-	28	29(1985)
United Kingdom	15	13	10	14
West-Germany	33	26	21	22

Source: OECD data

At the moment just one community rule allows penetration of a foreign market in this sector. This is the 1973 directive on 'freedom of establishment'. But tomorrow the task of insurers will be much easier with the 'free provision of services'. With the new directive they will no longer need headquarters or branches within another Member State to sell their products there. Germany remains an exception. They have succeeded in upholding the principle of specialization for health insurance, thus effectively preventing market penetration by foreign insurers.

Possible expansion of the private insurance sector is not without risk to the effectiveness of social insurance systems and national health policies. It can produce an inflation of costs by covering excessive reimbursements - even illegal supplements. It also erodes the principle of solidarity on which social cover is based, by selection of risks. In the long term these practices can undermine the financial base of public schemes and penalise the sick, the invalids and the aged, because the characteristic of health expenses for the individual is that it is very concentrated in time.[5] This is just the situation we can see in the USA where the cost of health care continues to grow rapidly (nine percent increase in 1987 to reach in 1990 about twelve per cent of the GNP). Despite this increase the population covered is steadily decreasing (37 million people are now totally excluded from any coverage and about 53 million people are under-insured, of which 40 million are 'dangerously undercovered'. It is also interesting to note that in the early 80s the cost increase started to accelerate at the time when ADS's (Alternative Delivery Systems) became more widely applied to introduce more competition.[6]

8.4.5 Mutualities - Sickness Funds - Provident Associations

The changes that can be expected as a consequence of the Single market can exert an important influence on the position of all those involved in the field of health insurance and health care. We can read today the strategies which are being prepared:

Private insurers are hoping to win new market segments; public authorities are trying to contain the growth of costs to stabilize their budgets; some health care providers are aiming to make profits from free circulation while others wish to attract funds for it; UNICE (Europe's employer's federation) is opposed to regulated social rights, and wants lower employer's contributions to improve the competitiveness of European enterprises. In high GNP countries, unions defend what they have won in social protection and seek levelling up of the social protection of workers in other countries. As for mutualities, supporting the principle of convergence of the level of social protection according to a calendar defining the stages of improvement for the countries with less coverage. They also claim for specific and European legal status to offer common transnational services. This would also correct the imbalance existing in the present directives, which until now are exclusively intended for commercial companies. Non-for-profit associations, cooperatives and mutualities are until now not mentioned.

To understand the nature of this position, we must recall the role played by mutualities in Europe and in health care in particular. Historically it was a form of mutual aid, depending on solidarity, which inspired all our models of social protection. Bismarck built his compulsory protection regime in the mutualist style of the times. This type of solution was introduced in many Member States of the European community, right up to the Second World War.

In all the countries we can see the originally of mutualism. There are five main characteristics: freedom of membership, elected self-governments, independence with regard to public authorities, absence of lucrative motives and above all responsible solidarity. It is because of these five principles that mutualities are operating differently from commercial insurance companies. Mutualities do not select risks, do not limit continuity of membership, do not allow no-claim bonuses and forbid any form of personal profit from distribution of surpluses. In this way mutualities supply their services direct without intermediaries, to subscribers who are also members in order to secure the most favourable terms possible.

To sum up, mutual benefit funds have both social and economic functions within the Community.

The social function is expressed as insurance protection for members against the great uncertainties of life (sickness, handicap, disability) while the economic function works mainly through a variety of enterprises with social objectives. These funds have taken the initiative in service sectors (care centres, domiciliary aid services, campaigns on sickness prevention, health eduction training of the young, and so on). Today more than a third of the population of Member States is represented by this movement, making it undeniably one of the most important social movements in the Community. This fact cannot be ignored.

It certainly seems that the Single Market of 1992 must produce increased mobility of highly-qualified executives. Contrary to commercial insurers the mutualities cannot today operate transnationally. To extend their services across national borders, a specific legal status is essential. Necessary but not by itself sufficient. We must carefully preserve what is unique about mutualism if we are to avoid building an uni-dimensional economic Europe. Social cohesion is also a clear objective of the Single Act according to the new article 130A.

Mutualities, sickness funds and provident associations are important players and it is vital for the future that they can compete with the private, commercial insurances to improve their products and services offered to the subscribers or consumers of health insurance and health care.

The mutualities of Europe do not request any protectionism but they simply want the same space as transnational development, as do the commercial insurers and that through a European legislation adapted to their specific way of operating on a non-for-profit base.

As far as harmonization of the level of social protection is concerned we might ask, since the Council of Europe is updating the Code of Social Security with precise definitions of guaranteed coverage, whether the EEC wouldn't better rely on this new Code of Social Security to fix the minimum rights to guarantee to the citizens of all the member countries according to a time scheme rather than to look for new definitions.

8.4.6 Conclusion

We must not allow the debate on the politics of health insurance to focus on a simple dilemma between the public sector and private profit. That could raise ideological hackles and damage the main objective, which is to give everyone access to health care services.

Of course the dangers of bureaucracy always threaten public systems. That is certainly why in every Community country today there are forms of cooperation which link mainly non-for-profit private players with public policies for social protection. These working public/private models certainly are the most efficient in that area we currently have available. The constant improvement of our managerial techniques is the absolute condition for preserving a high level of efficiency.

Newcomers to the scene, whether producers of medical goods or private insurers, should not be allowed to upset this social consensus simply to generate extra profits or oversupply of technology or facilities.

For legal protection systems, the natural territorial entity for the time being is the Member State. It is the national unit which best represents the expression of the cultural diversity in our Community - and culture is the structural foundation of our systems. We should remember Jean Monet in his famous phrase, 'Et si c'était à refaire je recommencerai par la culture ...' ('And if we had to start again, I would start with culture ...').

The European Mutualities and provident associations are convinced supporters of a stronger Europe - more coherent economically, politically but also socially. A Europe whereby removing trade barriers but also by cutting down inequalities, 'social humanism' will continue to prevail and develop and this by guaranteeing to *all* it's citizens the possibility of access to these goods, services and values such as social security - 'freedom of want and of fear' - health and eduction.

For they determine the quality of life and ensure the dignity of every person.

8.4.7 Notes

1 That is, till the necessary decrees according to the new legislation are enforced.
2 The Dekker Plan was amended by the new government.
3 Hurwitz, Léon, 'La libre circulation des médecins dans la C.E.E.', in *Revue Française des Affaires Sociales*, 3/88, juillet septembre, 15 - 25.
4 Gottely Jacqueline, 'La mobilité des médecins en Europe', in *Solidarité Santé*, Etudes statistiques n. 1/1989.
5 'Three per cent of the sick consume half of the care and ten per cent threequarter', D'après Poullier J.P. (1987), 'Les dépenses de santé: une croissance inéluctable?', in *Revue Française des Finances publiques*, **18**, 55 à 78.
6 See for example Figure 1, page 20 of Professor J.M. Graf v.d. Schulenburg's paper on 'Competition, Solidarity and Cost Containment'.

8.5 Inter-State Variation in Medical and Health Insurance Regulation: Implications of American Experiences for Health Insurance in the European Community
B.L. Kirkman-Liff and S. Lewis

8.5.1 Introduction

My approach to the topic of 'Public and Private Health Insurance in Europe After 1992' is to ask the following questions: First, is it *necessary* to have a single social health insurance system in the European Community after 1992?   Second, is it *necessary* to have a harmonized system for the regulation of private health insurance in the Community after 1992?   Must the European Community move towards a harmonized structure, or can it prosper with separate social health insurance systems (or national health services), diverse private health insurance markets, and separate national regulation of these markets?

I do not intend to address the issue of the desirability of a harmonized structure for health care.   That involves a complex trade-off of the projected advantages of continental-wide competition, some degree of central regulation from Brussels, and conflicts with local providers, insurers, regulators, traditions and culture.   Nor will I address the concern of some that the Treaty of Rome mandates a single health insurance market.   That issue is far beyond my expertise.

My answer involves an examination of social and private health insurance in the US.   In my view the US does not have a single, harmonized system.   Rather, it is composed of many separate state-operated social insurance programmes, with an uneven system of subsidies from the federal government, a large number of separate markets for private health insurance, with little regulation or intervention by the federal government, and a small number of federal government insurance programmes.   This structure of many programmes and markets with state regulation and control provides some indication of the advantages and disadvantages of retaining non-harmonized markets for social and private health insurance and programmes in the European Community after 1992.

My comments will be in three parts. The first section will review the variation among the states in the provision of social health insurance through the Medicaid programme. The second section will present a discussion of the respective roles for the state and federal government in the regulation of private health insurance, especially Health Maintenance Organizations (HMOs). Last, I will draw some suggestions for Europe after 1992 from this analysis of the variation within the US health insurance programmes and markets. My goal is to stimulate thought, not to give any specific recommendations. An appendix reviews the overall structure of the markets for private health insurance and the programmes for social health insurance in the US.

8.5.2 Medicaid: Variations in America's Social Health Programme for the Poor

Medicaid is an attempt at a federal state programme to assure that some of the poor have adequate access to essential health care services. Unlike Medicare, the federal health insurance scheme for the elderly, Medicaid is composed of 56 distinct state and territorial programmes, with some federal efforts at uniformity.[1] Medicaid was intended to provide insurance to low-income single mothers with children receiving welfare and destitute elderly, blind or disabled persons (some of whom might be covered by Medicare, the federal insurance programme for the elderly, but would have limited access to care due to the Medicare deductibles and co-payments). In recent years more than fifty per cent of the Medicaid expenditures have gone to nursing home residents and other long-term care patients who have depleted their own assets and now qualify as impoverished.

Table 8.5
Structural Differences Between Medicare and Medicaid

	Medicare	Medicaid
Financing:	Federal social security tax	Federal and state general tax revenues Inter-state variation in method
Benefits and Co-payments:	Uniform across US	Some federal mandate of minimum benefits Inter-state variation in total benefits
Eligibility:	Uniform across US	Some federal mandate of minimum eligibility Inter-state variation in optional eligibility
Fee Structures:	Hospital payment method: DRGs Hospital payment variation: urban versus rural Physician payment method: Fee-for-service Physician payment variation: local market	Inter-state variation in hospital payment method: DRG's, charges, per diem rates, contracts Inter-state variation in physician payment method: Fee-for-service, contracts
Cross-subsidy between states?	Not generally considered as Medicare is a federal programme with benefits going directly to the individual	Political process at federal level; subsidy ranges from fifty to nearly eighty per cent
State autonomy	None - no participation by states in Medicare	High - states design their own programme, subject to federal approval

As seen in Table 8.5, Medicare and Medicaid differ in their uniformity across the states. Compared to Medicare, Medicaid contains a high degree of variability in benefits, co-payments and eligibility. Provider reimbursement varies in both method and payment levels between states. As Medicare bypasses the states and provides a direct benefit to its members, the issues of cross-subsidy from wealthy to poor states and of state autonomy in programme design do not arise. Medicaid is different. Explicit political decisions are made about the level of subsidy from the federal government to each state, which represents a form of cross-subsidy. There is a constant political and bureaucratic tension between federal and state levels over programme design: the states constantly want more autonomy to modify Medicaid, while the federal level is concerned with cost-containment and equitable care.

Eligibility for Medicaid depends on eligibility for a more general welfare programme, Aid to Families with Dependent Children, which is usually limited to single mothers with children. As the income eligibility for this programme varies by state, so does Medicaid eligibility. As seen in Table 8.6, the difference between lowest (most restrictive) and highest (most generous) eligibility is greater than six hundred per cent. States can expand eligibility to include persons who have become impoverished due to catastrophic illness costs, and such programmes can serve as a 'safety-net' for the uninsured. Thirty-six of the fifty states have such a programme, but again the eligibility varies by state. The maximum income through this mechanism can be eight times higher in some states as in others. The result of this variation is that in a few states one hundred per cent of the poor are covered, while in some states less than twenty-five per cent of the poor are covered. Length of eligibility varies, and many Medicaid recipients find themselves without coverage due to small changes in their income.[2] [3]

Table 8.6
Variations in Medicaid Eligibility

Eligibility Criterion (Maximum Monthly Income)	State Definition of Maximum Monthly Income ($)			
	Lowest	Highest	Average	Weighted Average
Of all 50 states:				
Single Mother and 1 Child	88	692	300	334
Single Mother and 2 Children	118	779	368	413
Single Mother and 3 Children	144	866	433	490
Of 36 states:				
Impoverished Individual	68	550	314	356
Impoverished Family - 2 Members	167	684	410	469
Impoverished Family - 3 Members	217	850	479	549
Impoverished Family - 4 Members	267	1 009	552	627

N.B.: Excludes the US territories

Source: Medicaid Source Book: Background Data and Analysis

There is a great deal of variation in the benefits provided under Medicaid. Data from all 56 programmes is seen in Table 8.7. Access to several forms of organ transplantation varies by state, as does access to occupational, physical and rehabilitative therapies. Even such essential items as eye glasses and hearing aids are unavailable in some Medicaid programmes. Several states require recipients to pay co-payments for drugs, physician office visits, and other services. These co-payments are minimal (between 0.5 and 2 dollars), and many providers will not refuse care if a recipient does not have the co-payment.

Table 8.7
Variations in Medicaid Coverage

Service:	Number of States Excluding Coverage:
Hospice Services	50
Pancreas Transplants	48
Heart-Lung Transplants	41
Occupational Therapy	31
Heart Transplants	23
Speech and Hearing Services	23
Physical Therapy	21
Rehabilitative Services	19
Dentures	19
In-patient Psychiatric Services for Children	19
Liver Transplants	15
Eyeglasses	9
Hearing Aids	7
Service:	Number of States With Service Co-Payments:
Drugs	19
Eyeglasses	7
Physician Office Visit	7
Hearing Aids	6
Service:	Number of States Limiting Coverage:
Number of Physician Visits	29
Length-of-Stay of Hospitalizations	21
Review of Referrals to:	Number of States With Programmes for Prospective Review of Referrals:
Nursing Home	31
Surgery	13

N.B.: Out of 56 states and territories.

Source: Medicaid Source Book: Background Data and Analysis

More than half of the states and territories limit the total number of physician visits per recipient that Medicaid will pay: further visits must be paid by the individual, or the physician must write-off those costs. Some twenty-one states have maximums on the length-of-stay of hospitalization: hospitals in these states generally write-off as bed debt any excess days. A growing proportion of states conduct prospective review of referrals to nursing homes and surgery, as part of the increased use of managed care within Medicaid.

There is much variation in the methods used by the state programmes to pay providers, as seen in Table 8.8. Some states pay providers based upon historic costs or current provider-determined charges, while others use complex rate-setting programmes that incorporate negotiation, selective contracting, or prospective budgets.[4] While twenty-two states do not enroll medicaid recipients in HMOs, twenty-six give recipients this option. Only nine states require Medicaid recipients to join HMOs; these programmes generally operate in the urban areas of state, and rural recipients remain in a more conventional Medicaid programme.

Table 8.8
Variations in Medicaid Reimbursement Methods

	Number of States	
Hospital In-patient Reimbursement		
Retrospective costs	8	
Prospective costs	42	
Flat rate (per day or per admission)		21
DRGs (per admission)		14
Budget systems		4
Negotiation and selective contracting		3
Hospital Out-patient Reimbursement		
Retrospective costs	23	
Fee Schedules	11	
Prospective prices	9	
Negotiation	2	
Other Method	5	
Physician Reimbursement		
Fee schedules	27	
Prevailing charges	19	
Relative value scales	4	
Use of HMOs		
No Use	22	
Voluntary Use	26	
Mandatory Use (selected areas)	9	

Source: Medicaid Source Book: Background Data and Analysis

The last area to be examined is Medicaid expenditures and the role of federal subsidy. The federal subsidy varies from fifty per cent of programme costs to nearly eighty per cent. The subsidy rate is based on a comparison of each state's *per capita* income with the US *per capita* income. In table 8.9 the states have been grouped by the subsidy rate. The states with the lowest rate (fifty per cent) account for forty-eight per cent of Medicaid expenditures and forty-three per cent of recipients, while the states with the lowest *per capita* incomes and highest matching rates only account for eight per cent of expenditures and ten per cent of recipients. The high income states have a total cost per recipient that is fifty-two per cent higher than that in the low income states. However, the federal subsidy in dollar terms per recipient is almost equal between high and low incomes states. The lower subsidy rate for high income states is balanced by the higher costs in those states to give an almost equal federal contribution as in the low income and high subsidy states.

Table 8.9
Variations in Medicaid Expenditures

	State Groupings by Federal Matching Rate				
	50%	>50% and <60%	>60% and <70%	70%	Total
Number of States	14	16	13	8	51
Expenditures ($1 000 000s)	21 331	14 273	5 270	3 409	44 283
Percent of Total	48%	32%	12%	8%	
Recipients (1 000s)	9 002	7 019	2 655	2 197	20 873
Percent of Total	43%	34%	13%	10%	
Expenditures per Recipient	$2 369	$2 033	$1 985	$1 552	$2 122

Source: Medicaid Source Book: Background Data and Analysis

The great deal of inter-state variability in Medicaid has made this programme the subject of much research, and several detailed analyses of this variation have been completed.[5] [6] [7]

8.5.3 Federal and State Regulation of Private Health Insurance

The regulation of all forms of insurance in the United States, including health insurance, has remained in the domain of the individual states and has generally not come under the jurisdiction of the federal government. This situation was the result of a Supreme Court decision in 1868 that the business of insurance was not inter-state commerce.[8] At that time insurers were organized within the political boundaries of each state and only insured local risks. The lack of federal involvement in insurance regulation lead to the development of state-level regulatory mechanisms. However, these mechanisms were inadequate to deal with insurance cartel arrangements in the early twentieth-century. In 1944 a Supreme Court decision reversed the 1868 ruling and held that insurance was inter-state commerce and therefore subject to federal anti-cartel acts.[9] The insurance industry and the state regulators responded with pressure on Congress, which passed the McCarren-Ferguson Act, which returned regulation of insurance to the states.[10] Since then the Federal Trade Commission has gained jurisdiction over false insurance advertising, while the Securities and Exchange Commission has gained regulatory jurisdiction over variable annuity insurance products that involve equity funding.[11] Outside of these limited areas, the states have jurisdiction over all insurance, including health insurance.

1) State Regulation There is a great deal of variation between the states in their regulation of health insurance. All states regulate the solvency of health insurers, through requirements for annual filings and financial examinations and audits. However, the time period between audits varies among the states. The magnitude and definition of capital and reserve requirements vary. Minimum capital is $100 000 in some states, and $1 000 000 in others. Some states define reserves as a fixed number of dollars per enrolled person, while others define these requirements in terms of a fixed amount, regardless of the number of enrollees. In some states detailed criminal investigations of the directors of an insurance firm are required before it will be licensed to operate in the state, while others require a simple listing of these individuals. All states have passed laws defining and providing penalties for fraudulent and deceptive advertising and practices.[12]

Regulation of insurance rates varies across the states. Approximately one-third of the states do not require commercial insurers to file their rates. Some states require a review of the rate structure, which usually focuses on the proposed rate increases. In most states the rate review is concerned with insurer solvency: it is not possible to lower a reduction in excessive rates. Some states do monitor the proportion of benefit dollars paid out in claims, and can require insurers to make future adjustment in order to reach a minimum benefit-cost ration.[13]

States vary in their taxation of premiums. The highest rate of taxation is four per cent, while some states do not apply any insurance tax. In some states these revenues are allocated by law for the operation of pools for medically uninsurable residents. Under this system, individuals who cannot obtain health insurance due to a severe pre-existing condition that is undergoing active treatment - such as cancer or AIDS - can obtain health insurance from these pools. Alternatively, some states use these revenues for their Medicaid programmes.

Many states have mandated that all health insurers include certain benefits. Sometimes these benefits are intended to encourage more competition in the provision of health services. For example, insurers are required to cover the costs for psychiatric social workers and clinical psychologists as well as for psychiatrists, if the latter is covered, in order to encourage substitution of a lower-cost professional. Sometimes these mandated benefits are intended to encourage the provision of health promotion and disease prevention services. For example, insurers may be required to provide various cancer screening tests with no deductibles to their members. Lastly, these mandated benefits may be intended to improve access to care. For example, insurers may be required to include prenatal care as a benefit, or may be prohibited from applying deductibles or co-payments to prenatal care.

The states are able to establish their own regulation of alternative insurance arrangements. This regulation often takes the form of an independent review of the medical care delivery system of the HMO, as well as its financial viability. In some states this licensure is a function of the insurance regulators, while in other states the regulators of health facilities and programmes are involved. The regulation of HMOs is sometimes shared between these different agencies. Table 8.10 provides a summary of the different state strategies for HMO licensure.[14] As with conventional health insurance, financial regulation of HMOs varies between states. The results from a survey of 29 states revealed that working capital requirements varied from $100 000 to $1 500 000, net worth requirements varied from $100 000 to $1 200 000, and special deposit requirements varied from $50 000 to $500 000. At least seven states regulate the rate that HMOs are allowed to charge, and four states regulate HMO advertising and marketing campaigns.[15]

2) Federal Regulation The major area of federal regulation of health insurance involves HMOs. This regulation is voluntary, and entails the certification that the HMO complies with a set of guidelines established by the federal government. The vast majority of HMO members are in such federally-certified plans. Current law requires that an employer offer at least one federally-certified HMO to their employees, if a federally-certifies HMO insists (or mandates) such an offering. (However, the employer can choose to offer another federally-certified HMO, and not the one that brought the demand.) Federal certification generally does not exempt the HMO from tighter state regulations.

Table 8.10
Variations in State Strategy for HMO Regulation
(Number of States with Selected Strategy - Total of 51)

	State Strategy Regulating Agency:			No Regulation
	Department of Insurance	Department of Health	Joint Responsibility	
Delivery System	6	22	3	20
Quality of Care	6	23	4	18
Financial Requirements	32	4	1	14
Approval of Contracts with Members	29	5	4	13
Approval of Agreements with Providers	16	12	8	15
Consumer Complaints	17	9	14	11

A second area of federal involvement in regulation is an exemption given under federal law to self-insured employers. This law prohibits states from exercising regulatory authority over the health plans of such employers. Instead, the self-insured employers must comply with relatively less stringent federal regulations, which generally pertain to reporting requirements. Self-insured employers under these laws are exempt from state mandated benefits and from state insurance premium taxes. These exemptions are some of the powerful incentives behind the movement towards self-insurance.

A third area involves requirements (only passed in 1988 and weakened in 1989) for tax-exempt status for employer-provided health insurance. These regulations go into effect in 1991, and require an equitable offering of health insurance to all employees, if the employer desires to retain the tax exemption for insurance plans. This exemption will be lost when such insurance is only offered to highly-paid employees.

3) Trends in Regulation The system of health insurance regulation is also undergoing a transformation in response to the events within the health care system. A recent stimulus to change has been the bankruptcy of Maxicare, a chain of HMOs that once operated in more than twenty states. This bankruptcy has revealed the lack of clear jurisdiction of multiple state regulators. Conflicts between the states and the federal bankruptcy court have already lead to problems in the protection of past enrollees. A National Association of HMO Regulators ('NAHMOR') has proposed the enactment of legal devices within each state that would reduce these complications in the future. Overall, the current trend is to harmonize state regulation, but this process will be slow. The European Community is already ahead of the US in the harmonization of regulations on financial reserves.

8.5.4 Conclusions

The many differences among the health care systems of the European Community and the even greater differences between these systems and America make it difficult to venture any firm conclusions. Instead I put forward some tentative suggestions.

There appears to be no necessity to move the regulation of private health insurance from the national level to the Community level. Current EC regulations on reserve requirements already represent greater harmonization then we have achieved in the US.

A reliance on national regulation would require adequate participation by all parties in such matters as fee negotiations. For example, a British private insurer operating in the Netherlands would want to have representation in one of the Dutch associations in order to have input in the fee negotiations with physicians.

The EC could promote flexibility in the provision of health insurance. Just as self-insured employers in the US are regulated under federal laws, and are exempt from state regulation, the EC could develop a form of licensure and registration for health insurance programmes provided to the employees of EC-chartered corporations. Under this approach, such corporations would provide a uniform health insurance benefit to all of their employees across the EC, subject to EC regulations and exempt from national regulation. These regulations might allow selective contracting, which would aid corporations seriously interested in health care cost-containment. Such a development would allow large EC firms to emulate the self-insured managed-care programmes in the US. Of course there are numerous technical and legal issues surrounding such an idea.

Turning to the area of social insurance, the American experience with Medicaid indicates that there can be sizeable variation in benefits, eligibility and reimbursement under social insurance programmes. There can also be large variations in the cross-subsidy between high-income and low-income regions. The paradox emerges that high-income states tends to have high health care costs, reducing the magnitude of the cross-subsidy. There is no intrinsic necessity for uniformity within a continent-wide system: uniformity is not essential from a macroeconomic perspective.

However, one lesson from Medicaid should be clear: a lack of uniformity means a lower level of social equity and solidarity within members of the same continent-wide community. Most Americans accept this lack of solidarity. It is up to you to decide whether a poor person in Amsterdam or Barcelona will have better or worse access to care than an equally poor person in Athens or Birmingham. Depending upon that decision, uniformity may be essential from an equity perspective.

8.5.5 Appendix: US Health Insurance Markets

The US is unique in all of the industrial world in that we continue to use voluntary insurance as a major component for the financing of our health care delivery system. Under this approach most individuals receive health insurance either through their employer or through the employer of someone in their family. As will be discussed in more detail, employer-provided insurance involves varying level of employee contribution to the cost of insurance, as well as various deductibles, co-payments, limitations, and requirements. These schemes are supplemented by various governmental entitlement or welfare programmes which provide insurance (or occasionally direct services) to various categories of beneficiaries.

Proposals for a federal health insurance system or a compulsory-but-private insurance system have emerged repeatedly in the past forty years. While the elderly and poorest of the poor were covered in 1965 under Medicare and Medicaid, no further expansion of private or social insurance has occurred in the past twenty-five years. In recent years there has been a reduction in coverage, such that there are estimated to be more than 30 million uninsured.

1) Employer Provided Insurance   There are a variety of different forms of employer-provided insurance. Blue Cross & Blue Shield Associations are organized as non-profit organizations, usually within the boundaries of one state. These associations were created by enabling laws passed separately in each state, not by federal laws. The hospital sector was the original advocate for these organizations during the 1930s, in order to create a mechanism to provide insurance for the costs of hospitalization (and later physician fees).[16] They are exempt from state and federal income taxes (although the federal tax exemption was limited in 1986), state insurance premium taxes and local property taxes. In exchange for these tax benefits and their unique position in each state, they are generally required to operate in the public interest. This has traditionally taken the form of community rating, in which there is one premium rate for all insured, as well as coverage for small employers and individuals.

Commercial insurers are explicitly for-profit, with no favourable tax exemptions. They have tended to use experience rating, in which the premium rate varies with the past experience of the employees of each employer. Commercial insurers have tended to avoid covering small employees or individuals, or only at very high rates, due to risk of self-selection.

Health Maintenance Organizations (HMOs) have existed in the US since the 1930s, but until the 1970s never covered more than three per cent of the US population. These organizations integrate insurance with the provision of medical services. They are characterized by selective contracting with a limited panel of providers, and using a variety of incentives and bureaucratic mechanisms to manage the delivery of medical care. Traditionally they used community rating.

Preferred Provider Organizations (PPOs) are a creation of the early 1980s. They are similar to HMOs, in that there is a limited panel of 'preferred' providers, and in their use of incentives and other mechanisms to manage medical care. However, they preserve fee-for-service payment and some insurance benefit to use of providers who are not 'preferred'.

The last category consists of self-insured employers. These firms do not buy insurance coverage for their employees, but establish a mechanism by which medical bills will be reimbursed. This approach in effect provides the same experience rating as with commercial insurers, while obtaining an exemption from state insurance premium taxes, as with Blue Cross plan. These programmes are also exempt from other forms of state insurance regulation, because formally there is no purchase of insurance.

2) Government-Provided Insurance The largest governmental insurance programme is Medicare, which covers the over-65 population, as well the disabled and those with end-stage renal disease. It is the closest that the US comes to a 'national' health insurance programme, in that there is nationally uniform eligibility, benefits and co-payments. Payment rates (especially for physicians) vary by region, and the programme is administered through private contractors (frequently Blue Cross Associations). Medicare has substantial deductions and co-payments and requires a contribution from the beneficiary for the supplemental insurance for physician fees. The Medicaid programme has been extensively discussed in the body of the paper.

Lastly there are several federal programmes that involve the direct provision of medical care to categorical groups, such as military veterans, Native Americans and Inuits (American Indians and Eskimos), and migrant agricultural workers.

3) Trends in the Health Insurance Market   In the last ten years there has been a significant restructuring of the health insurance markets within the US. Table 8.11 presents a crude estimate of the distribution of insurance coverage. Compared to the late 1970s, Blue Cross and commercial insurers now account for significantly smaller share of the privately insured market. This shift is mostly due to the lower costs of self-insured employers, HMOs, and PPOs. HMOs now cover about twenty per cent, with PPOs at twelve per cent of the market. The largest increase has been in the proportion of the privately insured population which now receives coverage from self-insured employers. This segment may reach forty per cent by 1990.[17] [18] [19] [20] [21]

A major spur to the growth of self-insured employers has been the development of selective contracting and managed care activities within a self-insured structure. Self-insured employers can now obtain many of the advantages of HMOs (lower utilization rates and low costs per unit of service) by the operation of utilization review programmes. Components of managed care programmes have also been adopted by Blue Cross and commercial insurers. These usually involve efforts to reduce the use of hospital care, through pre-admission certification, concurrent review, and discharge planning. Expanded use of economic incentives and bureaucratic controls to encourage the use of ambulatory surgery and free-standing urgent care are also part of the managed care activities of indemnity insurers.

These estimates contain a significant amount of duplicate coverage and counting. Some of the duplication is in households in which both adults work and receive employer-provided insurance. There is also some double counting involving members of HMOs or PPOs owned by Blue Cross Associations or commercial insurers.

4) Variation in Coverage   There is a great amount of variation in the coverage of these different forms of health insurance, both between different forms of coverage and within each category. The individual's share of the insurance premium can vary from none to fifty per cent. Eligibility for employer-provided insurance varies by employer. Some employers require an employee to work for six months before they are provided with insurance coverage; others provide insurance from date of employment. Traditionally, some employers only covered full-time employees, while others only covered permanent employees and excluded seasonal workers. Lastly, some employer would only extend coverage to executive or managerial level employees, or would only insure salaried employees.

Table 8.11
Estimated Distribution of US Population Among Insurance Arrangements
(Millions of Covered Persons)

Employer-Based or Individual Purchase Insurance	156	
(Primary Insurance):		
Blue Cross	48	
Commercial Insurance	97	
Self-Insured Employers	72	
Health Maintenance Organizations	31	
Preferred Provider Organizations	18	
Duplicate Coverage or Counting	110	
Government-Sponsored Insurance (Primary Insurance):	52	
Medicare (Elderly or Disabled)	31	
With Blue Cross supplements:		9
With Commercial Insurance supplements:		6
With Medicaid		3
Enrolled in HMOs:		<1
Medicaid (Poor)	21	
With Medicare		3
Enrolled in HMOs:		1
Military	2	
Indian Health Service	1	
Uninsured:	37	
Total US Population	245	

Sources: Health Insurance Association of America, *Source Book*, 1986-1987; Interstudy, *National HMO Census*, 1985; US Government Printing Office, *Medicaid Source Book: Background Data and Analysis*, 1988; DiCarlo and Gabel, 'Conventional Health Insurance: A Decade Later', *Health Care Financing Review*.

Deductibles and co-payments vary across and within all forms of insurance. Front-end deductibles can range from $200 to $2 000 dollars per family per year. There is a large variation in co-payments. Some insurers only require a ten per cent co-payment, while some PPO plans require a fifty per cent co-payment for use of a 'non-preferred' provider. Co-payments are increasingly found within HMOs: while most range from $2 to $5 per physician visit, other have $10 co-payments.

Equally important are the exclusions in coverage. Dental care is generally excluded from employer-provided insurance, although many employers offer optional dental insurance. Coverage of mental health services and alcohol and drug treatment is not always present (although such coverage is increasing). Some insurance excludes prenatal care, and a few policies continue to only cover hospitalization.

The great variation in coverage and forms of insurance, when combined with the large inter-state variation in health care costs, results in substantial differences for employers in their insurance premiums. This creates a competitive advantage for employers to locate in 'low premium' states. However, health care insurance costs are just one of many factors influencing such decisions. Access to markets, union militancy, transportation infrastructure, workforce eduction, climate, land costs: all of these can be far more significant than health insurance premiums.

8.5.6 Notes

1   Congressional Research Service (1988), *Medicaid Source Book: Background Data and Analysis*, U.S. Government Printing Office, Washington, D.C., November.
2   Short, Pamela Farley, Cantor, Joel C., Monheit, Alan C. (1988), 'The Dynamics of Medicaid Eligibility', *Inquiry*, 25, Winter, 504 - 16.
3   Burwell, Brian O., Rymer, Marilyn P. (1987), 'Trends in Medicaid Eligibility: 1975 To 1985', *Health Affairs*, Winter, 30 - 45.
4   Buchanan, Robert J. (1984), 'A National Survey of Medicaid Reimbursement Factors', *Hospitals*, 58, 1 September, 60 - 4.
5   Cromwell, Jerry, Hurdle, Sylvia, Schurman (1987), 'Defederalizing Medicaird: Fair to the Poor, Fair to Taxpayers?', *Journal of Health Politics, Policy and Law*, 12, Spring, 1 - 34.
6   Perloff, Janet D., Kletke, Phillip R., Neckerman, Kathryn M. (1987), 'Physicians' Decisions to Limit Medicaid Participation: Determinants and Policy Implications', *Journal of Health Politics, Policy and Law*, 12, Summer, 221 - 35.
7   Joe, Thomas C. W., Meltzer, Judith, Yu, Peter (1985), 'Arbitrary Access to Care: The Case for Reforming Medicaid', *Health Affairs*, Spring, 59 - 74.
8   Paul v. Virginia, 75 US (8 Wall.) 168 (1868).
9   US v. Southeastern Underwriters Association, 322 US 533 (1944).
10 Caddy, Douglas (1986), *Legislative Trends in Insurance Regulation*, College Stations, TX, Texas A & M Press.
11 Kimball, Spencer L., and Denenberg, Herbert S. (eds) (1969), 'An Overview of Federal Interest in Insurance', in *Insurance, Government and Social Policy: Studies in Insurance Regulation*, Chapter 16, Richard D. Irwin, Homewood, IL.
12 Shaughnessy, Peter, Updegraff, Gail, Grayson, Harriet, Hoffman, Nancy (1975), *Regulation of Private Health Insurers*, Spectrum Research, Inc., Denver, CO, 26 - 7.
13 Shaughnessy, Peter, Updegraff, Gail, Grayson, Harriet, Hoffman, Nancy (1975), *Regulation of Private Health Insurers*, Spectrum Research, Inc., Denver, CO, 28.
14 *Preliminary Results of the Multi-State Licensing Study group As Reported to the NAIC-NAHMOR Joint Committee*, June 22, 1987 (mimeograph).
15 LeBoeuf Consultants, *Findings and Recommendations Based on the 1988 Survey on Regulation of HMOs and HMO Solvency for the NAIC HMO Solvency Working Group*, (no date) (mimeograph).
16 Eilers, Robert D. (1963), *Regulation of Blue Cross and Blue Shield Plans*, Richard D. Irwin, Homewood, IL.
17 Health Insurance Association of America, 'Employer-Sponsored Health Insurance in America: Preliminary Results from the 1988 Survey', *Research Bulletin*, HIAA, Washington, DC, 1989.
18 Goodwin, Thomas G. (1989), 'A Roundtable Discussion - Business Looks at Health Care', *Federation of American Health Systems Review*, January/February, 24 -32.
19 Kennedy, Cheryl (1989), 'Group Health Insurers Speak Out About Skyrocketing Premiums', *Federation of American Health Systems Review*, January/February, 34 - 8.

20 French, H.E., III, and Ginsburg, Paul B. (1988), 'Competition Among Health Insurers, Revisited', *Journal of Health Politics, Policy and Law*, **13**, (2), Summer, 279 - 91.
21 DiCarlo, Steven, Gabel, Jon (1989), 'Concentional Health Insurance: A Decade Later', *Health Care Financing Review*, **10**, (3), Spring, 77 - 89.

9 General Conclusions

Discussions on 'Health Care in Europe after 1992' have shown that slowly but surely health questions are becoming part of the main issues in the European Community. There will be a growing need for the development of common approaches; the reduction or at least the slowdown of the increase in health care costs is important.

EC law plays an important role also in opening possibilities for citizens and Member States to benefit from free trade and traffic in the health care sector. Community law is binding upon both citizens and Member States and the creation of a proper national legislation in due time should be stressed, taking account of restrictions on the national margins of action. The real margins under a Community directive may be broader if the directive is properly implemented in the national legislation, but in case of conflict between Community and national law, Community law will prevail in order to guarantee uniform legislation throughout the Community.

The rights and obligations under EC law are limited. Any Member State should respect the non-discrimination rule; it covers specific situations with regard to, for example, professional activities. The scope of the rights of the self-employed is even wider than the mere rule of non-discrimination; the exceptions in the Treaty allowing restrictive measures are very small. National authorities have no discretionary power, for example, to investigate or to decide whether an applicant fulfils the national professional qualifications. National licence-regimes for the building of hospitals should not imply any discrimination. National measures intended to control the increase of the price of for example pharmaceutical products, and discriminating between domestic and imported products, are not compatible with the EC Treaty. The national health care systems can be affected by the Community's social security legislation and by the rules on the free movement of goods and the free provision of services. Patients can also invoke certain rights as customers. Altogether, however, it is still not completely clear what the implications will be of Community legislation in the health insurance sector.

Most of the activities of the European Community aim at balancing the economic objectives of the Community with the right to protection of health and safety of the consumer. It is to be expected that in the field of immaterial aspects related to health technology, a common approach will develop from the common market.

Four patterns of intra-European developments with regard to health and health policy come to mind; a comparison has been made in this book with trains travelling on railway tracks which allow for four unequal speeds. One of the lessons the European Community could learn from the experiences in the United States is how to utilize the new pathways that federalism offers for desirable changes in the health care field. European integration may create room for emerging competition. It will probably depend on decisions made by the European Court of Justice. Many recommendations to the Member States tend to generate a policy of 'wait and see'; more speedy progress is to be expected in the private sector because it is in the position to experiment with new methods, which, once proven to be sound, could be applied in the public sector as well. These unequal speeds and possibilities raise the need to put ethical questions on the agenda; the statement has been made that 'there is no positive contribution to be expected to European integration from an explicit debate on ethical issues between governmental representatives of the Member States', but on the other hand it was stated that 'the increasing international cooperation within medical ethics has made it possible to begin answering the question whether larger global differences in relation to informed consent can be detected'. It could be an interesting idea to found an international ECPE, a European Council of Professional Ethicists, to advise the politicians in Europe about the ethical implications of the progress in medical sciences. Teaching of medical ethics is also very important for many reasons, one of them being that doctors should be made aware that medical practice is repeatedly facing 'value judgements' and not only technical problems. If the ethical guidelines will be soon translated into laws, the danger of polarization could emerge; the actual communication between doctor and patient will then not be promoted, but influenced by juridicalization that is not accepted in the medical field. On the other hand there should be legislation that gives positive incentives to the improvement of communication: the professional's expertise and the patient's experience and knowledge must be brought into balance. That is one way to improve the quality of health care; the measurement of patients' opinions is another. In most of the European countries there is no special legislation on the quality assessment sector; legislators should support all attempts to establish institutions for quality assessment on a voluntary basis of the parties involved. A more intensive exchange of knowledge and data on quality assessment in the different countries has also to take place.

In the pharmaceutical sector European harmonization has made substantial progress; it enables the Community to exercise international responsibilities. The tension between the harmonising process on the one hand, and the diversity on the other, could be seen as the prime challenge to the EEC with regard to the pharmaceutical industry. Here the transparency directive plays an important role in keeping a balance between the need for the national governments to keep the costs of health care under control and some experts have stated that the pricing process of the pricing should be left to markets and market forces: a supra-national European bureaucracy in matters of application for, and admission of, drugs should be avoided.

In the hospital sector an increasing number of privatizations and commercial initiatives will take place in the years forthcoming. Many 'hospital consultancies' will appear. The increasing influence of employers and the constantly developing process of unification of the European market will cause changes in the health care decision-making process. In the European hospital world there is currently no consensus on possible political actions in the health care field. The growing shortage of health care personnel in many European countries leads to the question of a European approach; also the question of European medical Centres of Excellence beyond the country borders has to be answered, as well as that of minimum quality norms. Last but not least, workers' participation will receive a new impetus after 1992.

The European internal market will also be an opportunity for health care professionals. They are already and will be more able to practise in every Member State. Maintaining the high quality of care training and specialization will be one of the most urgent questions for the health care sector in Europe; the free admittance to professions in health care requires specific attention for manpower planning at a national level. Mutual assistance by rendering services without going to another Member State, offers major possibilities for combining highly specialized techniques in health care. For nurses, 1992 could mean new challenges; they can play an important role in the organizational process and a specific Nurse Management Development programme could be a useful instrument.

In health insurance, and especially in the social health insurance, the contributors do not expect immediate changes. It is difficult to give a formal definition of social health insurance. However there are some important aspects such as insurance based on public law, a contribution related to wage or income and benefits fixed by the government.

The compulsory nature of the schemes is not a necessary condition, because in Germany, for example, voluntary private health insurance could have far-reaching consequences for Europe after 1992. Social health insurance in the European perspective will be dominated by the European Community Regulation 1408/71; article 22 enables publicly insured persons to receive medical care in another Member State, and they are then covered for the services and benefits as applicable in the country in which they stay. The future will show us to what degree 'medical tourism' will take place and to what consequences it will lead.

For private health insurance companies, Europe 1992 means a more competitive environment. They have to consider the so-called European directives on non-life insurance business; it makes possible for insurers to launch cross-border operations from their own headquarters into any other EC Member State. Existing differences in national practices are to be harmonized. Existing solidarity aspects could get into difficulties, especially in those countries with a substantial voluntary (supplementary) health insurance.

There is, among the authors, a general agreement that compulsory health insurance cannot be expected in a short time. In the long run harmonization may be accomplished as a result of the evolution of the common market. The experiences in the United States have taught that there is no intrinsic necessity for uniformity within the system. However it is important to realise that a lack of uniformity could lead to a lower level of social equity and solidarity within the European Community as such.

This brings us back to the starting point of this book. 'Europe 1992' will bring a lot of freedom: the freedom to move goods, services, and capital and the freedom to move as persons within the European Community. The EC lacks at this moment authority to decide on health (services) policies and it lacks operational responsibilities to implement policy decisions. National sovereignty is defended and national law applies to most health issues. In the future, after 1992, health care in Europe will become one of the most important sectors on the Community scene.